p 28 Jurors stereotypes vs actual eye
info during hypnosis —

Peary recall (actual)
correct incorrect memories
priming w/ 4 cases/
1 minute each —

? cross seek to elicit accounts

Prz Reg — Checkable

# HYPNOSIS AND MEMORY

The Guilford Clinical and Experimental Hypnosis Series
*Michael J. Diamond and Helen M. Pettinati, Editors*

HYPNOSIS AND MEMORY
Edited by Helen M. Pettinati

HYPNOSIS, WILL, AND MEMORY:
A PSYCHO-LEGAL HISTORY
Jean-Roch Laurence and Campbell Perry

CLINICAL PRACTICE OF HYPNOTHERAPY
M. Erik Wright with Beatrice A. Wright

# HYPNOSIS AND MEMORY

*Edited by*

Helen M. Pettinati

THE GUILFORD PRESS
*New York     London*

© 1988 The Guilford Press
A Division of Guilford Publications, Inc.
72 Spring Street, New York, NY 10012

Printed in the United States of America

Last digit is print number: 9 8 7 6 5 4 3 2 1


Library of Congress Cataloging-in-Publication Data

Hypnosis and memory.

(The Guilford clinical and experimental hypnosis series)
Includes bibliographies and index.
1. Hypnotism. 2. Memory. 3. Amnesia—Treatment.
I. Pettinati, Helen M. (Helen Marie) II. Series.
[DNLM: 1. Hypnosis. 2. Memory. WM 415 H9963]
RC497.H96 1988 154.7 87–7597
ISBN 0–89862–338–3

# Contributors

Henry L. Bennett, Ph.D., Department of Anesthesiology, University of California–Davis Medical Center, Sacramento, California

Kenneth S. Bowers, Ph.D., Department of Psychology, University of Waterloo, Waterloo, Ontario, Canada

David F. Dinges, Ph.D., Unit for Experimental Psychiatry, The Institute of Pennsylvania Hospital, Philadelphia, Pennsylvania; Department of Psychiatry, University of Pennsylvania School of Medicine, Philadelphia, Pennsylvania

Joyce D'Eon, Ph.D., Department of Psychology, Concordia University, Montréal, Québec, Canada (Present affiliation: Department of Psychology, Royal Ottawa Regional Rehabilitation Centre, Ottawa, Ontario, Canada)

Matthew Hugh Erdelyi, Ph.D., Department of Psychology, Brooklyn College of the City University of New York, Brooklyn, New York; The Graduate Center of the City University of New York, New York, New York

Frederick J. Evans, Ph.D., Department of Psychiatry, University of Medicine and Dentistry of New Jersey–Robert Wood Johnson Medical School, Piscataway, New Jersey

Fred H. Frankel, M.B.Ch.B., D.P.M., Department of Psychiatry, Beth Israel Hospital, Boston, Massachusetts; Department of Psychiatry, Harvard Medical School, Boston, Massachusetts

Ernest R. Hilgard, Ph.D., Department of Psychology, Stanford University, Stanford, California

Marc H. Hollender, M.D., Department of Psychiatry, Vanderbilt University School of Medicine, Nashville, Tennessee

Lawrence C. Kolb, M.D., Veterans Administration Medical Center, Albany, New York; Department of Psychiatry, Albany Medical College, Albany, New York

Jean-Roch Laurence, Ph.D., Department of Psychology, Concordia University, Montréal, Québec, Canada

Emily Carota Orne, Unit for Experimental Psychiatry, The Institute of Pennsylvania Hospital, Philadelphia, Pennsylvania; Department of Psychiatry, University of Pennsylvania School of Medicine, Philadelphia, Pennsylvania

Martin T. Orne, M.D., Ph.D., Unit for Experimental Psychiatry, The Institute of Pennsylvania Hospital, Philadelphia, Pennsylvania; Department of Psychiatry, University of Pennsylvania School of Medicine, Philadelphia, Pennsylvania

Campbell W. Perry, Ph.D., Department of Psychology, Concordia University, Montréal, Québec, Canada

Helen M. Pettinati, Ph.D., Carrier Foundation, Belle Mead, New Jersey; Department of Psychiatry, University of Medicine and Dentistry of New Jersey–Robert Wood Johnson Medical School, Piscataway, New Jersey

Peter W. Sheehan, Ph.D., Department of Psychology, University of Queensland, Brisbane, Queensland, Australia

Beverlea Tallant, M.A., Department of Psychology, Concordia University, Montréal, Québec, Canada

Wayne G. Whitehouse, Ph.D., Unit for Experimental Psychiatry, The Institute of Pennsylvania Hospital, Philadelphia, Pennsylvania; Department of Psychiatry, University of Pennsylvania School of Medicine, Philadelphia, Pennsylvania

# Acknowledgments

The following people should share in the credit for the publication of this book. I believe it was Fred Frankel who conspired with Seymour Weingarten, the editor-in-chief of The Guilford Press, in encouraging me to edit this volume as well as in inviting me to be a series editor with Michael Diamond for the Guilford Clinical and Experimental Hypnosis Series, which includes this book. I especially thank the contributors to this volume for making my job easy and sharing my enthusiasm for this project. I am particularly indebted to the generous advice I received from Dr. Martin Orne and Emily Orne in facilitating the planning of the book. In addition, I wish to express my grateful admiration to Julie Wade for helping me edit some of the more challenging parts and to Mary Anne Hinz for organizing me during the years it takes from the inception to the completion of such a project. Also, a special thank-you to my husband, Joseph, and my three children, Lisa, Anne, and Joseph, for their unwavering love, confidence in my abilities, and patience.

Preparation of the volume was supported in part by the Carrier Foundation.

Helen M. Pettinati

# Preface

For over a century, there has been a widely held belief that hypnosis is a powerful tool for bringing back forgotten memories. Clinically, a number of cases have been published describing the use of hypnosis in recovering traumatic, repressed events (e.g., Raginsky, 1969). Over the last 20 years, hypnosis has been used in the forensic setting to improve the memory of witnesses and victims for gaining information to solve crimes, with reportedly high success (Reiser, 1976). Yet knowledgeable opponents to the use of hypnosis in the forensic setting underscore its dangers in this context (Orne, 1979).

In the past, opinion on hypnosis and memory had to rely on beliefs, clinical reports, and fantastic claims; over the past decade, however, a wealth of empirically sound research on the topic of hypnotic hypermnesia has emerged. Thus, the time is ripe for a systematic compilation of this work that seriously speaks to the potential for hypnosis to aid recall, and this volume is the first of this kind.

The title *Hypnosis and Memory* conjures up a number of different images. It may prompt many to picture hypnosis as it is seen in the movies— as a tool to replay what were thought to be long-lost traumatic memories. Others will wonder about the use of hypnosis in penetrating the amnesia seen in some war veterans. Still others will wonder whether hypnosis can be used in criminal investigations where details have been hopelessly lacking, or where the crime was so heinous that the victim has blocked memories of it. Finally, others will perhaps think of the rare but dramatic reports of reincarnation experiences under hypnosis. The relative diversity of images is the very reason that such a book is needed: to consolidate into one source a variety of topics relating to hypnosis and memory. To achieve this end, special care has been taken to select experts in the various areas.

It is particularly relevant that the Council of Scientific Affairs of the American Medical Association (1985) recently published a report addressing the highly controversial area of using hypnosis in refreshing recollection by witnesses and victims of crime. Four contributors to the book were part of the committee that produced the report: Drs. M. T. Orne, Erdelyi, Evans, and Frankel. While the report is focused solely on the present scientific status of hypermnesia in the forensic setting, and the present volume is multifocused, it is no accident that a section of this book (Chapters 2–5) reports on research that has major implications for the forensic issues. Also timely is the continual introduction into a number of State Supreme Courts of the important legal question of the admissibility of hypnotically refreshed memories in court cases.

The comprehensive nature of this book should allow the professional seeking to study hypnosis and memory in depth the opportunity to gain the perspective of many experts in the field. Its scope, however, does not preclude the relative newcomer to the fields of hypnosis or memory from gaining information as well.

H. M. P.

## REFERENCES

Council on Scientific Affairs, American Medical Association. (1985). Scientific status of refreshing recollection by the use of hypnosis. *Journal of the American Medical Association, 253*, 1918–1923.

Orne, M. T. (1979). The use and misuse of hypnosis in the court. *International Journal of Clinical and Experimental Hypnosis, 27*, 311–341.

Raginsky, B. B. (1969). Hypnotic recall of an aircrash cause. *International Journal of Clinical and Experimental Hypnosis, 27*, 1–19.

Reiser, M. (1976). Hypnosis as a tool in criminal investigation. *Police Chief, 43*, 36, 39–40.

# Contents

# INTRODUCTION

# 1

## Some Complexities in Understanding Memory

KENNETH S. BOWERS
*University of Waterloo*
ERNEST R. HILGARD
*Stanford University*

Hypnosis can affect memory in a number of ways. It can engender interference with recall (as in hypnotic amnesia); it may enhance recall through age regression and related techniques; and it frequently produces memory distortions, such as confabulation and unwarranted increases in confidence. This book addresses these issues, and, in doing so, attempts to correct some of the erroneous notions that so readily infect the entire domain of hypnosis. The complexities of memory in the context of hypnosis can be understood, however, only if the vagaries of memory outside of hypnosis are kept in mind. Hence, in this introductory chapter we address some general problems of memory, with only minor reference to the role of hypnosis; we leave to subsequent chapters a detailed account of the ways in which hypnosis and memory interface.

### UNCONSCIOUS PLAGIARISM: THE HELEN KELLER EPISODE

When a person is in the midst of solving a problem, or engaging in creative writing, memory is obviously called upon, for people can only have ideas that derive in some manner from what they already know. The appearance of complete originality is thus an illusion; every novel idea or creative endeavor has a past. What interests us at the moment are those instances in which memory may intrude something into a thought sequence that the thinker believes to be original, when in fact it is based on specific memories that are not identified as such.

In Helen Keller's (1905/1961) autobiography, she reports an incident that had a profound impact on her and her teacher, Anne Sullivan. Helen was 11 years old when she wrote a short story entitled "The Frost King," as a birthday present for Michael Anagnos, then the director of the Perkins

Institution for the Blind, and a close friend and confidant of Anne Sullivan. It was an altogether delightful story, clearly the work of a precocious and imaginative child, and so full of visual imagery that it was hard to believe that it was written by a girl who had been blinded and deafened by a childhood disease suffered when she was only 19 months old. So delighted was Anagnos with the story that he published it in one of the Perkins Institution reports. Soon thereafter, it was reprinted in a weekly magazine, with full recognition of its remarkable qualities.

What happened next is quite extraordinary. It soon became clear that Helen Keller's opus was closely patterned after a short story entitled "The Frost Fairies," written before Helen was born, by one Margaret Canby. So close were the theme and some of the passages of the two stories that Helen's tale was incontestably informed by the earlier work. This state of affairs constituted a serious embarrassment for everyone concerned, and Helen, now 12 years old, was made to appear in front of a "court of investigation composed of the teachers and officers of the Institution" (Keller, 1905/1961, p. 66). The issue was not so much *whether* as *when* Helen had "heard"[1] the story—the suspicion being that Anne Sullivan had in fact "read" it to her gifted protegée, thus encouraging her, perhaps unwittingly, on the course of plagiarism. This charge was rejected vociferously and tearfully by a distraught young girl, and indignantly by her teacher, who, in addition, denied any knowledge of Canby's original story.

Still, it was clear that Helen must have "heard" the story somewhere, and the likely source, according to Miss Sullivan, was one Mrs. Hopkins, a family friend whom Helen had visited in the summer of 1888. Mrs. Hopkins owned a copy of the book in which Canby's "The Frost Fairies" appeared, along with other short stories by the same author. Mrs. Hopkins was confident that she had "read" to Helen from the book, though Helen herself had no memory of having "heard" the story. Assuming that this episode was the true inspiration of "The Frost King" implies that a story "heard" by 8-year-old Helen was forgotten *qua* memory, but was retained in her fertile mind sufficiently to inform her own short story written 3 years later.

If Anne Sullivan's version of this episode is correct,[2] it is a most remarkable example of "cryptomnesia" (Reed, 1974). Essentially, cryptomnesia in-

---

1. Helen "heard" stories by having the letter of each word spelled into the palm of her hand via the manual alphabet for the deaf. We place such words as "heard" and "read" in quotation marks here to help the reader remember that Helen Keller did not literally hear what she was told, and that people did not actually read aloud to her.

2. In his biography of Helen Keller, Lash (1980) demurs from the account of the "Frost King" episode offered by Sullivan and Keller. Lash's view of the incident seems heavily influenced by an anonymous report written by a teacher at the Perkins Institute, which recounts a conversation she had had with Helen. In the course of the conversation, Helen allegedly revealed that Anne Sullivan, not Mrs. Hopkins, had read the original story to her.

volves remembering something without recognition of it *as* a memory. Reed gives several examples of this phenomenon, while indicating that little work has been done in memory research that bears directly on it. However, recent literature dealing with previously unfamiliar topics such as source amnesia (Evans & Thorn, 1966; Perry, Laurence, D'Eon, & Tallant, Chapter 5, this volume) and remembering without awareness (Jacoby & Witherspoon, 1982) implies that people can retrieve recently acquired information from memory without experiencing the information as the recall of something recently learned. So, under the right circumstances, it seems quite possible for a person to mistake the memory of previously acquired information for an original idea. Given this mental possibility of mistaking something old for something new, unconscious plagiarism becomes a phenomenon that must be taken seriously.

The incident of "The Frost King" implies that the *experience* of remembering something can be cut off or dissociated from the fact of something remembered—that there is, in other words, an important distinction to be made between something remembered and the experience of remembering something. Once this distinction is recognized, we are confronted with a possibility that the experience of remembering can occur in the absence of something remembered. And in fact, the experience of remembering can infest fantasies, thoughts, and images that have no correspondence to actual historical events. This is the problem of "confabulation," or false memories. Since confabulation involves the unwarranted experience of memory, and cryptomnesia involves its unwarranted absence, confabulation and cryptomnesia are, so to speak, opposite sides of the same coin.

Both of these mnemonic aberrations can create serious difficulties. We have seen how Helen Keller was victimized by memory without an associated experience of remembering. Confabulation, on the other hand, is currently a problem of considerable concern to investigators studying eyewitness testimony (see especially Orne, Whitehouse, Dinges, & Orne, Chapter 2, this volume; Perry *et al.*, Chapter 5, this volume).

## BIASED RECALL: FALSE RECOLLECTIONS

Although the biasing of testimony in the courtroom has been a topic of special interest to those using hypnosis, there has been a long-standing interest in the influence of leading questions outside the hypnotic context,

---

The fact that there was considerable jealousy among the other teachers toward Sullivan and her relationship with Helen might weigh more heavily with another authority. What is clear is that Helen Keller, who had an "almost holy feeling about telling the truth" (Lash, 1980, p. 145), denied for the rest of her life that Sullivan had "read" Canby's story to her.

partly because courtroom practices tend to value testimonial evidence very highly despite its known inadequacies and dangers. For example, a professor of law at Yale University, in the early days of the Institute of Human Relations there, published an account of 65 criminal prosecutions and convictions in which the convicted person was obviously innocent (Borchard, 1932). He indicated that mistaken identity was the major source of the miscarriage of justice in the cases reviewed. In 29 of these cases, mistaken identity was almost exclusively responsible for the result. In 8 of these cases the convicted person did not resemble at all the guilty person, later unmistakably found to have been the criminal. In 12 cases there was a certain resemblance, but it was not at all close, and in only 2 cases did the convicted person and the true culprit resemble each other sufficiently for the resemblance to be called striking.

What are the causes of such distortions of memory, when there is no attempt to deceive? Students of memory have shown that distortion can occur at the time the information is acquired and encoded—perhaps because the events are taking place at a distance and/or in dim light, or because there is confusion about where or when the crime is being committed. Then there is a retention period between the time of acquisition and recall, during which memories fade or become reworked for various reasons. Finally, there is the retrieval stage, during which time, in criminal testimony, various forms of interrogation may introduce bias in memory. Each stage is important, but studies tend to focus largely on the final stage because there is the one that is most apt to have social consequences.

Testimony experiments that did not use hypnosis showed a number of circumstances that could bias recollections. Among these is the form of question. Even a direct question can yield different answers, depending on how it is put. For example, the question "Did you see a [gun]?" led to more reliable answers in an early experiment than did the question in the form "Didn't you see a [gun]?" (Muscio, 1916). The matter of leading questions is discussed further in Chapter 2. In any case, the impact of leading questions is not limited to hypnosis; the point addressed in several chapters that follow is whether or not hypnosis *accentuates* the force of a leading question. (For an earlier review, see E. R. Hilgard & Loftus, 1979.)

## CORRESPONDENT AND EXPERIENTIAL ASPECTS OF MEMORY

Both cryptomnesia and confabulation derive from the same fundamental fact of human memory—namely, that it involves *both* the degree to which a mental representation corresponds to some earlier event, *and* the degree to which the person experiences the mental representation as a memory. Thus, we can refer to the "correspondent" and "experiential" aspects of memory.

When a mental representation has a high correspondence to a past event, but is unaccompanied by the experience of it as a memory, we have the conditions for cryptomnesia; when a mental representation is experienced as a memory, even though it has low or no correspondence to a past event, we have the conditions for confident confabulation. In addition to these two problematic combinations of correspondent and experiential aspects of memory, there are, of course, two other combinations: (1) A mental representation is highly correspondent to a past event and is accompanied by the experience of that representation as a remembrance; and (2) a mental representation has low or no correspondence with a previous event, with no associated experience of it as a memory. Figure 1-1 represents the various combinations of correspondent and experiential aspects of memory.

There are a couple of points to be made in connection with this representation of memory. In the first place, it is quite different from a signal detection analysis of memory, in which an analogous $2 \times 2$ layout for recognition memory would show the presence and absence of information arrayed along one axis, and a subject's responses (e.g., yes–no) along the other axis. Nothing along either axis would refer to how a person experienced a mental representation—a consideration that signal detection treats with indifference. It focuses instead on the pattern of hits and misses in the four cells, from which indices of sensitivity ($d'$) and report criterion ($\beta$) can be calculated. As indicated by Erdelyi in Chapter 3 of this volume, lowering the report criterion will increase the number of mnemonic "hits," but at the cost of an increased number of "false alarms." An increase in false alarms should *not*, however, be confused with an unwarranted (i.e., noncorrespondent)

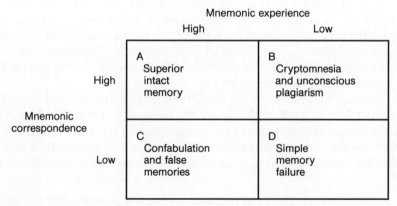

Figure 1-1. The relationship between correspondent and experiential aspects of memory.

increase in experiential memory, which cannot even be represented in a signal detection analysis. The consequence of an unwarranted increase in mnemonic experience is confident confabulation. One consequence of a decreased report criterion, on the other hand, is *less* (not more) confidence in the resulting false alarms—a state of affairs psychologically quite distinct from confabulation.[3]

The second feature of Figure 1-1 that bears emphasis concerns the difference between cells A and D. Both cells represent an appropriate fit between the correspondent and experiential aspects of memory, and in that sense, one could argue that both cells represent a mnemonic intactness quite different from the situation in cells B and C. However, while cell A implies an excellent memory, cell D represents a poor one. A memory in which mental representations are frequently noncorrespondent, and experienced as such, is a failing memory—even if it is not one suffering the additional indignities of confabulation or cryptomnesia.

Before we pursue the correspondent and experiential aspects of memory any further, it may be useful to consider them in the context of other distinctions that have recently emerged in the literature concerned with memory and cognitive psychology. Two major categories have recently come to prominence in discussion of memory: first, a distinction between "short-term memory" and "long-term memory"; and, second, a distinction between "episodic memory" and "semantic memory." The first of these distinctions need not concern us here, but the second is relevant. Episodic memory consists of experienced events in the life of the person engaged in the recollection of these events. It is part of the personal biography, recognized as such, and thus overlaps with what we have been calling "experiential memory," although they are not exactly alike. Experiential memory is that aspect of recall that *identifies* it as a memory. Hence, experiential memory applies to both episodic and semantic memory, for either kind of memory may or may not be recognized for what it is. For example, there is a form of memory in hypnosis in which factual information taught in hypnosis is recalled, although the source of the memory is forgotten. The material can be classified as semantic memory, but the recall is a distortion of both episodic and experiential memory, provided that the recall corresponds to what was taught in hypnosis (Evans & Thorn, 1966).

Tulving, who proposed the distinction between episodic and semantic memory (Tulving, 1972, 1983), has carried his analysis a few steps further in relating the categories of memory to consciousness (Tulving, 1985). His first step is to add "procedural memory" to the other two classes. In a skilled habit, for example, there is a minimum of consciousness involved, even

3. It should be noted that a lowered report criterion may generate recall errors of low confidence that are, on a subsequent occasion, recalled again with much higher confidence that they are correct (e.g., Dywan, 1983).

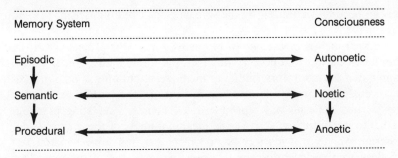

Figure 1-2. Memory systems and varieties of consciousness (after Tulving, 1985).

though there is some conscious activity going on as the demands of the feedback are reacted to in the skilled act. He then goes on to relate the three types of memory systems to three varieties of consciousness (see Figure 1-2).

Tulving's "autonoetic consciousness" is self-knowing, and is related to episodic memory that recognizes events as belonging in the personal past. "Noetic consciousness" is the kind represented in thinking about objects and events (and relationships among them) in their absence, and hence implies semantic memory. Finally, "anoetic consciousness," or nonknowing, is still consciousness because it permits appropriate behavioral responses to relevant aspects of the environment. Tulving's discussion shows how far the interest in consciousness has advanced in the 1980s, encouraged by the acceptance of cognitive psychology. Because modifications in hypnosis are commonly conceived as alterations in consciousness, the new climate in psychology is more favorable to recognizing the significance of the changes brought about by hypnosis.

## EXPERIMENT AND THEORY: FORCED RECALL AS AN EXAMPLE

There is a subtle interplay between the theoretical concepts and methodology employed in scientific investigation. It is the nature of experiments to select from a larger domain of knowledge certain limited aspects that can be subjected to measurement and used to establish lawful relationships among selected variables. This is an advantage in producing results that can be replicated by others, thereby meeting standards of objectivity. However, caution is needed in generalizing from any one series of experiments because of their selective nature—a selectivity often determined by the theoretical orientation of the investigator. Unless such dangers are kept in perspective, we can become victimized by the so-called "cult of empiricism" (Toulmin & Leary, 1985).

Experimental investigations of memory make the problem clear. During the three-quarters of a century in which the Ebbinghaus type of experiment dominated the laboratory studies of memory, attention was paid primarily to the correspondent aspects of memory—that is, the faithfulness with which the learned material was reproduced. Of course, interesting psychological variables were studied, such as the meaningfulness of the materials, but the criterion was that of mastery based on the original subject matter learned. Modern studies do not escape this same danger—that is, of being factually correct but limited in reference to the richness of the memorial experience. To illustrate this point, we give a rather full account of one of the favored methods in the recent study of memory: the method of forced recall.

Suppose a subject is exposed, one at a time, to 60 line drawings that depict common household objects, animals, plants, and so forth. And then suppose that the subject is asked to remember as many of the drawings as possible. Under free-recall conditions, the average person will record about 30 of the 60 drawings, and will only rarely be incorrect (e.g., Dywan, 1983). However, if our average person is instead required to record 60 responses (the so-called forced-recall procedure), about half of his or her responses will not be experienced as correspondent to the previously presented drawings; indeed they will be experienced as guesses. Nevertheless, some of these guesses will in fact correspond to previously viewed line drawings, so that people frequently achieve more mnemonic "hits" under this forced-recall procedure than they would under free-recall conditions.

Adopting a forced-recall procedure eliminates the impact of report criterion on the assessment of memory. In free-recall procedures, a person who adopts a conservative report criterion is ordinarily reluctant to list a somewhat vague or uncertain mental representation *as* a memory (i.e., as correspondent to one of the previously viewed line drawings). Another person adopting a more liberal report criterion under free-recall conditions typically lists this same vague and uncertain mental representation as a memory (i.e., as correspondent to a previously viewed line drawing). Consequently, the first person may list fewer correct memories than the second person. However, this difference may well be due almost entirely to the fact that the first person records fewer responses reflecting vague and uncertain mental representations—some of which are doubtless correspondent to line drawings previously viewed. The forced-recall procedure, on the other hand, requires everyone, regardless of his or her preferred report criterion, to record the same number of responses, the better to index the extent to which vague and uncertain mental representations are in fact correspondent. In sum, forced-recall procedures prevent differences in report criterion from differentially influencing this "correspondence index."

Erdelyi (Chapter 3, this volume; Erdelyi & Kleinbard, 1978) has been an apologist for forced-recall methodology in his research on hypermnesia outside of hypnosis. His preference for this paradigm emphasizes a conceptual commitment to a particular view of memory—namely, that what really counts as memory is its correspondence to previously encoded information when individual differences in report criteria are eliminated by the forced-recall procedure. However, this identification of memory with correspondence ignores the experiential component of the human memory system.

The best way of indicating the potential problems introduced by a forced-recall procedure is revealed by a thought experiment. Imagine three subjects, each of whom makes a "perfect" score on some aspect of the 60-picture problem introduced above, but whose memories are nevertheless quite different. Utilizing the forced-recall paradigm, Alan achieves a perfect correspondence index, which is to say that each and every one of his responses corresponds to one of the previously presented line drawings. Furthermore, he experiences each and every response as a "mnemonic hit." Betty, like Alan, achieves a perfect correspondence index; however, unlike Alan, she experiences each and every one of her responses as a guess (i.e., as a "mnemonic miss"). Carol, unlike both Alan and Betty, has a zero correspondence index—not one of her responses corresponds to a line drawing. However, she, like Alan, experiences each of her responses as a "mnemonic hit," even though this experience is in every case unjustified.

What do we learn from this implausible thought experiment? Consider first Alan and Betty, both of whom have a perfect correspondence index, but totally opposite scores on mnemonic experience. According to a strict application of the forced-recall methodology, the memories of these two people are identical. Furthermore, the fact that Alan and Betty are so different in how they experience their mnemonic success becomes the best possible justification for exploiting the forced-recall procedure, because without it, Betty would have recorded nothing at all, whereas Alan would have recorded 60 responses, all of them correct. Carol's mnemonic difficulties are of course very well revealed by the forced-recall method, since she confidently reports 60 memories, each of which is demonstrably noncorrespondent.

If we refer this cast of characters back to Figure 1-1, Alan, Betty, and Carol occupy cells A, B, and C, respectively. A fourth character, Dave, occupies cell D, and is suffering from a failing memory; however, for what it is worth, his experience of memory matches his low level of mnemonic correspondence. Only Alan, securely ensconced in cell A, has what we might refer to as a "superior intact" memory.

If we focus for a moment of Betty and Carol, it should be clear that they are going to have considerable trouble in an ecologically complex world, though for quite different reasons. Betty, with perfect recall but zero experience of her mental representations as memories, will be the archetypal cryptomnesic—remembering all sorts of things that are experienced and forwarded as novel and original. Carol, on the other hand, is the archetypal confabulator, whose fantasies or wishes are experienced as having already occurred. While Betty has the mnemonic grounds for action, she does not experience them as such, and so *does not* act appropriately. Carol, on the other hand, has the experience of remembering in the absence of any mnemonic justification for it, so she *cannot* act appropriately. In either case, there is a serious deficiency in memory.

In sum, the forced-recall procedure as typically employed is interested only in the correspondence of subjects' responses to line drawings they have seen earlier; it is indifferent to how a person experiences the relationship between memory reports and the stimuli he or she is trying to recall. While this quality of the forced-recall paradigm has some advantages for some purposes, it provides a somewhat truncated concept of memory. In real life, experiencing mental representations as memories increases the likelihood that they will be forwarded, and regarded, as such. Accordingly, the reason hypnotically "enhanced" memory is often so convincing to onlookers is that the person subjected to such procedures may confidently experience various mental representations as correspondent, even though they are often confabulations that were not previously represented at all, or were originally experienced with such uncertainty and vagueness that they were not reported as memories. It would be far less problematic if hypnotic procedures merely lowered a person's report criterion, so that an increased number of mental representations would be reported as memories, but with considerably greater hesitancy and lowered confidence.

The important point here is that the forced-recall procedure, in controlling for differences in report criterion, overlooks the extent to which experiential memory contributes to everyday life. Ordinarily, the experience of memory serves as an important basis for action, and surely such mnemonic experiences (and the actions that flow from them) are typically warranted by the correspondent aspects of memory. On the other hand, overreliance on free-recall procedures to assess hypnotically refreshed memory has erroneously led some people to accept a confidently asserted memory experience as a convenient and suitable substiute for an index of correspondence. As Perry *et al.* indicate in Chapter 5 of this book, the results of this error can be tragic.

## THE CONFIDENCE FACTOR IN MEMORY AND ASSOCIATIVE CLOSENESS

Clearly, the experiential aspect of memory is closely tied to the issue of mnemonic confidence—a topic that is central to Sheehan's discussion in Chapter 4 of this book. In general, what we mean by "confidence" is the degree of subjective certainty that a mental representation corresponds to something that actually happened.[4] We assume that confidence is at least in part generated out of underlying mnemonic processes such as encoding, storage, and retrieval, and to the extent that this is true,[5] it is reasonable to examine the issue of confidence in terms of these underlying processes.

The experiment testing memory for line drawings of familiar objects, previously introduced, also includes a condition in which memories for the line drawings are "hypnotically refreshed." While we are leaving the presentation of hypnotic data primarily to the chapters that follow, it may be noted that a significant number of hypnotically refreshed responses, especially when offered by highly hypnotizable subjects in a hypnosis treatment condition, have been found to be misremembrances (Dywan & Bowers, 1983). Thus, it is evident that hypnosis is not a truth serum. However, the main point we wish to underscore has little to do with hypnosis per se, and can in fact be illustrated by the following unpublished finding (by K. S. Bowers).

In this supplementary experiment, it was demonstrated that recall errors made by subjects were influenced or informed by the line drawings they had actually seen. This state of affairs was determined by a two-stage procedure. First, recall errors generated by a hypnotized subject were yoked with pseudo-errors of recall made by a control subject who had *not* viewed the line drawings. Instead, a yoked control subject was told in general terms about the kinds of line drawings viewed by actual subjects, and then was asked to fill in the 60 blanks of the recall protocol with plausible responses. If a subject in the memory experiment made 9 recall errors, comparably located responses from the protocol of a yoked control subject were selected as pseudo errors. The list of 9 genuine errors of recall and the list of 9 pseudoerrors were paired, thereby constituting one of 34 similarly generated items on an Error Identification Test (EIT). The EIT was then presented to 47 independent judges in the second part of the experiment. These judges had themselves viewed the original 60 line drawings, and were enjoined to select which list of

4. Mnemonic confidence is not identical to the experience of memory, however. One can imagine circumstances in which mnemonic confidence is high when the experiential aspects of memory are low. Thus, one may not experience a correspondent mental representation as memory, while reasoning or inferring with some confidence that it must be. Moreover, the experience of memory may be high, but one may have little confidence in its correspondence to a real historical event. This occurs in instances of *déjà vu* in which a person may fully appreciate that a particular mnemonic experience cannot possibly correspond to anything in his or her past. Both of these possibilities we judge to be relatively rare, however, so that indices of mnemonic experience and confidence are ordinarily interchangeable.

5. It is true, of course, that the experience of memory is also fashioned out of other factors, such as attributional processes, social compliance effects, and so on. To the extent that nonmnemonic factors predominate in the experience of memory, correspondence is apt to deteriorate.

words in each EIT item were genuine errors of recall. This forced-recall procedure would generate a 50% success rate by chance alone, so that the obtained result of 61% was quite statistically significant ($t = 5.24, p < .001$).

These findings suggest that, compared to the protocols of yoked control subjects, the error protocols of people who had actually viewed the 60 line drawings contained an "associative residue" of what they had seen—in other words, that their misremembrances were associatively *informed* by the line drawings they were attempting to recall. For example, if a person is first presented with a line drawing of a tiger and then subsequently misremembers it, he or she is more likely to misremember it as a lion than as a teacup. This is true because "lion" and "tiger" are closely related in most people's associative networks, whereas the relationship between "tiger" and "teacup" is probably more remote. The yoked control subjects in this experiment, on the other hand, were never exposed to any information that would have biased their misremembrances toward "lion" instead of "teacup."

Notice that the very concept of informed error presupposes the existence of an associative network into which the line drawings must have been recieved and encoded. That is, it is only because "tiger" and "lion" are already close neighbors in a person's associative network that a line drawing of a tiger is apt to be misremembered later as a lion. Accordingly, someone who is familiar with tigers, but who has never heard of lions, will have a zero likelihood of misremembering a picture of a tiger as a lion. Thus, recall errors not only depend on the events a person is trying to remember, but will be influenced as well by the pertinent associative networks that the person brings to the task of recall.

This state of affairs introduces an important ambiguity into the assessment of memory. Unless the investigator has independent access to the events and information a person is trying to remember, it can be difficult to know in any given instance the degree to which the person's testimony corresponds to events previously witnessed, and the degree to which it is attributable to idiosyncratic characteristics of his or her associative network. In other words, for any particular recall attempt, it is important to ask how much the investigator has learned about the specific historical events a person is trying to remember, and how much the investigator has learned about the person's network of pertinent associations that has been activated by the *process* of remembering something previously perceived.

It seems plausible that the *experience* of memory (and the confidence with which a particular mental representation is asserted as a memory) is also influenced by associative closeness. In other words, if the event to be recalled and the person's misremembrance of it are closely linked in his or her associative network, perhaps the misremembrance will bring with it some of the confidence that ordinarily accompanies an accurately recalled event. If this turns out to be the case, a person who misremembers "tiger" as "lion" will be relatively confident in this recollection partly because "tiger" and "lion" are close neighbors in his or her associative network.

The ambiguities implicit in the assessment of memory contribute to the conviction, expressed by several contributors to this book, that hypnotically refreshed testimony should be corroborated by independent evidence and not simply used to confirm the suspicions of the interrogator. Hypnosis is known to activate imagination and fantasy (J. R. Hilgard, 1979). In effect, this means that under hypnosis a person's associative networks are activated in a manner that is minimally or remotely tied to external reality constraints, and maximally responsive to a person's idiosyncratic mnemonic themes, imaginings, and fantasies. In other words, it is precisely under hypnotic conditions that we are apt to learn more about a person's idiosyncratic and imaginal contributions to memory reports, and less about the specific external events he or she is trying to recall. As we shall see in the next section, there are circumstances in which it is desirable to tap these imaginal contributions to memory (e.g., Erdelyi, 1984; J. R. Hilgard & LeBaron, 1984), but the forensic use of hypnosis is not one of them.

## MEMORY IN THE CONTEXT OF CREATIVITY AND DISCOVERY

The relationship between memory and creativity has a long philosophical history, going back at least to Plato. Recall for a moment Plato's dialogue with Meno, in which the two men arrive at an apparent paradox that Plato summarizes as follows:

> I know, Meno, what you mean; but just see what a tiresome dispute you are introducing. You argue that a man cannot enquire either about that which he knows, or about that which he does not know; for if he knows, he has no need to enquire; and if not, he cannot; for he does not know the very subject about which he is to enquire. (Jowett, 1892/1937, Vol. 1, p. 360)

Plato's extended response to Meno's paradox is that all new knowledge is in fact a recollection of things already known. He proceeds to demonstrate his point by getting a shepherd boy of little learning to spout complex geometric insight simply by asking him a series of questions that "remind" the boy of knowledge already acquired, presumably in a previous life.

As bizarre as Plato's rebuttal seems to be, we would like to argue that he is at least partially correct. To be sure, he is wrong in the obvious sense that a truly novel or creative insight cannot, by definition, literally be something remembered. However, if we identify memory not with a particular correspondent report, but with a mnemonic process, we can begin to make more sense out of Plato's claim. Surely, the creative process must in part involve activation of appropriate mnemonic networks. Thus, an intuitive physicist must know a great deal of physics, and a creative artist must have considerable artistic knowledge and skill. In each case, this knowledge and skill must be mnemonically stored and appropriately activated if the person is to generate an elegant scientific breakthrough or a great work of art. Clearly, however, the criterion for success in the context of creativity and discovery differs from that for success in the context of remembering. Successful remembering involves producing a mental representation that corresponds to, or matches, a particular historical event. Successful creation or discovery involves something less definable that we can call, for want of a better term, "goodness of fit." Thus, the elements of a work of art or of a scientific theory somehow integrate and fashion themselves into a satisfying expression that reflects and reveals more than was previously realized about the world and/ or about the human condition.

In sum, we can resolve Meno's paradox as follows: The acquisition of new knowledge involves activation of mnemonic networks, but the emergent expression is not literally something remembered; rather, it represents novel recombinations of information precipitated out of one's mnemonic networks. It is perhaps of passing interest that hypnotic ability has been implicated in creativity (Bowers & Bowers, 1979), no doubt because people who are highly hypnotizable are characterized by their enjoyment of fantasy and absorbed imagining (J. R. Hilgard, 1979).

Occasionally, the results of mnemonic activation precipitate an outcome that is ambiguous regarding how it should be evaluated—whether as a remembrance or as a creative work of imagination. Such was the case in regard to Helen Keller's short story "The Frost King." It was clearly a work influenced by the earlier story of Margaret Canby, but Shakespeare, too, borrowed from all sorts of predecessors, dressing up earlier tales with his own unique additions and improvements to the originals.

Fortunately, unconscious plagiarism is typically distinguished by embellishments and emendations to the original version, and this was indeed the case with Helen Keller's "The Frost King." Margaret Canby, the plagiarized author in this case, was generous enough to state in a letter to Anne Sullivan:

> What a wonderfully active and retentive mind that gifted child must have! If she had remembered and written down, accurately, a short story, and that soon after hearing it, it would have been a marvel; but to have heard the story once, three years ago, and in such a way that neither her parents nor teacher could ever allude to it or refresh her memory about it, and then to have been able to reproduce it so vividly, even adding some touches of her own in perfect keeping with the rest, which really improve the original, is something that very few girls of riper years, and with every advantage of sight, hearing, and even great talents for composition, could have done as well, if at all. (quoted in Lash, 1980, p. 142)

Mark Twain was more emphatic: "[N]inety-nine parts of all things that proceed from the intellect are plagiarism, pure and simple. . . . To think of these solemn donkeys [the inquiry board] breaking a little child's heart with their ignorant damned rubbish about plagiarism!" (quoted in Lash, 1980, p. 147). Nevertheless, the great American humorist surely would not deny the difference between the kind of unconscious plagiarism perpetrated by Helen Keller and the deliberate, rote *copying* of someone else's original work. Unconscious plagiarism, as distinct from mere fraud, reflects some of the complexities of the human memory system, which constitute the *raison d'être* of this chapter.

## THE RANGE OF APPLICABILITY OF HYPNOSIS TO THE STUDY OF MEMORY

In the foregoing account, we have called attention to some of the complexities of memory more or less without respect to the additional issues raised by memory's interplay with hypnosis. Considerable care is needed to avoid attributing to hypnosis problems that really belong to the domain of memory per se. Only when the separate complexities of memory and hypnosis are appreciated are we apt to understand how they interact to engender specific mnemonic distortions and/or benefits. The remainder of this book is, of course, directed to elucidating some of these interrelationships between memory and hypnosis.

The four chapters of Section II (by Orne *et al.*, Erdelyi, Sheehan, and Perry *et al.*) address the potential for hypnosis to enhance memory while introducing necessary cautions against exaggerated claims in practical situations (e.g., forensic settings). The next section in the book describes three different types of amnesia that pose a challenge to hypnosis in recovering lost memories. One of the most fascinating aspects of hypnosis is the production of temporary amnesias and their reversal (Evans, Chapter 6). The nonverbal breaching of material learned under anesthesia without conscious awareness (Bennett, Chapter 7) underscores how much we still do not know about our memories. Finally, the differing memory disruptions that occur in different varieties of hysteria, to which hypnosis is historically related, are distinguished as to their nature and the roles they play in the various disorders (Hollender, Chapter 8). Section IV of the book gives case examples of how hypnosis has been utilized in psychiatry (Frankel, Chapter 9), and how related procedures (e.g., narcosynthesis) have been used in the rehabilitation of people whose memories have been damaged by traumatic stresses (Kolb, Chapter 10). In the final chapter, Pettinati integrates the findings presented in this volume and points the way to future research.

## ACKNOWLEDGMENTS

A Spencer Foundation Grant to Kenneth S. Bowers helped support the writing of this chapter. We would especially like to thank Dr. Jane Dywan for her comments on an earlier draft of this chapter. The order of authorship has been determined alphabetically.

## REFERENCES

Borchard, E. M. (1932). *Convicting the innocent: Errors of criminal justice.* New Haven, CT: Yale University Press.

Bowers, P. G., & Bowers, K. S. (1979). Hypnosis and creativity: A theoretical and empirical rapprochement. In E. Fromm and R. E. Shor (Eds.), *Hypnosis: Developments in research and new perspectives* (2nd ed., pp. 351–379). New York: Aldine.

Dywan, J. (1983). *Hypermnesia, hypnosis, and memory: Implications for forensic investigation.* Unpublished doctoral dissertation, University of Waterloo.

Dywan, J., & Bowers, K. S. (1983). The use of hypnosis to enhance recall. *Science, 222,* 184–185.

Erdelyi, M. (1984). *Psychoanalysis: Freud's cognitive psychology.* New York: W. H. Freeman.

Erdelyi, M., & Kleinbard, J. (1978). Has Ebbinghaus decayed with time?: The growth of recall (hypermnesia) over days. *Journal of Experimental Psychology: Human Learning and Memory, 4,* 275–289.

Evans, F. J., & Thorn, W. A. F. (1966). Two types of posthypnotic amnesia: Recall and source amnesia. *International Journal of Clinical and Experimental Hypnosis, 14,* 162–179.

Hilgard, E. R., & Loftus, E. F. (1979). Effective interrogation of the eyewitness. *International Journal of Clinical and Experimental Hypnosis, 27,* 342–357.

Hilgard, J. R. (1979). *Personality and hypnosis* (2nd ed.). Chicago: University of Chicago Press.

Hilgard, J. R., & LeBaron, S. (1984). *Hypnotherapy of pain in children with cancer.* Los Altos, CA: William Kaufmann.

Jacoby, L. L., & Witherspoon, D. (1982). Remembering without awareness. *Canadian Journal of Psychology, 36,* 300–324.

Jowett, B. (Ed. and Trans.). *The dialogues of Plato* (Vol. 1). New York: Random House. (Original work published 1892).

Keller, H. (1961). *The story of my life.* New York: Dell. (Original work published 1905).

Lash, J. P. (1980). *Helen and Teacher: The story of Helen Keller and Anne Sullivan Macy.* New York: Delacorte Press/Seymour Lawrence.

Muscio, B. (1916). The influence of the form of a question. *British Journal of Psychology, 8,* 351–389.

Reed, G. (1974). *The psychology of anomalous experience.* Boston: Houghton Mifflin.

Toulmin, S., & Leary, D. E. (1985). The cult of empiricism in psychology and beyond. In S. Koch & D. E. Leary (Eds.), *A century of psychology as science* (pp. 594–617). New York: McGraw-Hill.

Tulving, E. (1972). Episodic and semantic memory. In E. Tulving & W. Donaldson (Eds.), *Organization of memory* (pp. 381–403). New York: Academic Press.

Tulving, E. (1983). *Elements of episodic memory.* Oxford: Oxford University Press.

Tulving, E. (1985). Memory and consciousness. *Canadian Psychology, 26,* 1–12.

# MECHANISMS OF MEMORY ENHANCEMENT WITH HYPNOSIS

# 2

# Reconstructing Memory through Hypnosis: Forensic and Clinical Implications

MARTIN T. ORNE
WAYNE G. WHITEHOUSE
DAVID F. DINGES
EMILY CAROTA ORNE
*The Institute of Pennsylvania Hospital and University of Pennsylvania School of Medicine*

Historically, the phenomena of hypnosis that have aroused the greatest amount of popular and scientific interest are those that appear to transcend normal voluntary abilities. Attempts to experimentally validate claims of enhanced performance by hypnotized individuals not only have contributed conceptually to an understanding of hypnosis, but also have led to many important methodological developments (e.g., Barber, 1969; London & Fuhrer, 1961; Orne, 1959; Sheehan & Perry, 1976). Certainly, too, the possible potentiation of human abilities by hypnosis holds considerable pragmatic and therapeutic promise; some of this promise has already been realized, as in the clinical use of hypnosis in the control of pain (J. R. Hilgard & LeBaron, 1984; Orne & Dinges, 1984).

Consistent with this enduring interest in the "extraordinary" potential of hypnosis, a great deal of attention has turned recently to its purported effectiveness in reviving memories that seem to elude normal waking efforts at recollection. Much of the evidence for this hypermnesic effect of hypnosis derives from data obtained in the clinical context—highlighted by the early work of Breuer and Freud (1895/1955) in the treatment of hysteria. By the beginning of the 20th century, hypnotic hypermnesia was already being classified among the phenomena of hypnosis by major textbooks on the subject (e.g., Bramwell, 1903/1956; Janet, 1925; Moll, 1889/1958). Moreover, several pioneering laboratory experiments seemed to provide empirical evidence for these clinical impressions, documenting a tendency for enhanced recall of temporally remote memories in hypnosis as contrasted with ordinary waking recall (see Hull, 1933, pp. 111–127). Thus, the belief that hypnosis may aid in the recovery of lost memories is virtually contemporaneous with the disciplines of modern psychiatry and psychology.

Nevertheless, the major impetus to the present resurgence of interest in this topic has been the enthusiastic response by many law enforcement agencies to proposals and demonstrations of the usefulness of hypnosis in the forensic context. Proponents of the use of hypnosis in police investigation point confidently to a number of cases (e.g., the Chowchilla, California, kidnapping, reported in Kroger & Doucé, 1979) in which decisive evidence was apparently uncovered following the hypnotic interviewing of a witness or victim of a crime.

However, the use of hypnosis in the forensic setting has not been limited solely to the purpose of developing leads to physical evidence. In some instances, defendants have voluntarily submitted to hypnotic memory enhancement procedures in an effort to recall information that might help to reduce charges against them or to exonerate them. In other situations, hypnotic memory "refreshment" has been employed where there is a paucity of objective evidence to corroborate the fragmented, inconsistent, or vague recollections of a witness or victim. There is currently considerable controversy over the extent to which the use of hypnosis in an attempt to facilitate testimony in court is justified, given its potential to create a miscarriage of justice.

In this chapter, we examine the current scientific status of the facilitation of memory by hypnotic techniques. Our task begins with a conceptualization of the nature and characteristics of hypnosis, emphasizing possible mechanisms that are relevant to memory enhancement. This is followed by a critical evaluation of the clinical and laboratory evidence delineating the conditions under which hypnotic hypermnesia may be manifested. We also seek to assess whether the risks of false recollections, vulnerability to memory distortion, and unjustified confidence can be exacerbated by hypnosis to the detriment of the legal process. Finally, we consider the impact of such factors in the clinical setting. The discussion focuses on the distinction between forensic and clinical goals and procedures, and their implications for the use of hypnosis in the context of memory retrieval.

## HYPNOSIS: INTRINSIC FACTORS AND THEIR RELATION TO MEMORY ENHANCEMENT

### The Nature of Hypnosis

One of the more salient aspects of hypnosis to an observer is an apparent increase in the subject's willingness to accept and to respond to suggestions given by the hypnotist. What distinguishes true hypnotic responding, however, is not simple behavioral compliance, but rather the person's ability to experience suggested alterations in perception, memory, or mood (Orne,

1959, 1977). Whereas untrained nonhypnotized individuals can purposively feign the suggested distortions in a most convincing manner (Orne, 1959), the hypnotically responsive subject tends to experience the change as phenomenally real. These observations underscore the basic unreliability of overt behavioral compliance as a criterion of hypnosis. At the same time, they emphasize that the profound alterations in subjective experience (e.g., involuntariness, belief in the reality of the suggested event, etc.), which accompany attempts to respond to suggestions, constitute the essential characteristic of hypnosis.

A prerequisite for hypnosis is the willingness to adopt the role of "hypnotic subject," with its implicit social contract for uncritical acceptance of appropriate suggestions administered by the hypnotist (Orne, 1959; Sarbin, 1950; White, 1941). This requires the individual temporarily to relinquish reality orientation (Shor, 1959) and critical judgment and to allow the hypnotist to orchestrate the subject's experiences, with little concern for the inherent sense or nonsense of the suggestions or of his or her reactions to them.

The ability to experience hypnosis (i.e., hypnotizability) is a relatively enduring attribute of persons (Morgan, Johnson, & Hilgard, 1974), which has a near-normal distribution within the population (E. R. Hilgard, 1965). Consequently, all but a very few persons are capable of experiencing at least some of the effects of hypnosis when it is carried out in a facilitating context. Among the several factors that are important in this regard are the level of trust placed in the hypnotist by the subject; the subject's motivation to cooperate; and the kind of preconceptions the subject has concerning the nature of hypnosis and its effects. Thus, the induction of hypnosis actually begins with the hypnotist's efforts to establish rapport, while attempting to maximize the subject's expectations to respond and to allay any apprehension about the procedures to follow. Subsequently, any one of a variety of formal induction procedures can be used to promote the hypnotic condition.

## General Effects of Hypnosis on Memory

Once an individual has been exposed to a hypnotic induction for the purpose of restoring memory concerning some earlier incident, a number of factors—including the expectancies and motivations of all parties involved, and the very context of hypnosis (apart from the nature of specific suggestions)—may conspire to shape the content and/or quality of the memories that are reported. In view of the importance of this issue, particularly in the legal context, it seems useful to summarize these factors from the perspective of their implications for the validity and credibility of hypnotically accessed memories.

1. Hypnosis usually takes place in a calm, relaxed atmosphere that invites the subject to relinquish normal reality-monitoring activities, as well

as responsibility for behaviors manifested during hypnosis. Such a context may be particularly well suited for the elicitation of additional details or novel information in memory reports, much of which the subject may otherwise have been too uncertain about to have reported. Thus, it is possible that hypnosis may not enhance memory per se; instead, it may simply lower the threshold for *reporting* uncertain items of information.

2. Involvement in imagination or fantasy is an integral component of hypnosis (e.g., J. R. Hilgard, 1970), and one that is instrumental in producing many of the positive effects obtained with the technique in psychotherapeutic and medical applications. Indeed, hypnosis has been defined as "believed-in imaginings" (Sarbin & Coe, 1972). It is therefore reasonable to anticipate that fantasy productions may intrude upon and enmesh with historically valid portions of the memory reports of hypnotized persons.

3. Following the induction of hypnosis, individuals manifest an increase in suggestibility (Hull, 1933), in part as a direct consequence of their willingness to put aside critical evaluative functions while in hypnosis. As a result, memories accessed during hypnosis may be contaminated—wittingly or unwittingly—by the way in which suggestions are given, as well as by casual remarks or subtle cues of the hypnotist or others present during the session. Subsequently, it may be impossible for the subject to distinguish such "implanted" details from true memories.

4. When the subject has a belief about an incident in the past, but lacks full recollection of the events that occurred, hypnosis may serve as a catalyst to transform this belief into what is experienced as an actual memory. The increased tendency toward fantasy and the decrease in critical judgment, coupled with the conviction that hypnosis will produce accurate recall, may allow the subject to visualize what he or she believes might have happened and to accept the hypnotic visualization as a true memory of what actually occurred.

5. Without any special knowledge or training, individuals can successfully simulate being hypnotized, and it is exceedingly difficult to detect such purposive simulation (Orne, 1977).[1] Moreover, subjects who are in fact deeply hypnotized are still able to lie. Thus, it would be possible for a subject to *willfully* distort recollections in hypnosis (or while feigning hypnosis), in an effort to enhance the appearance of cooperation or otherwise to serve his or her own interests (Orne, 1961; Orne, Dinges, & Orne, 1984b).

6. Separate from the matter of the veridicality of memories retrieved with hypnosis, there are also characteristics of hypnotic experience that more

---

1. Without specially designed procedures, as well as blind observation of many hypnotized and simulating subjects followed by subsequent feedback as to their status, even highly trained clinicians and/or researchers cannot reliably identify individuals who are simulating hypnosis.

directly affect the *credibility* of the subject's memory reports. The subject's willingness to accept fantasy as reality during the hypnotic experience, together with the often dramatic vividness of recollections in hypnosis, may inspire great confidence that the recalled material is true to fact. In turn, the subject's conviction that these memories are accurate, and the greater number of details reported subsequent to hypnosis, confer credibility upon his or her memory reports in the minds of others, regardless of their factual status. These processes are often reinforced by the popular misconception that persons are unable to lie when hypnotized and/or by the widely held belief that hypnosis can produce increases in accurate memory (Orne, Soskis, Dinges, & Orne, 1984).

In conclusion, the hypnotic *context* provides a number of nonspecific influences that may underlie the apparent utility of hypnosis in restoring memory. However, we are particularly interested in assessing the nature and extent of effects that are specific to, or a direct consequence of, the hypnotic *process*. For example, posthypnotic amnesia is a hypnotic phenomenon in that it requires an appropriate suggestion administered to a hypnotizable person following the induction of hypnosis. Similarly, a demonstration that hypermnesia is specific to hypnosis would require that it result from appropriate suggestions given to a hypnotizable individual after induction. Another possibility is that an effect may be due to the trait of hypnotizability, independent of hypnotic induction. In subsequent sections of this chapter, we try to determine the extent to which the effects of hypnosis on the facilitation of memory can be demonstrated and which specific and nonspecific effects may contribute to the phenomenon.

## POTENTIAL MECHANISMS OF HYPNOTIC MEMORY ENHANCEMENT

Our consideration of hypnosis and the role of the hypnotic context in promoting increased memory has focused thus far on processes extraneous to memory that nevertheless can have an important influence on the apparent recovery of forgotten information. In this section, we briefly examine several theoretically relevant cognitive processes purportedly involved in normal memory, which can be assumed to covary with or be made more accessible by hypnosis. Thus, one might reasonably inquire, "What aspects of normal memory are likely to be influenced by hypnosis?" Or, to phrase it another way, "Why should memory be affected by hypnosis at all?"

Our approach to such questions begins with the almost universal conceptualization of memory as a three-stage process involving the acquisition, retention, and later retrieval of information (e.g., Bourne, Dominowski, &

Loftus, 1979; Gleitman, 1981). Moreover, in considering the processes by which hypnosis might facilitate recovery of memories, our discussion is confined to mechanisms of retrieval. It is likely, in any case, that deficits related to the acquisition or storage of information would prove unresponsive to attempts at memory remediation by hypnotic or any other means, since in such instances the memory "trace" either was never encoded or was physically ablated, as through organic disease or physical insult. Hypnosis may prove valuable, however, in cases involving retrieval failure, where certain cognitive mechanisms activated by hypnosis may reinforce normal retrieval functions or provide alternate access to the unrecovered memories. Here we consider several hypotheses that posit mechanisms of this sort in the effects of hypnosis on memory.

### Posthypnotic Amnesia

A purely intuitive basis for anticipating that hypnosis might make contact with mechanisms necessary for the enhancement of memory derives from the phenomenon of suggested posthypnotic amnesia among individuals who have experienced deep hypnosis (L. M. Cooper, 1972; Kihlstrom & Evans, 1979). What is striking is the apparent ease with which such amnesia can be induced and subsequently lifted in hypnotically responsive subjects, simply by administering the relevant suggestion. The reversible nature of posthypnotic amnesia provides assurance that the target memories have not decayed but are merely temporarily inaccessible (Orne, 1966). More importantly, the potential of the amnesia suggestion to render specific memories inaccessible to recall, coupled with the ease of reinstating these recollections by simple suggestion, indicates a pliancy to hypnotic suggestion of some critical substrate of information recovery from the memory store. Thus, it is possible that a direct suggestion for hypermnesia may also activate this substrate in a manner analogous to the cancellation of posthypnotic amnesia, and thereby may breach nonsuggested spontaneous amnesia as well (Nace, Orne, & Hammer, 1974).

### Functional Amnesias

Another class of memory retrieval failures consists of those commonly precipitated by an experience involving severe psychological trauma. Amnesias of this nature involve motivated forgetting or repression—that is, the active exclusion of unacceptable memories from conscious awareness. In extreme cases, however, the inaccessible memories have an etiological role in certain serious clinical disorders (e.g., hysteria, fugue states, and multiple personality). Interestingly, it was the striking similarity of certain hypnotic phenomena (e.g., limb catalepsy, sensory anesthesias, and spontaneous amnesia) to the symptomatology of hysteria—noted in the experiments carried out by Charcot at the Salpêtrière and by Bernheim at Nancy—that suggested a possible relationship between the two conditions to many 19th-century students of psychopathology (Janet, 1925; see also Ellenberger, 1970). Recent clinical evidence (Frankel, 1976; Spiegel & Spiegel, 1978) confirms that some of these dissociative disorders share characteristics common to hypnosis and are often associated with hypnotizability. Given this long-standing conceptual intimacy between naturally occurring dissociative states and their hypnotic analogues, the use of hypnosis in the treatment of psychogenic amnesia followed logically. Indeed, there are now numerous clinical case reports describing recoveries of repressed memories, and the abatement of corresponding psychological symptoms, following either spontaneous or suggested age regression in the context of hypnotherapy (e.g., Cedercreutz, 1972; Conn, 1960; Frankel, 1976; Garver, Fuselier, & Booth, 1981; MacHovec, 1981; Raginsky, 1969; Spiegel, Shor, & Fishman, 1945; Twerski & Naar, 1976).

Unfortunately, the absence of control procedures in such case studies leaves the mechanism(s) involved in the breaching of amnesia by age regression largely unilluminated. Perhaps the commonality between characteristics of hypnosis and dissociative symptoms is indicative of a common cognitive substrate providing access to ideas and emotions blocked from awareness. Alternatively, hypnosis, via age regression techniques, may be successful in restoring inaccessible memories by mentally reinstating conditions present at the time of the original incident, thereby increasing the availability of relevant retrieval cues. Finally, it is useful to consider the possibility that the memories that are "recovered" following hypnotic age regression may not be the same ones that were "lost"; that is, the hypnotically recovered memories may consist of an indeterminable ratio of fiction to fact. Nevertheless, this lack of historical accuracy need not diminish the therapeutic value of the recollections. The significance of this possibility is taken up in greater detail in a later section.

## Imagery-Mediated Recall

Mental imagery has been recognized as an important factor in human cognition and memory (e.g., Neisser, 1967; Paivio, 1969). The use of imagery during encoding is thought by many researchers (e.g., Paivio, 1969) to facilitate later recall of certain types of verbal information. For example, the recall of paired-associate nouns can be significantly improved when, during study, subjects imagine the referents of each such pair interacting in some way (Bower, 1970).

Imagery also appears to play a role in the representation of events in memory (e.g., Kosslyn, 1981; Paivio, 1971), as suggested, for example, by studies involving the mental rotation of objects (L. A. Cooper & Shepard,

1973), image scanning (Kosslyn, 1973), and comparative judgments between images of objects (Paivio, 1975). Moreover, it has specific relevance for the storage of personal experiences in "episodic memory," where items are characterized solely by their perceptible properties and their temporal–spatial relations to other experienced events (Tulving, 1972). Finally, experimental data (e.g., Sheehan, 1972) indicate that imagery production may be a particularly useful strategy for the retrieval of incidentally acquired information—the kind of information that is often of considerable importance in both the clinical and forensic contexts.

Whatever advantage hypnosis may confer upon the retrieval of episodic experiences from memory can reasonably be linked to its capacity to increase image utilization and vividness (K. S. Bowers, 1976; Crawford & Allen, 1983; S. Sanders, 1969; Sheehan, 1979). In this connection, there is considerable evidence indicating a positive relationship between hypnotizability and vividness of imagery (P. G. Bowers, 1978, 1982; Shor, Orne, & O'Connell, 1966; Spanos, Valois, Ham, & Ham, 1973; Sutcliffe, Perry, & Sheehan, 1970; 't Hoen, 1978)—a finding that is consistent with the purported tendency for hypnosis to affect imagery. However, this relationship also suggests the possibility that in some circumstances where hypnosis appears to enhance the production of imagery, it does so in a permissive fashion, giving expression to a trait that is associated with the ability to experience hypnosis. In such cases, any corresponding memory enhancement, rather than implying a role for imagery-mediated *retrieval*, may conceivably reflect a bias in the manner by which events were originally *encoded* in memory (i.e., "holistic" vs. "detail-oriented" or "deep" vs. "superficial" processing), which is correlated with the individual's imagery ability.

It is well established that encoding strategies that favor deep processing (Craik & Lockhart, 1972) result subsequently in better recall and recognition performance. Moreover, there is some evidence (Crawford & Allen, 1983) that hypnotically responsive subjects are more likely to employ deep-level (imagistic or holistic) processing of visual stimuli, particularly during hypnosis, with the result that performance on tasks dependent upon visual memory is significantly facilitated. Thus, there is support for the view that imagery-mediated retrieval mechanisms evoked during hypnosis, or possibly information-processing biases associated with imagery ability and hypnotic responsiveness, may play some role in the effects of hypnosis on memory.

## Reinstatement of Encoding Context and Mood

One way in which hypnotic age regression procedures may interact with imagery processes aroused during hypnosis to facilitate memory is by elaborating images of the context in which the forgotten information was originally encoded. Mentally reconstructing the contextual cues present during encoding may then permit those same cues to guide the process of retrieval, much as an experimenter's explicitly providing an appropriate retrieval cue at test reliably enhances a subject's recall relative to an uncued test (Tulving & Pearlstone, 1966).

Compelling evidence for the effectiveness of mentally reinstating the context at acquisition was provided by S. M. Smith (1979), who showed that memory for verbal material was enhanced by recalling the material in the same room in which it was learned. Furthermore, he demonstrated that even when recall was attempted in a different room, memory could be improved simply by visualizing the original learning environment. A related finding was reported by Malpass and Devine (1981), using a "guided-memory" procedure with witnesses to a staged vandalism that had occurred 5 months earlier. Essentially, this technique consists of a series of specific questions that provide considerable correct information and then ask the subject for additional related details. Subjects were instructed to visualize aspects of the original environmental setting, including others present and their activities, as well as to remember whatever thoughts, feelings and reactions they might have experienced at the time of the critical events. Following the detailed guided-memory interview, witnesses were more accurate in identifying the vandal in a photographic lineup than were witnesses who were simply asked to identify the vandal's photograph. Similar findings with eyewitnesses have been reported using a "cognitive interview" technique that also relies upon context reinstatement, as well as repeated attempts to mentally review the events from different perspectives and in different temporal orders (Geiselman *et al.*, 1984).

Cognitive retrieval strategies of this nature, if part of the hypnotic procedure, may account for memory improvement (e.g., Shaul, 1978; Stager & Lundy, 1985). However, such results may not invariably be obtained (see Loftus, Manber, & Keating, 1983; Sturm, 1982), due, among other factors, to situational variability in the degree to which contextual cues become associated with the critical events during encoding or in the degree to which they can be reinstated at recall.

The "context" associated with an event may also include effects that the situation produces on the affective experience of an observer. Research indicates, moreover, that a person's mood or level of autonomic arousal while experiencing a particular event may determine the subsequent accessibility of memory for that event; accessibility is generally improved when the mood state during retrieval is similar to the mood state at acquisition (M. S. Clark, Milberg, & Ross, 1983; Teasdale & Fogarty, 1979). The capacity to alter an individual's mood by hypnotic suggestion (Hodge, Wagner, & Schreiner, 1966; Orne & Hammer, 1974) appears to provide a potentially effective technique for the recovery of mood-specific memories, as demonstrated by the research of Bower and his associates (Bower, 1981; Bower, Monteiro, & Gilligan, 1978).[2] Thus, hypnotic reinstatement of the affect uniquely associated with certain episodic events may possibly increase the availability of relevant retrieval cues, and consequently may improve an individual's memory for such events.

## Multiple Retrieval Attempts and Nonhypnotic Hypermnesia

An alternative process to those considered above, which has nothing to do with hypnosis per se, may occur as the product of allocating extended time and effort to memory retrieval. Laboratory studies suggest that the amount of information retrieved from memory on any given recall trial is often not exhaustive of the total set of items available in storage (e.g., Brown, 1923; Tulving & Pearlstone, 1966). Moreover, particularly in circumstances where pictorial or imagistic stimuli have served as input material (Erdelyi & Becker, 1974; Erdelyi, Finkelstein, Herrell, Miller, & Thomas, 1976; Erdelyi & Kleinbard, 1978; Popkin & Small, 1979; Roediger & Payne, 1985), repeated memory testing has been found to yield progressive increases in accurate recall over trials. This effect (referred to as "hypermnesia") appears to involve a true increase in memory accessibility as opposed to a change in report criterion[3] (e.g., reporting an increasingly higher proportion of guesses over successive trials), since intertrial increments in correct recall occur even when subjects are required to produce a constant high output across trials (Erdelyi & Becker, 1974; Erdelyi & Kleinbard, 1978).

Some researchers (e.g., Roediger & Payne, 1982) have suggested that hypermnesia occurs specifically because of repeated testing (whether conducted at an overt or a covert level), which conceivably leads to better organization of recall and hence to more efficient retrieval strategies over trials. Regardless of the underlying mechanism, however, the phenomenon is robust and reliable under a variety of multitrial-recall conditions (Erdelyi, 1984;

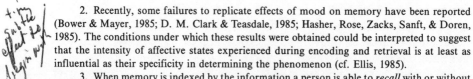

2. Recently, some failures to replicate effects of mood on memory have been reported (Bower & Mayer, 1985; D. M. Clark & Teasdale, 1985; Hasher, Rose, Zacks, Sanft, & Doren, 1985). The conditions under which these results were obtained could be interpreted to suggest that the intensity of affective states experienced during encoding and retrieval is at least as influential as their specificity in determining the phenomenon (cf. Ellis, 1985).

3. When memory is indexed by the information a person is able to *recall* with or without the aid of retrieval cues, it seems to us useful to refer to the subjective standard that the individual invokes to distinguish information retrieved from memory as the "*report* criterion." In a *recognition* task, where the person is not required to produce information, but merely to judge (typically by responding "yes" or "no") whether some currently presented information is the same as that which was previously encoded in memory, we refer to the level of subjective certainty required for a "yes" response as the "*response* criterion."

Roediger & Payne, 1985), given appropriate imagistic or meaningful stimulus materials.

The significance of this phenomenon for understanding the potential enhancement of memory by hypnosis resides in the simple fact that the efficacy of hypnosis is assessed in many situations by the uncovering of *previously inaccessible* memories. That is, one or more overt or covert attempts to retrieve the elusive memories in the normal waking condition precede the use of hypnosis to aid recollection. This pattern is probably characteristic of the majority of cases in which clinical hypermnesias with hypnosis have been observed, and is true of virtually every instance in which hypnosis has been used for investigative purposes by law enforcement officials. These same issues also apply to laboratory studies of hypnotic hypermnesia where a hypnotic recall follows a waking test.

Thus, what is taken as support for the efficacy of hypnosis in aiding memory retrieval may at times be a true hypermnesic process, but one that has little to do with hypnosis per se. Of course, the ubiquity of nonhypnotic hypermnesia resulting from repeated recall attempts does not preclude effects in hypnosis of the kinds of cognitive processes that we have discussed above. Indeed, nonhypnotic hypermnesia can be thought to subsume a variety of such effects, as suggested, for example, by its apparent dependence on imagery processes. However, the phenomenon of nonhypnotic hypermnesia requires that apparent memory enhancement effects attributed to hypnosis be evaluated against the proper baseline control procedure—one that takes account of the role of repeated testing, retrieval time, and effort in facilitating recall.

This section has reviewed certain mechanisms of normal memory that conceivably may be optimized by the hypnotic process. Our objective in selecting representative mechanisms has been to highlight those that may readily (perhaps unwittingly) be brought into play, even in nondirective applications of hypnotic procedures. For example, it does not necessarily require a specific suggestion to alter mood; age regression to a psychologically disturbing episode in a person's life can be quite effective! Then, too, the list is not exhaustive, and other possible mechanisms could be appended, such as anxiety reduction (cf. Erdelyi, 1985, pp. 240–242) or memorial "focusing" (Loftus, 1982).

Consequently, it should be clear that many of the procedures utilized during hypnosis incidentally involve the kind of cognitive strategies discussed above. Since these strategies can be shown to affect recall without hypnosis, it becomes relevant to ask whether hypnosis or hypnotizability adds to, or interacts with, these processes to yield hypermnesia. We turn our attention now to the rapidly accumulating scientific literature to evaluate the evidence bearing on this issue.

## EMPIRICAL STATUS OF THE FACILITATION OF
## MEMORY BY HYPNOSIS

### Hypnotic Age Regression

Near the end of the 19th century, psychiatry had become alerted to the pathogenic influence of persistent memories (both conscious and unconscious) of early traumatic events as an etiological factor in many psychological disorders. Pierre Janet, in reviewing the clinical evidence for this prevalent viewpoint, outlined the rationale for the use of hypnosis in certain cases:

> [I]t soon became apparent to me that many of the most important traumatic memories might be imperfectly known by the subject. . . . Sometimes we had to look for them when the patient was in a special mental condition; sometimes, lost memories would crop up in the somnambulist state, in automatic writing, in dreams. (1925, p. 594)

In an earlier work (*L'Automatisme Psychologique*, 1889, cited in Ellenberger, 1970), Janet described the hypnotic treatment of a patient, Marie, who during a previous hypnosis had attributed her present convulsive attacks and delirium to a childhood experience that occurred at the time of her menarche:

> . . . I tried to take away from somnambulic consciousness this fixed and absurd idea that the menstruation was stopped by a cold bath. At first, I could not manage to do it; the fixed idea persisted. . . . I was able to succeed only thanks to a singular means. It was necessary to bring her back, through suggestion, to the age of thirteen, put her back into the initial circumstances of the delirium, convince her that the menstruation had lasted for three days and was not interrupted through any regrettable incident. Now, once this was done, the following menstruation came at the due point, and lasted for three days, without any pain, convulsion or delirium. (Ellenberger, 1970, p. 365)

This was one of the earliest reports of a psychotherapeutic use of hypnotic age regression, in this case for the purpose of hypnotically modifying the traumatic memories that subserved a hysterical illness; in other instances, Janet employed the technique to elicit the unconscious memories and emotions themselves, if they were not spontaneously forthcoming when the patient was questioned in hypnosis (cf. Ellenberger, 1970, p. 364). The issue of whether such hypnotically elicited memories had historical validity was not of relevance to Janet; his use of age regression involved supplanting whatever disturbing memories (veridical or not) the patient reported with psychologically more tolerable ones.

Freud's use of hypnosis was for a different purpose—namely to explore the emotionally stressful childhood events that were thought to be the basis of patients' psychological symptoms (Breuer & Freud, 1895/1955). The phenomena that emerged in the course of this work endowed these hypnotic remembrances with an aura of credibility. Thus, the intense emotional reactions and the wealth of detail that characterized the hypnotic reminiscences of his patients, as well as the often dramatic alleviation of their symptoms subsequent to the hypnotic reliving of painful life events, originally had misled Freud to suppose that such recollections corresponded to true autobiographical occurrences.

But clinical experience soon caused Freud to question the historical accuracy of the recollections reported in hypnosis; he eventually came to recognize that while emotionally valid, these memories were not necessarily veridical relivings of traumatic childhood experiences (cf. Freud, 1906/1953, p. 274). Rather, the hypnotically elicited memories of such early events were often comprised of various proportions of fact, fantasy, and confabulation.

Laboratory research into the mechanisms of hypnotic age regression has typically concerned itself with whether age regression produces a genuine reviviscence—an actual reliving of earlier developmental stages accompanied by behavioral, psychological, and physiological responses appropriate to such stages. Thus, several studies reported, with varying rates of success, the elicitation of the neonatal Babinski reflex to plantar stimulation when subjects were regressed to an age of 5 months or less (Gidro-Frank & Bowers Buch, 1948; McCranie, Crasilneck, & Teter, 1955; True & Stephenson, 1951). However, Barber (1962) reviewed evidence from three studies observing over 500 normal infants, and concluded that, contrary to popular belief, the Babinski sign was *not* the modal response to plantar stimulation among infants less than 7 months of age. Carefully controlled studies (e.g., McCranie *et al.*, 1955) have also failed to document the claimed occurrence of spontaneous characteristic changes in electroencephalographic (EEG) patterns when adult subjects are age-regressed to infancy.

Similarly, a systematic replication and extension of the classic monograph study of Reiff and Scheerer (1959), carried out by O'Connell, Shor, and Orne (1970), revealed that many of the apparent developmental changes in cognitive functioning reported in the original investigation resulted from experimenter bias and situational demand characteristics. Of particular relevance to the present evaluation, however, was the failure of O'Connell *et al.* (1970) to find any evidence of hypermnesia during age regression for remote autobiographical information, such as the name of a subject's second-grade teacher or fellow classmates, as was apparently obtained in the original study of Reiff and Scheerer (1959). Other dramatic claims for hypermnesia during hypnotic age regression (e.g., True, 1949) also could not be replicated (Barber, 1961; O'Connell *et al.*, 1970; Orne, 1951). In summary, the weight of experimental evidence from carefully controlled studies of hypnotic age regression fails to provide convincing support for a literal revivification process, at least in the domains of memory, physiological functions, and perceptual/cognitive development.

Some recent work (Nash, Johnson, & Tipton, 1979; Nash, Lynn, Stanley, Frauman, & Rhue, 1985) has demonstrated apparent age-dependent changes of an affective nature involving interpersonal and object relations (i.e., toward a transitional object), which occur in hypnotized, but not in simulating, subjects who are regressed to age 3. These findings suggest a possible link to mechanisms of the kind that occasion intense emotional abreaction when age regression is employed in the context of dynamic hypnotherapy. However, an interesting and highly germane footnote to the research program of Nash and his colleagues is that despite the more characteristically childlike affective response exhibited by hypnotizable subjects during age regression, the same subjects were significantly *less* accurate in recalling their own childhood transitional objects than were simulators, when retrospective reports by parents served as a criterion (Nash, Drake, Wiley, Khalsa, & Lynn, 1986). Of course, parental memory surely cannot constitute an infallible standard; hence this finding should be regarded merely as suggestive, but, as we shall see, it does not stand alone.

## Hypnotic Effects on Recall and Recognition of Verifiable Facts

One common methodological weakness associated with research on hypnotic age regression, and illustrated in the aforementioned study by Nash *et al.* (1986), is the difficulty of obtaining reliable corroborative evidence with which to determine the veridicality of the subject's apparent memories (see also O'Connell *et al.*, 1970; Reiff & Scheerer, 1959). The issue is not peculiar to the research laboratory; indeed, it is a crucial and persistent concern in the forensic use of hypnosis, and although the validity of memory may be of lesser importance to the psychotherapeutic process, its verification in the clincial setting is no less problematic. Consequently, when the evidence for hypnotic hypermnesia is being evaluated, those studies in which there is explicit foreknowledge of or control over the to-be-remembered stimuli must be weighted more heavily, because they are able to identify confabulations and pseudomemories. Due to space limitations, a critical review of each of these studies is not possible here. Instead, we focus discussion on certain key investigations and draw generalizations, where warranted, from other related experiments.

### Meaningful versus Nonmeaningful
### Stimulus Material

With only a single exception (Augustynek, 1978, 1979), attempts to demonstrate memory enhancement by hypnosis have failed when the stimulus items have been devoid of either inherent or contextual meaning. Although the studies whose findings give rise to this conclusion vary considerably in methodological sophistication, they are nevertheless remarkably consistent on this score. Among the memory materials found to be intractable to hypnotic enhancement procedures are nonsense syllables (Baker, Haynes, & Patrick, 1983; Barber & Calverley, 1966; Dhanens & Lundy, 1975; Eysenck, 1941; Huse, 1930; Mitchell, 1932; White, Fox, & Harris, 1940); lists of unrelated words or word pairs (Das, 1961; Salzberg & DePiano, 1980; Young, 1925); and ostensibly irrelevant, incidental, or peripheral details (Baker *et al.*, 1983; Young, 1926; but see DePiano & Salzberg, 1981, and Sheehan & Tilden, 1984, for exceptions involving meaningful peripheral materials).

On the other hand, the various stimulus materials that tend to be conducive to apparent memory enhancement by hypnosis are those that can be characterized as more or less personally, intrinsically, or contextually *meaningful*. Thus, pictures, poetry, stories, films, and other thematic materials have been found to give rise to greater recall during hypnosis than during the nonhypnotic condition (DePiano & Salzberg, 1981; Dhanens & Lundy, 1975; Rosenthal, 1944; Stager & Lundy, 1985; Stalnaker & Riddle, 1932; White *et al.*, 1940). However, stimulus meaningfulness is not a sufficient condition to ensure the superiority of the hypnotic treatment over waking memory. Thus, the impact of the hypnotic intervention may be greater with subjects high, rather than low, in hypnotizability (Dhanens & Lundy, 1975; Dywan & Bowers, 1983; Stager & Lundy, 1985); or it may fail to differentiate hypnotic and nonhypnotic recall (McConkey & Nogrady, 1984; Nogrady, McConkey, & Perry, 1985; Putnam, 1979; Sheehan & Tilden, 1983), particularly when hypnosis is compared with motivating instructions (L. M. Cooper & London, 1973; Nogrady *et al.*, 1985; Shaul, 1978).

The influence of stimulus meaningfulness on the expression of hypnotic hypermnesia may be attributable to differential constraints on the extent of spontaneous perceptual processing of meaningful and nonmeaningful materials (Shields & Knox, 1986). This conceptual outlook derives from the levels-of-processing framework of Craik and Lockhart (1972), which holds that retention is a positive function of the depth of analysis or extent of encoding elaboration an item receives. Accordingly, nonmeaningful materials, by definition, lack semantic attributes that are necessary for deep-level processing and hence are poorly registered and poorly retained in memory. In constrast, meaningful stimuli can (but need not) be more readily submitted to deep-level analysis (i.e., processed semantically and/or associated with existing cognitive structures) to ensure their persistence in memory and accessibility during retrieval. Support for the view that hypnosis may improve memory for deeply, but not shallowly, processed stimuli that have been equated for meaningfulness has been reported by Shields and Knox (1986; see also Crawford & Allen, 1983), but was not found in a face recognition task (Redston & Knox, 1983). Further experimental work is needed to determine whether this alternative conceptual approach provides better clarification of the conditions under which hypnotic memory enhancement may occur.

## Recent versus Remote Memories

Laboratory studies of the effects of hypnosis on memory have generally confined themselves to assessing the retention of comparatively recently presented information. This bias has arisen and is maintained largely because of the difficulty in controlling variability of longer retention intervals, as well as other methodological considerations (e.g., the control of stimulus content and acquisition factors) and pragmatic issues (e.g., minimizing subject attrition). Unfortunately, such studies can be criticized from the perspective of their external validity for failing to adequately reconstruct the conditions around which real-life claims of the utility of hypnosis to improve memory often revolve. Thus, when hypnosis is employed in a police investigation or in a therapeutic setting, it is often for the purpose of helping individuals to remember the details of an autobiographical episode thought to have transpired days, weeks, months, or even years previously.

A good deal of the evidence relevant to this issue has already been taken up in the discussion of hypnotic age regression. On the basis of available data from properly controlled experiments and studies in which the researchers had access to biographical records, there is no support for the view that hypnotic age regression improves accurate recollection of childhood memories (cf. O'Connell *et al.*, 1970).

In a classic investigation, Stalnaker and Riddle (1932) used subjects of high hypnotic responsivity to study the capacity of hypnosis to improve recall for poetry and prose selections learned at least 1 year previously. In terms of the total number of words from these selections that were correctly recalled by all subjects combined, hypnosis accounted for a gain of approximately 54% over ordinary waking recall. However, word counts and excerpts from some of the subjects' protocols obtained in both the waking and hypnotic conditions revealed the likely source of the superiority of hypnotic recall: As summarized by Stalnaker and Riddle, "the subjects wrote more of both correct and incorrect words in the trance state than in the waking" (p. 439). This indicates that the effect of hypnosis was primarily to increase the number of responses produced (correct as well as incorrect) over the number proferred during waking recall trials. In reviewing these findings in 1933, Hull already suggests the mechanism whereby the hypnotic enhancement effect might have been realized:

> Moreover, there is strong indication in the Stalnaker–Riddle results that the standard of material which the subjects were willing to offer as satisfactory recall in the trance was considerably lower than that characteristic of the waking

condition. It is conceivable that this difference in standard of certainty or accuracy may be entirely responsible for the increased amount of recall characteristic of the trance state. (p. 115)

These observations by Stalnaker and Riddle (1932) and by Hull (1933) directly pertain to what is now termed the "response criterion problem" (Klatzky & Erdelyi, 1985). Very simply, the "problem" is that an increase in correct recall does not distinguish whether hypnosis actually improves the accessibility of information in memory, or instead merely liberalizes the subject's criterion for *reporting* such information. The qualitative evidence highlighted by Stalnaker and Riddle and by Hull is, however, more consistent with the latter possibility.

The Stalnaker and Riddle (1932) study was also the first to focus on the increased tendency toward confabulation in hypnotic recollection. For example, one subject, who was unable in the waking condition to furnish the second stanza of Longfellow's "The Village Blacksmith," once hypnotized, "recalled" the following:

> *The smithy whistles at his forge*
> *As he shapes the iron band;*
> *The smith is very happy*
> *As he owes not any man.*

Considered on its own merits, the subject's reproduction appears quite plausible—a common characteristic of confabulation. It possesses a realistic quality that results partly from the careful attention to structure (i.e., rhyme, meter) and style. But, with the exception of the final line, it bears only the faintest resemblance to Longfellow's original second stanza:

> *His hair is crisp, and black and long,*
> *His face is like the tan:*
> *His brow is wet with honest sweat,*
> *He earns what e'er he can,*
> *And looks the whole world in the face,*
> *For he owes not any man.*

Stalnaker and Riddle (1932) provide several other examples of the increased willingness of their subjects to confabulate or improvise verses of poetry while recalling in hypnosis—an inclination that was relatively slight in the waking condition. It is not difficult to see how, in the absence of a source of verification, such confabulations can masquerade as true recollections, thereby appearing to confirm the effectiveness of hypnosis in restoring lost memories. The study by Stalnaker and Riddle, although interpreted by them to have clearly established hypnotic hypermnesia for meaningful material learned more than a year previously, remains, paradoxically, one of the most instructive sources of evidence available concerning *pseudo*hypermnesic effects of hypnosis.

More recent studies have investigated the effects of hypnosis on memories of approximately 1 week's vintage. Some of these have been concerned with the effects of hypnosis on eyewitness recognition memory for photographs of faces, videotaped crime sequences, and staged enactments. In all such cases, hypnosis failed to increase recognition accuracy beyond that of nonhypnotic performance (G.S. Sanders & Simmons, 1983; Wagstaff, 1982; Wagstaff, Traverse, & Milner, 1982), and actually led to fewer correct (G.S. Sanders & Simmons, 1983) as well as more incorrect identifications (Wagstaff, 1982; Wagstaff *et al.*, 1982). L.M. Cooper and London (1973), using a within-subjects design involving immediate and delayed (2 weeks) cued-recall tests for meaningful information, found no significant improvement over waking recall due either to hypnosis or to hypnotizability. However, a significant nonspecific hypermnesia effect was obtained, in that all treatment groups exhibited greater recall on the second (delayed) test than they had on the first test.

A notable exception to the outcomes of the preceding studies is an experiment by Stager and Lundy (1985). These investigators found an increase in cued recall for information presented in a film 1 week earlier among hypnotizable subjects given a hypnotic treatment. What is striking about these results is that the increase in correct recall apparently occurred without a concomitant increase in errors—a finding that would seem unlikely if hypnosis had merely augmented subjects' productivity. In view of the singular status of this pattern of findings and its implications for the hypnotic improvement of memory, two independent attempts (Lytle & Lundy, 1986; Whitehouse, Dinges, Orne, & Orne, 1987) to replicate these results were carried out, but neither could reproduce the hypnotic hypermnesia reported by Stager and Lundy (1985).

## Impact of Emotionally Arousing Stimuli

The success of hypnosis in the therapeutic situation probably owes much to the fact that, whatever experiences are remembered during hypnosis, they often involve intense emotions of which the patient was previously unaware. Such "abreaction" is generally followed by clinical improvement. This covariation of memory and emotion leads naturally to debate over which process is responsible for the patient's improvment—insight from the memory, or experience of the intense emotion, or both.

On other grounds, the relationship can be seen to exemplify notions of "encoding specificity" (Tulving & Thomson, 1973) or "mood-state dependency" (Bower, 1981), which have been proposed as determinants of the efficacy of memory retrieval processes. As we have seen, the work of Bower and his associates provides some indication that hypnosis can be utilized to modulate mood to provide greater access to memories characterized by similar affective tone (Bower, 1981; Bower *et al.*, 1978). It should be noted, however, that failures to find mood-dependent retrieval with hypnosis have also been reported (e.g., Bower & Mayer, 1985), just as more generally applicable nonhypnotic procedures of mood induction (e.g., Velten, 1968) have successfully yielded mood-specific retrieval effects (Teasdale & Fogarty, 1979).

The characteristic of hypnosis that many consider instrumental to the uncovering of traumatic memories is its ability to diminish anxiety (e.g., Schafer & Rubio, 1978; Spiegel, 1980). Typically, hypnotic induction and deepening procedures are replete with suggestions for calmness, security, pleasantness, and profound relaxation. When accepted by the patient or eyewitness to a crime, these suggestions may coalesce to form a powerful antagonist to the fear and anxiety that otherwise may be aroused by remembering emotionally charged events, thereby making the individual more willing to think about and recall these events.[4]

Laboratory studies of the impact of hypnosis on memory for emotionally stressful events have yielded inconclusive results. An early investigation by Rosenthal (1944) found that hypnosis produced a significant increase (relative to nonhypnotic retrieval) in the recall of poetry and nonsense material that was learned in, and made relevant by, an experimentally induced anxious state. However, several more recent studies (Baker & Patrick, 1987; DePiano & Salzberg, 1981; Helwig, 1978; Shaul, 1978; Zelig & Beidleman, 1981) have failed to provide support for these findings. In view of the procedural differences among such a small number of studies, however, and the difficulties inherent in effectively controlling manipulations of stress and arousal, further experimental work is necessary before firm conclusions on the matter can be justified.

## Forensic Simulation Studies and Case Illustrations

A number of researchers have assessed the effects of hypnotic procedures on memory for stimuli and events that share certain features with actual forensic cases. It is fair to say, however, that no laboratory studies successfully mimic, in all details, the circumstances confronting an eyewitness or victim of a crime (DePiano & Salzberg, 1981; M. C. Smith, 1983). Nevertheless, attempts to investigate these ecologically more relevant variables, albeit often in isolation, have yielded remarkably consistent observations.

In an investigation reported by Putnam (1979), subjects of equivalent

4. The restoration of inaccessible traumatic memories as the result of a reduction in anxiety brought about by hypnosis is distinctly antithetical to the theoretical basis for mood-dependent retrieval, according to which hypnosis would be employed to *reinstate* the individual's emotional reactions at the time of the original trauma, in an effort to revive effective mood-relevant retrieval cues.

hypnotizability viewed a videotape depicting a traffic accident. Subsequently, half of the subjects received a hypnotic induction while the remaining subjects did not, and all were questioned about details of the event while mentally reviewing the episode on an imaginary television set (cf. Reiser, 1976). Hypnosis did not increase the amount of correctly remembered information over the amount obtained in the nonhypnotic condition. However, 6 of the 15 questions that were put to all subjects were misleading questions, in that they were designed to subtly suggest a specific incorrect answer. Putnam found that hypnotized subjects were significantly more susceptible to making errors in response to these leading questions than were nonhypnotized control subjects. In addition, despite making more errors, hypnotized subjects were just as confident in the accuracy of their memories, both correct and incorrect, as were control subjects. A more recent study by Zelig and Beidleman (1981), using an emotionally upsetting accident film as a stimulus, obtained the same pattern of findings. Thus, hypnotized subjects made more errors in response to leading questions and exhibited misplaced confidence in the accuracy of their responses, compared with subjects tested in the waking condition. Again, though, hypnosis did not increase the quantity of accurate information beyond that provided by nonhypnotized subjects.

The failure of hypnosis to enhance memory under controlled conditions has been observed in several other investigations that have some generalizability to the forensic domain, such as studies involving films or slide sequences of vehicular accidents and criminal acts (Buckhout, Eugenio & Grosso, 1981; Helwig, 1978; G. S. Sanders & Simmons, 1983; Sheehan, Grigg, & McCann, 1984; Sheehan & Tilden, 1983, 1984; Sturm, 1982; Yuille & McEwan, 1985); studies involving staged incidents and mock crimes (Timm, 1981; Wagstaff *et al.*, 1982); and most significantly, a major field study of hypnotic interviews by police officers of witnesses and victims of actual crimes (Sloane, 1981). Nearly as common is the finding that these hypnotically acquired memories are less reliable than nonhypnotic memories (G. S. Sanders & Simmons, 1983; Sheehan & Tilden, 1983; Sturm, 1982; Tallant, 1984; Wagstaff, 1982; Wagstaff *et al.*, 1982), and incommensurate in accuracy with the degree of confidence that is placed in them (G. S. Sanders & Simmons, 1983; Sheehan *et al.*, 1984; Sheehan & Tilden, 1983, 1984; Timm, 1982; Wagstaff, 1982; Wagstaff *et al.*, 1982).

The aspects of hypnosis that make hypnotic recall less accurate and the subsequent memories less reliable are not mere laboratory curiosities, but have been demonstrated in a very considerable number of court cases in which hypnotically created testimony played a significant role (for an extended discussion of such cases, see Orne, Soskis, Dinges, Orne, & Tonry, 1985). Increased errors and confabulation in hypnotic recall were illustrated, for example, in *People v. Kempinski* (1980), where, during hypnosis, a witness "remembered" the facial characteristics of someone under conditions that vastly exceeded the limits of the human eye. Similarly, in *State v. Mack* (1980), a hypnotized person remembered eating a pizza in a restaurant that did not serve pizza, seeing tattoos on someone who had none, and having been stabbed with scissors or a knife where there was no evidence that a weapon was involved. The effect of leading questions was dramatically illustrated in *State v. Forney* (1984). In this case, a suspect was hypnotized and asked leading questions about a rake, which only the police, the hypnotist, and the assailant knew had been used on the murder victim. Subsequently, the suspect's hypnotically created "recollection" of a rake was used as proof of his guilt, since the fact could only have been known by the true perpetrator. Finally, dangers associated with hypnotically augmented confidence are exemplified in numerous cases where a witness was originally uncertain about what had occurred, but subsequent to hypnosis became convinced, and in turn provided convincing testimony leading to an indictment and conviction of an individual (e.g., *Commonwealth v. Kater*, 1983; *People v. Shirley*, 1982; *State v. McQueen*, 1978).

## Modification of Subjective Report Criteria

Regardless of whether a particular study shows an increase in correct recall or, alternatively, an escalation of inaccurate recall following a hypnotic induction, such evidence cannot tell us directly whether hypnosis has its effect on memory accessibility or upon the criterion that subjects adopt in reporting their remembrances. If hypnosis has a true effect on memory accessibility, it should act upon the same processes that are affected by variables such as the allocation of attention, stimulus familiarity and meaningfulness, rehearsal strategy, retention interval, and so on—in short, mechanisms of information processing, storage, and retrieval. If, on the other hand, hypnosis modulates the threshold for acceptable recall, the effect may be brought about exclusively by performance factors, motivation, and incentives. Thus, for example, altering the consequences (i.e., payoffs and risks) for correct relative to incorrect memories can substantially change the amount of uncertain information an individual may be willing to report. Deciding between these alternatives requires special methodology, such as the application of signal detection theory (Green & Swets, 1966) to data obtained in the recognition memory paradigm, or the control of report criteria in free recall by requiring both hypnotized and nonhypnotized subjects to produce responses to the same (usually high) output level (Klatzky & Erdelyi, 1985). The critical evidence in all such studies relies on the concurrent evaluation of correctly recalled or recognized information (hits) and incorrect recalls (distortions, confabulations) and recognitions (false alarms). (For an expanded discussion of these issues and methodological procedures, see Erdelyi, Chapter 3, this volume.)

Unfortunately, laboratory studies of the effects of hypnosis on recognition memory almost universally show no enhancement or a decrement compared with nonhypnotic recognition performance (e.g., Redston & Knox, 1983; G. S. Sanders & Simmons, 1983; Sheehan *et al.*, 1984; Sheehan & Tilden, 1983; Timm, 1981; Wagstaff, 1982; Wagstaff *et al.*, 1982). To our knowledge, the only contradiction to this general pattern was a study reported by Shields and Knox (1986), in which words studied at a semantic level of analysis were recognized more accurately by hypnotized subjects than by their nonhypnotized counterparts. This was a statistically significant but modest effect. On the whole, however, the amenability of recognition memory data to signal detection analyses for the purpose of separating potential hypnotic effects on memory from response bias or criterion effects appears to be quite beside the point; typically, there are no such effects of hypnosis to warrant analysis.

Very few studies have attempted the alternative strategy of controlling subjects' report criteria in the context of the free-recall paradigm. The first such study sought to evaluate the effects of hypnosis on memory for pictorial stimuli (Dywan & Bowers, 1983), using a modification of the forced-recall procedure developed by Erdelyi (Erdelyi & Becker, 1974; Erdelyi & Kleinbard, 1978). Using this technique, Dywan and Bowers repeatedly tested recall of a set of line drawings over a 1-week interval that culminated in a final forced-recall session in which half of the subjects were given a hypnotic induction procedure and half were given task-motivating instructions for enhanced recall. With potential differences in report criteria ostensibly controlled, both between treatments and within subjects, Dywan and Bowers (1983) found that highly hypnotizable subjects recalling in hypnosis retrieved significantly more additional correct items than did control subjects; however, they also produced three times as many errors!

Thus what appears to be a true memory-enhancing effect of hypnosis is dwarfed by the magnitude of recall intrusions elicited by the procedure. However, because the analysis was based only on *novel* correct and incorrect responses that the subjects confidently "presented as memories" (Dywan & Bowers, 1983, p. 184), the resulting data set was equivalent to one produced by a free-recall procedure (i.e., one dependent on report-criterion rather than that produced by the forced-recall method). Consequently, the data that were reported fail to identify the locus of the effect of hypnosis on recall. They are, nonetheless, fully consistent with the possibility that hypnosis merely liberalized the report criteria of the hypnotically responsive subjects.

This study is unique, however, in providing a quantitative estimate of the effects of hypnosis on recall following repeated concerted efforts to remember—conditions that virtually exhaust normal waking hypermnesia (e.g., Erdelyi & Kleinbard, 1978). This provides a conceptual parallel to the life situation of witnesses or victims who repeatedly try to remember what occurred in the course of a crime and are highly motivated to do so. Under such circumstances, hypnosis appears to allow the individual to tender previously unreported items as confident memories, even though most of them are incorrect. It is this aspect of hypnosis that makes it seem to an observer that the procedure brings forth totally new information, and thus makes it attractive as a technique to elicit inaccessible memories, particularly when they cannot be checked.

We have recently completed a study (Whitehouse *et al.*, 1987) using the forced-recall methodology to assess the effects of hypnosis on interrogatory recall of filmed material. The focus of this study was to understand the nature of the hypnotic enhancement of correct recall reported by Stager and Lundy (1985). Although the positive effect observed in the Stager and Lundy study occurred without a concomitant increase in errors, the effect may nonetheless have been due to a shift in report criterion. This is possible because some of their subjects apparently availed themselves of a third response category— effectively, "I don't know"—or simply omitted responses to some questions (cf. Stager, 1974, p. 67). Thus, if hypnosis produced a shift in report criterion (i.e., an increased willingness to offer responses), then some of the "I don't know" responses given prior to hypnosis inevitably would be replaced by correct responses during the hypnotic recall, creating the appearance of enhanced memory. The fact that hypnotized subjects did not also produce more erroneous responses may have been due to the use of questions that provided an extensive amount of *accurate* description and detail to serve as retrieval cues for the target information.

To determine the viability of this interpretation, we employed the same materials and procedures that had been used by Stager and Lundy (1985), but in addition we required subjects to *answer each question* (by guessing if necessary), and to rate their confidence in the accuracy of each response. Two such forced-recall tests were carried out, the first of which occurred in the waking condition for all subjects. Half of the subjects were exposed next to a hypnotic induction and received suggestions for improved recollection, while the remaining subjects performed an irrelevant task, prior to being tested for recall a second time. Both groups of subjects recalled additional correct information on the second test, but the magnitude of improvement was no greater for hypnotized subjects than it was for waking subjects. Moreover, during this second recall, hypnotized subjects were more likely than were waking subjects to increase confidence ratings for responses previously identified as guesses, irrespective of their accuracy. This finding, that *previously uncertain* responses (which are not likely to be reported in the absence of a forced-recall requirement) were endowed with greater certainty in hypnosis, is consistent with the occurrence of a shift in report criterion.

A second forced-recall study by our laboratory (Dinges, Orne, Whitehouse, Orne, Powell, & Erdelyi, 1987) compared the efficacy of hypnosis to

motivated waking recall using a multitrial hypermnesia paradigm (e.g., Erdelyi & Kleinbard, 1978). Subjects viewed a set of pictorial stimuli and, following a 1-week retention interval, they received a series of eight forced-recall
trials. Although the complexity of the experimental design prohibits a detailed description, the important findings were: (1) All subjects (without
regard to hypnotic versus waking treatment) continued to produce additional
correct recall on each successive trial; (2) The recall improvement (i.e.,
hypermnesia) observed in hypnotized subjects was *less* than that seen in
waking subjects; and (3) Although there was a significant general pattern
among subjects to become more confident of their recall productions over
trials, this effect was particularly evident in the confidence that highly hypnotizable subjects invested in their erroneous recall.

Each of these studies from our laboratory (Dinges *et al.*, 1987; Whitehouse *et al.*, 1987) relied on forced-recall procedures to prevent the occurrence of a shift in report criterion when hypnosis was induced. Neither found
hypnosis to be superior to the waking treatment in eliciting further accurate
recall; in fact, Dinges *et al.* (1987) observed a decremental influence of
hypnosis on the hypermnesia normally observed with repeated attempts to
remember. Although further research using this methodological approach is
needed, these findings of no enhancement of recall by hypnosis when report
criterion is controlled raise serious doubts about the reality of hypnotic
hypermnesia.

## Vulnerability to Memory Distortion by Postevent Information

Loftus and her colleagues (e.g., Loftus, 1979; Loftus, Miller, & Burns, 1978)
have suggested that information encountered after a witnessed event has the
potential to revise an individual's memory concerning specific details of the
target event. Although this "integration" viewpoint has aroused theoretical
controversy (Bekerian & Bowers, 1983; McCloskey & Zaragoza, 1985), the
empirical phenomenon itself has been well established under conditions
much like those of the typical eyewitness situation. Thus, when subjects are
presented with subtle misinformation following a stimulus such as a slide
sequence of a traffic accident, the incorrect postevent information can often
be more readily elicited than the originally perceived details in subject's
subsequent recognition memory reports.

In the context of hypnosis, where imagination, fantasy, and the uncritical acceptance of the hypnotist's suggestions are strongly encouraged and
socially reinforced, there is a good possibility that the tendency to incorporate postevent information into memory may be exaggerated, particularly
among highly hypnotizable persons. Studies germane to this topic have
investigated the effects of two techniques known to induce memory distortion: the use of subtle leading questions (Loftus & Zanni, 1975), and the
interpolation of misinformation between the target event and the memory

test (Loftus, 1979). Following visual presentations depicting a traffic accident and a series of shop accidents, respectively, Putnam (1979) and Zelig and Beidleman (1981) exposed hypnotized and nonhypnotized subjects to leading questions such as "Did you see the stop sign at the intersection?" (Putnam, 1979) or "Did you see Lucky take off his hat after his friend died?" (Zelig & Beidlemen, 1981), which tended to suggest an affirmative response as being correct. Both studies found that subjects in the hypnosis groups responded significantly more often in the direction implied by the misleading questions, and therefore were more frequently incorrect, than nonhypnotized control subjects. These findings suggest that hypnosis served to sensitize the subjects to subtle cues that communicated the nature of the "memories" that were ostensibly being sought, rather than increasing the accessibility of the subjects' true memories. In fact, on nonleading questions, no difference in the accuracy of responses by hypnotized and nonhypnotized subjects (i.e., no hypnotic hypermnesia) was found in either of the two studies.

Using the paradigm of interpolated misinformation, recent studies conducted at Sheehan's laboratory (Sheehan & Tilden, 1983, 1984) have found no differential effect of hypnosis or of hypnotizability. That is, hypnotized subjects were neither more nor less likely than nonhypnotized subjects to incorporate earlier misleading information into their memory reports. These null effects for susceptibility to misleading postevent information contrast with findings (Sheehan & Tilden, 1984) of increased distortion in free narrative recall by hypnotically responsive subjects given hypnosis. Recently, however, Sheehan *et al.* (1984) introduced misleading information *following* a hypnotic-induction procedure, carried out with highly hypnotizable subjects, and with relatively unhypnotizable subjects instructed to simulate hypnosis, and obtained significantly greater integration of the suggested false information among the hypnotized group.

Thus, the results of Sheehan *et al.* (1984) are consistent with those of Putnam (1979) and Zelig and Beidleman (1981). These investigations indicate that vulnerability of memory reports to distortion by intentional or unwitting cues and by counterfactual information is particularly acute for hypnotically responsive individuals while they are in the hypnotic condition.

A recent demonstration by Laurence and Perry (1983) bears out and extends the implications of the preceding studies of memory distortion in hypnosis. Highly hypnotizable subjects were interviewed to establish that they had slept uneventfully through a particular night of the previous week. Following this, they were hypnotized and age-regressed to the night in question. During the hypnotic reliving of the night's sleep, the subjects were asked whether they had heard some loud noises that had awakened them. Out of 27 subjects, 17 responded to the suggestion implicit in the leading question and reported hearing noises that aroused them from their sleep. When hypnosis was terminated, some subjects were tested immediately, whereas the remaining subjects were tested 7 days later, for spontaneous (i.e., nonsuggested) posthypnotic retention of the pseudomemory created in hypnosis. Overall, 13 subjects (6 with utter certainty) now recalled the noises and insisted that they had actually occurred and had awakened them during the night in question. Even when confronted with the fact that the noises had been suggested to them in hypnosis, they remained unshakeable in their conviction.

This demonstration by Laurence and Perry (1983) illustrates the malleability of memory in hypnosis; more importantly, it shows the persistence and seeming reality following hypnosis of such hypnotically created (distorted) memories. This point is crucial when the hypnotically "refreshed" memory of an eyewitness or victim forms the basis for courtroom testimony. Apart from the heightened susceptibility of hypnotized persons to sources of memory bias and distortion, their relative inability to distinguish between hypnotic memories (whether accurate or not) and prior waking recollections renders any such testimony incompetent (cf. Diamond, 1980).

### Confidence, Accuracy, and Credibility

The demeanor of a witness, and particularly the level of confidence the witness conveys regarding his or her testimony, are major determinants of perceived credibility (Lindsay, Wells, & Rumpel, 1981; Wells, Lindsay, & Ferguson, 1979). At the same time, however, displayed confidence need have little to do with the accuracy of eyewitness information (Wells *et al.*, 1979); many witnesses truly believe their incorrect memories.

It is a natural corollary to the "report-criterion shift" hypothesis of hypnotic hypermnesia that a consequence of the procedure will be an increase in confidence about one's memory productions (Orne, 1979). Those studies in which subjects' confidence in their reported memories was assessed between hypnotic and nonhypnotic treatments provide an overwhelmingly consistent confirmation of this view. Thus, for example, Dywan (1983) and Nogrady *et al.* (1985)—both employing the multitrial-recall paradigm of waking hypermnesia (e.g., Erdelyi & Becker, 1974; Erdelyi & Kleinbard, 1978), with forced-recall and free-recall response formats, respectively—found significant increases in both correct items over trials (i.e., productivity). This effect was greater for hypnotized subjects with high hypnotic ability in Dywan's study (see Dywan & Bowers, 1983), but was found not to differentiate groups in the Nogrady *et al.* study. Importantly, however, Dywan (1983) reported a corresponding increase in confidence due to hypnosis in highly hypnotizable subjects. Nogrady *et al.* (1985) similarly observed an increase in confidence for subjects high (but not for those low) in hypnotizability who were tested in the hypnotic condition—an effect that was significantly associated with incorrect items during the last three recall tests. In both studies, therefore, the increase in confidence produced by hypnosis was attended by a parallel increase in intrusions, and hence was unjustified.

Analogous findings have been reported in the memory distortion studies carried out by Sheehan and his colleagues (Sheehan & Tilden, 1983, 1984; Sheehan *et al.*, 1984). Sheehan and Tilden (1983) found that highly responsive subjects displayed increased confidence in their recognition memory in the hypnosis condition, while hypnotizable subjects in the waking condition did not. Similarly, highly hypnotizable subjects asserted significantly greater confidence in memories elicited during hypnosis than they assigned to responses given on a subsequent waking test (Sheehan *et al.*, 1984; see also Perry & Laurence, 1983). Sheehan and Tilden (1984) reported, however, that unhypnotizable subjects who were instructed to simulate hypnosis also exhibited increased confidence, even in regard to their distorted recognition responses. It appears, therefore, that the increase in confidence or certitude produced by hypnosis is consistent with subjects' preconceptions about the effects of hypnosis in retrieving accurate memories (e.g., Orne, Soskis, *et al.*, 1984; Putnam, 1979).

In the domain of eyewitness identification, the confidence of a witness is often a key variable in determining whether a suspect can be charged and prosecuted successfully. Accordingly, many forensic simulation studies of hypnotic effects on memory have incorporated measures of confidence. Putnam (1979) and Zelig and Beidleman (1981) reported, not an increase in confidence during hypnosis, but rather a persistence of confidence despite an increase in errors due to leading questions. A similar pattern was obtained by G. S. Sanders and Simmons (1983): Both hypnosis and control subjects tended generally to be conservative in the degree of confidence they awarded to their recollections, but, for those items about which subjects were willing to testify in court, hypnosis subjects were significantly more often incorrect. In addition, in the Zelig and Beidleman (1981) study, a small but significant positive correlation ($r = .33$) was obtained between subjects' hypnotizability and their confidence ratings across treatment conditions, reflecting the tendency for highly hypnotizable subjects to place greater overall confidence in their remembrances. Finally, the use of hypnosis to enhance memory in lineup recognition tasks consistently fails to improve memory but often succeeds in escalating eyewitness confidence (G. S. Sanders & Simmons, 1983; Timm, 1982; Wagstaff, 1982; Wagstaff *et al.*, 1982).

Another factor known to influence the credibility of a witness's testimony is the amount of peripheral detail he or she provides in recounting the events in question (see the analysis of John Dean's Watergate testimony in Neisser, 1982; see also Wells & Leippe, 1981). A shift in report criterion caused by hypnosis is one mechanism through which hypnotically accessed memories can differ from normal recollections in terms of a greater quantity of detail. Similarly, the inclination to confabulate and to draw inferences to fill in missing information is apparently greater in hypnosis, and, as a consequence, can render the memory reports of hypnotized individuals deceptively more believable than normal recall (e.g., Stalnaker & Riddle, 1932).

In this regard, the studies of Sheehan *et al.* (1984) and Sheehan and Tilden (1984) showed that highly hypnotizable subjects who provided a free narrative recall during hypnosis introduced significantly more peripheral details—both correct and incorrect—and errors of inference than did unhypnotizable subjects simulating hypnosis. It is not clear, however, whether this was an effect of hypnosis or of hypnotizability, since the two variables were confounded in these experiments. An independent experiment by McConkey and Nogrady (1984) found a decrease in the number of correct inferences related to story recall; this was a function of hypnotic ability, but not of hypnosis. On the other hand, when subjects unselected for hypnotizability were exposed to either task-motivating instructions or hypnosis plus task-motivating instructions for hypermnesia of specifically cued peripheral details, there was a significant recall advantage for the hypnosis condition (DePiano & Salzberg, 1981). Thus, there is evidence that either hypnotic responsiveness or the effect of a hypnotic induction procedure, or both, serve to encourage the reporting of inferential and peripheral information. A consequence of this additional detail in the memory report is to endow such testimony with greater credibility.


## SIGNIFICANCE OF EMPIRICAL FINDINGS FOR CONTINUED INVESTIGATION AND USE OF HYPNOSIS IN THE SERVICE OF MEMORY RECONSTRUCTION

### Forensic Implications

Forensic Relevance in Research Designs

The continuing controversy over the utility of hypnosis for enhancing the memories of witnesses and victims of crimes (e.g., Diamond, 1980; Orne, Soskis, *et al.*, 1984; Perry & Laurence, 1983; Reiser, 1985) has inspired vigorous research activity. Thus far, this research has begun to elucidate the promises, perils, and limitations of hypnosis in the legal context. However, there is a pressing need for properly designed studies that have high ecological validity, while possessing adequate methodological power to isolate the source of effects despite the limitations of the typical forensic setting.

There are numerous anecdotal reports (e.g., Block, 1976; Reiser, 1976) claiming to document increased recall as a consequence of hypnosis. Although in some of these cases it appears that hypnotically obtained information may have provided the clues essential to the apprehension of a suspect, it is generally impossible to determine the specific role, if any, that hypnosis played in eliciting this information. Some of the most widely cited statistics (e.g., Reiser & Nielson, 1980) are based upon ratings by the senior investigating officer about how useful hypnosis was, without providing any criteria on which these ratings were based; such data in consumer surveys are called "happiness reports."

Any laboratory investigation that hopes to elucidate the processes underlying this phenomenon must involve a context in which at least apparent hypermnesia—analogous to what is claimed in the field—is produced. Such "apparent" hypermnesia need not consist of an increase in accurate memory; it might involve either more details or changes in what is remembered, or more overall novel information, in some combination or other. The failure to produce at least an ostensible hypermnesia may, like any null finding, help raise questions about the existence of hypermnesia, but it does not permit inference about other consequences of hypnosis (e.g., increased confidence) that might occur in situations where apparent hypermnesia is produced.

In addition, studies should attempt to distinguish whether the hypnotic treatment produces a bona fide increase in memory accessibility as opposed to a change in subjective report criterion. From a practical perspective, such a distinction might seem inconsequential. What difference should it make why novel memories become available in hypnosis, so long as they do? The answer is that hypnosis, as we have seen, has multiple effects (e.g., susceptibility to memory distortion, heightened confidence, etc.), many of which contraindicate its use in the legal context. Accordingly, analysis of the mechanisms of hypnotic memory enhancement will determine whether equally effective substitute procedures can be developed that do not entail the risks associated with hypnosis.

Efforts along these lines have already begun in the development of techniques such as "guided memory" (Malpass & Devine, 1981) and the "cognitive interview" (Geiselman et al., 1984); in fact, studies typically find no statistically significant differences in recall output between such procedures and hypnosis (Geiselman, Fisher, MacKinnon, & Holland, 1985; Sturm, 1982; Yuille & McEwan, 1985). Of course, it is important to consider that these retrieval mnemonics may be as efficacious as hypnosis in sponsoring increased memory productivity for the simple reason that they are not mere surrogates, but, like hypnosis, actively invite the subject to alter his or her standard of judgment. Furthermore, such techniques may explicitly tap some of the critical processes that inhere in hypnosis (see also E. R. Hilgard, 1984; Perry & Nogrady, 1985), including fantasy, imagery, and confabulation. It will be necessary for further research to decide whether these procedures provide viable alternatives to hypnosis or whether they share critical features of hypnosis, albeit in disguise.

Finally, research is needed on the role of perceived consequences as a motivational factor determining memory reports in the context of hypnosis. In reviewing the nonhypnotic literature on this topic, M. C. Smith (1983) concluded, "The results . . . do not support the hypothesis that processes underlying recall differ when there are perceived serious consequences associated with that recall" (p. 398). However, Orne (1961) suggested that the hypnotic context (independent of the condition of hypnosis) can serve as a facilitator of information that an individual may be fearful or embarrassed to report, or motivated by guilt to suppress. The function of the hypnotic context implicated here is the subject's abrogation of responsibility for information that is revealed in hypnosis, with the resulting perception of immunity from serious consequences. Thus, some of the differences in evidence for hypnotic hypermnesia that have been found between laboratory studies of hypnosis and its forensic use in the field may reside in the illusion of freedom from reprisal and/or legal sanctions that might ordinarily motivate witnesses to "forget" certain details of actual crimes. While this possibility has received some theoretical consideration (e.g., Perry & Nogrady, 1985; Timm, 1982), systematic research on the topic has yet to be inaugurated.

Contraindications for Courtroom Testimony

Elsewhere, we have reviewed evidence pertinent to the use of hypnosis for investigative purposes and in the preparation of a witness's testimony for trial (including the consequential hazards to justice), as well as the history of judicial posture on the admissibility of hypnotically "refreshed" testimony in court (Orne, Dinges, & Orne, 1984a; Orne, Soskis, *et al.*, 1984; Orne *et al.*, 1985). In the present chapter, we have cited evidence from a number of scientific studies that establishes (1) the fundamental unreliability of recollections elicited in hypnosis; (2) the persistence of these recollections in the waking condition, whereupon they may be impossible for the individual to distinguish from memories that existed prior to hypnosis; and (3) the unwarranted increase or maintenance of confidence in the accuracy of hypnotically elicited recall, which thereby reinforces its credibility. These considerations compel the conclusion that hypnotically induced memories should *never* be permitted to form the basis for testimony by witnesses or victims in a court of law.

To the degree that hypnosis may prove useful in searching for leads,[5] risks are likely to be reduced in those investigative circumstances in which neither the person to be hypnotized, the authorities, the general public, nor the media have any substantive or presumptive knowledge or beliefs about facts relating to possible perpetrators. In the absence of any such preconceptions that could influence the nature of the memories reported, hypnosis remains an unreliable procedure, but it is less dangerous in the sense that it does not lead an individual to confirm his or her own beliefs or the suspicions of the hypnotist. It should be clear, however, that in such cases the purpose of the hypnotic intervention is to develop leads that result in *new independent physical evidence*, not to elicit testimony. Accordingly, the possible increases in inaccurate information that may attend any accurate recollections reported in hypnosis have the principal disadvantage of wasting time and effort, but if

5. It is, of course possible that other similar techniques, such as repeated recall, cognitive manipulations, or even asking individuals to guess in order to lower report criterion, may be equally effective.

the investigative hypnotic session is carried out properly (see Orne, 1979; Orne, Soskis, *et al.*, 1984), and it is recognized that the individual cannot subsequently testify, it need not threaten the interests of justice.

Recently, the Council on Scientific Affairs of the American Medical Association (1985) has issued a report on hypnosis and memory based on a comprehensive review of the extant scientific literature.[6] It concludes as follows:

> [H]ypnosis can be useful during the investigative process, when even a single correct recall may lead to important new evidence and where it matters relatively little if the hypnotized subject also produces many incorrect responses. This use of hypnosis is in stark contrast to its use with a witness who is to testify in court. . . . The value of [the] investigative use of hypnosis must be balanced against the potential testimonial incapacitation or restriction of evidence by the hypnotic subject as a trial witness. (1985, p. 1922)

The Council's report recognizes that hypnosis may be of some benefit in an investigative context, although it emphasizes the lack of scientific evidence to document a memory-enhancing effect of hypnosis, and it recommends procedural safeguards to protect the integrity of the memory report as well as the welfare of the subject and the public. Furthermore, the Council warns of the potential dangers to the judicial process of the use of hypnosis with witnesses whose testimony will be used in court. The position outlined in the Council's report echoes the concerns enumerated in twin resolutions previously adopted by the Society for Clinical and Experimental Hypnosis (1979) and by the International Society of Hypnosis (1979). Accordingly, there is now consensus among major groups within the relevant scientific community regarding the unreliability of hypnosis as a memory-restoring technique, and the potentially grave legal implications associated with its use in the forensic context.[7]

## Relevance to Psychotherapy

In juxtaposition to the discouraging laboratory evidence for the hypnotic enhancement of memory are the clinical claims of dramatic memory recover-

6. This report is of particular interest because the official recognition of hypnosis as a therapeutic modality by the American Medical Association, and subsequently by the American Psychiatric Association and the American Psychological Association, has been taken as evidence in forensic areas for the acceptance of hypnosis to "refresh" recall, which has therefore justified its use as a basis for testimony in court. However, although the relevant scientific community considers hypnosis appropriate for therapy, it has *never* accepted the technique to be a reliable method of enhancing recall—an issue that is clarified by the Council's (1985) report.

7. The American Medical Association's position (which was ratified by its House of Delegates in December 1984) was also adopted as the official position of the Society for Clinical and Experimental Hypnosis in 1985 and of the International Society of Hypnosis in 1986.

ies brought about through hypnosis. We now consider some of the reasons that may account for this discrepancy.

The autobiographical memories retrieved with the aid of hypnosis in the clinical setting often deal with intense, meaningful experiences, some of which may be inaccessible to consciousness and involve material that is unacceptable to the individual. Laboratory studies of the efficacy of hypnosis in aiding recall of emotionally charged materials have thus far yielded equivocal results. However, it must be kept in mind that the laboratory rarely if ever reproduces the intensity of emotion associated with some autobiographical memories, and certainly does not approximate the guilt-related, highly personal, traumatic experiences that are often involved in treatment. Unless the stimulus material concerns experiential memories unacceptable to the individual and dynamically kept out of awareness, the relative ease of nonhypnotic recall would mitigate against positive findings.

Another possibility, acknowledged by Freud (1906/1953), that may have even greater generality and relevance is that the recollections of patients in hypnosis often include some measure of fantasy and confabulation that is not identified as such. As we have discussed above, the concomitants and sequelae of hypnotic recollections—particularly the reporting of vivid details, the intense affect, and the therapeutic improvement resulting from abreaction—tend to be accepted as convincing evidence that the patient's recollections are accurate. Moreover, the therapist is interested in the meaning, rather than the historical accuracy, of the abreacted experiences or other memories related during hypnosis. In age regression, for example, the therapist is not apt to challenge the veridicality of what is reported (except in a case of obvious anachronisms), since to do so, especially prematurely, may undermine treatment. For these reasons, together with the assumption that the patient would not jeopardize clinical improvement by deliberately inventing fictitious memories, the therapist's role involves accepting the patient's statements as historically accurate. Thus, the operational criteria for the validity of a "memory" in the context of psychotherapy are orthogonal to those of the laboratory and the forensic setting.

*Reconstruction in Hypnotic Memory Retrieval*

As we have seen, the task of the therapist is not to establish the accuracy of historical events recounted by the patient, but to help the patient to work through his or her own version of history, which may involve valid memories mixed with condensation, confabulation, and fantasy. At times, the therapeutic strategy of choice has been one that facilitates the "reconstruction" of that history. The early work of Janet (1889, cited in Ellenberger, 1970), and more recently the work of Erickson (1935; Erickson & Rossi, 1980) and others (e.g., Lamb, 1985), explicitly reveal the considerable therapeutic benefit that accrues from such constructions when ego-syntonic endings can be grafted onto memories of earlier traumatic experiences.

Many therapists feel that suggesting an ego-syntonic ending to earlier traumatic experiences is manipulative and therefore an inappropriate strategy. It is reasonable to assume, however, that when hypnosis is used in an attempt to reinstate traumatic memories, historical reconstruction takes place "spontaneously." One of the major advantages to the use of hypnosis as an adjunct to dynamic psychotherapy may be precisely the ease with which patients can alter their memories in response to subtle or unwitting cues. Given the diminution of the patient's critical faculties while hypnotized that allows him or her to accept the re-experienced events as memories, and given the features of hypnosis that render it convincing to the observer, hypnosis allows a reconstruction of history in ways that may be compelling to both therapist and patient. In this way, the therapist becomes able to provide validation for the importance and the presumed accuracy of the patient's memory. To be sure, such processes need not be dependent on hypnosis for their occurence (see Spence, 1982), but they would seem to be facilitated by it. Thus, in the absence of hypnosis, some patients in psychotherapy may require more time and effort to work through the feelings associated with their memories in ways that make them acceptable.

In contrast to its utility in the reconstruction of "memory" in psychotherapy, the use of hypnosis in law enforcement is concerned with ascertaining the truth of the matter. Obviously, hard physical evidence is most desirable, but often it is simply not available. Eyewitness reports have a particularly vital status in the criminal justice system, but, unfortunately, these too are often not to be had. It is hardly surprising, therefore, that many law enforcement officials look to any potential scientific aid to make their difficult task more manageable. Just as the use of Amytal Sodium or Pentothal as a "truth serum" was once favored in law enforcement, so there is a tendency to accept a "new" investigative tool, such as hypnosis without adequate scientific data. A real danger is inherent in the willingness of investigators and prosecutors to accept the view that, because hypnosis yields additional details about which witnesses often tend to be certain after hypnosis, these novel recollections are likely to be accurate. The wish to believe in the accuracy of reports obtained during hypnosis is so strong that, in one case, a rape victim who had never seen her assailant because he wore a mask was instructed in hypnosis to remove the mask and look at his face! This "eyewitness" identification was actually used in an attempt to gain a conviction.

Obviously, in a forensic context, the accuracy of information is paramount; nevertheless, it may be impossible to ascertain what really happened in any specific instance. Despite the problems associated with recall induced by hypnosis, there is a temptation to argue that if the information obtained in hypnosis independently corroborates (or is corroborated by) other evidence, then the previously hypnotized witness should be permitted to testify. Unfortunately, this argument is seriously flawed, in that it is a simple matter to inadvertently create such corroborating "memories" in hypnosis. For example, the identification of a suspect may be corroborated by hypnotic recall created either by subtle cues that may be present during, or prior to (Alexander, 1971), the hypnotic interview, or by the translation of pre-existing beliefs into "recollections" via hypnosis. The "corroboration" thus obtained by the use of hypnosis is illusory. It is for such reasons that the overwhelming majority of courts that have ruled upon the matter have excluded testimony based on recollections of a witness following hypnosis, although some courts have permitted *pre*hypnotic statements, reliably recorded, to be offered in testimony.

With regard to the clinical setting, however, the ability of hypnosis to alter memories in a psychotherapeutically desirable fashion may be useful. Clearly, the fact that a patient improves does not speak to the accuracy of the memories that were obtained, since purposively created pseudomemories can be therapeutic. Nonetheless, in hypnotic age regression, it often *appears* as if there is an actual reliving of an early childhood event, with accompanying accurate recollections. But in a clinical context, it is no easier than in a forensic one to ascertain the origin of the memory for such events. Thus, for example, it is not uncommon for a 2-year-old child to do something that is considered cute or precocious by the family, and hence the deed becomes worthy of periodic mention at family gatherings thereafter. If, as an adult, the individual "relives" the particular event while in hypnosis, and the facts are corroborated by a parent, this would not permit one to distinguish whether the recollection truly dates from age 2 or is the consequence of later family recountings. In a therapeutic context, such a distinction is unimportant; in qualifying an eyewitness in the forensic context, however, the source of the memory is *the* crucial issue.

## CONCLUSIONS

We have sought to review the relevant scientific literature concerning the accuracy and consequences of memory elicited during hypnosis, and to discuss the implications of such evidence for the use of hypnosis in reconstructing memory in therapeutic and forensic settings. In the clinical context, the therapist and patient jointly define the events, realities, and "memories" that are relevant to the goals of psychotherapy, which involve helping the patient to cope more effectively and to feel better. The historical accuracy of remembered events is less important in determining the patient's therapeutic progress than is the manner in which the events are expressed, understood, and dealt with. On the other hand, in the forensic domain, an overriding commitment is made to the uncovering of "truth." Here, however, such truth cannot be determined by consensus of the witness and hypnotist.

Despite the well-known vagaries of normal human memory (Loftus, 1979), it is nevertheless considerably more reliable than are memories induced by the hypnotic process. It appears that the criminal justice system's traditional use of a jury as the trier of fact, of the adversarial process, and of cross-examination has served as the best available means of defining "truth." However, this process can be subverted by a technique, such as hypnosis, that greatly facilitates the reconstruction of history, that allows an individual to be influenced unwittingly, and that may catalyze beliefs into "memories." The resultant testimony may then be presented under oath by an honest individual who is convinced of the accuracy of what may well be pseudomemories. Paradoxically, then, the same attributes of hypnosis that make it a useful adjunct to psychotherapy also create the greatest obstacles to its use in the forensic domain.

At the present stage of scientific knowledge, we cannot distinguish between veridical recall and pseudomemories elicited during hypnosis without prior knowledge or truly independent proof. Perhaps future research will provide ways for making this crucial distinction. Until such techniques become available, testimony based on hypnosis or on any other procedures that invite fantasy, diminish critical judgment, and increase the risk of pseudomemories, should be prohibited.

## ACKNOWLEDGMENTS

Preparation of this chapter was supported in part by Grant No. MH 19156 from the National Institute of Mental Health, U.S. Public Health Service; in part by Grant No. 82-IJ-CX-0007 from the National Institute of Justice, U.S. Department of Justice; and in part by a grant from the Institute for Experimental Psychiatry Research Foundation. We are grateful to our colleagues Matthew H. Erdelyi, Germain Lavoie, Campbell Perry, Helen M. Pettinati, and David A. Soskis for their valuable comments. We also thank Mary Fleming Auxier for editorial assistance.

## REFERENCES

Alexander, L. (1971). The prehypnotic suggestion. *Comprehensive Psychiatry, 12,* 414–422.

Augustynek, A. (1978). Remembering under hypnosis. *Journal for Basic Research in Psychological Sciences, Studia Psychologia, 20,* 256–266.

Augustynek, A. (1979). Hypnotic hypermnesia. *Prace Psychologiczno-Pedagogiczne, 29,* 25–34.

Baker, R. A., Haynes, B., & Patrick, B. S. (1983). Hypnosis, memory, and incidental memory. *American Journal of Clinical Hypnosis, 25,* 253–262.

Baker, R. A., & Patrick, B. S. (1987). Hypnosis and memory: The effects of emotional arousal. *American Journal of Clinical Hypnosis, 29,* 177–184.

Barber, T. X. (1961). Experimental evidence for a theory of hypnotic behavior: II. Experimental controls in hypnotic age-regression. *International Journal of Clinical and Experimental Hypnosis, 9*, 181–193.

Barber, T. X. (1962). Hypnotic age regression: A critical review. *Psychosomatic Medicine, 24*, 286–299.

Barber, T. X. (1969). *Hypnosis: A scientific approach*. New York: Van Nostrand Reinhold.

Barber, T. X., & Calverley, D. S. (1966). Effects on recall of hypnotic induction, motivational suggestions, and suggested regression: A methodological and experimental analysis. *Journal of Abnormal Psychology, 71*, 169–180.

Bekerian, D. A., & Bowers, J. M. (1983). Eyewitness testimony: Were we misled? *Journal of Experimental Psychology: Learning, Memory, and Cognition, 9*, 139–145.

Block, E. B. (1976). *Hypnosis: A new tool in crime detection*. New York: David MacKay.

Bourne, L. E., Jr., Dominowski, R. L., & Loftus, E. F. (1979). *Cognitive processes*. Englewood Cliffs, NJ: Prentice-Hall.

Bower, G. H. (1970). Imagery as a relational organizer in associative learning. *Journal of Verbal Learning and Verbal Behavior, 9*, 529–533.

Bower, G. H. (1981). Mood and memory. *American Psychologist, 36*, 129–148.

Bower, G. H., & Mayer, J. D. (1985). Failure to replicate mood-dependent retrieval. *Bulletin of the Psychonomic Society, 23*, 39–42.

Bower, G. H., Monteiro, K. P., & Gilligan, S. G. (1978). Emotional mood as a context for learning and recall. *Journal of Verbal Learning and Verbal Behavior, 17*, 573–585.

Bowers, K. S. (1976). *Hypnosis for the seriously curious*. Monterey, CA: Brooks/Cole.

Bowers, P. G. (1978). Hypnotizability, creativity and the role of effortless experiencing. *International Journal of Clinical and Experimental Hypnosis, 26*, 184–202.

Bowers, P. G. (1982). The classic suggestion effect: Relationships with scales of hypnotizability, effortless experiencing, and imagery vividness. *International Journal of Clinical and Experimental Hypnosis, 30*, 270–279.

Bramwell, M. (1956). *Hypnotism: Its history, practice and theory*. New York: Institute for Research in Hypnosis Publication Society and Julian Press. (Original work published 1903)

Breuer, J., & Freud, S. (1955). Studies on hysteria. In J. Strachey (Ed. and Trans.), *The standard edition of the complete psychological works of Sigmund Freud* (Vol. 2, pp. 1–305). London: Hogarth Press. (Original work published 1895)

Brown, W. (1923). To what extent is memory measured by a single recall? *Journal of Experimental Psychology, 6*, 377–382.

Buckhout, R., Eugenio, P., & Grosso, T. (1981, August). *Is there life after hypnosis? Attempts to revive the memory of eyewitnesses*. Paper presented at the meeting of the American Psychological Association, Los Angeles.

Cedercreutz, C. (1972). The big mistakes: A note. *International Journal of Clinical and Experimental Hypnosis, 20*, 15–16.

Clark, D. M., & Teasdale, J. D. (1985). Constraints on the effects of mood on memory. *Journal of Personality and Social Psychology, 48*, 1595–1608.

Clark, M. S., Milberg, S., & Ross, J. (1983). Arousal cues arousal-related material in memory: Implications for understanding effects of mood on memory. *Journal of Verbal Learning and Verbal Behavior, 22*, 633–649.

Commonwealth v. Kater, 388 Mass. 519 (1983).

Conn, J. H. (1960). The psychodynamics of recovery under hypnosis. *International Journal of Clinical and Experimental Hypnosis, 8*, 3–16.

Cooper, L. A., & Shepard, R. N. (1973). Chronometric studies of the rotation of mental images. In W. G. Chase (Ed.), *Visual information processing* (pp. 75–176). New York: Academic Press.

Cooper, L. M. (1972). Hypnotic amnesia. In E. Fromm & R. E. Shor (Eds.), *Hypnosis: Research developments and perspectives* (pp. 217–252). Chicago: Aldine-Atherton.

Cooper, L. M., & London, P. (1973). Reactivation of memory by hypnosis and suggestion. *International Journal of Clinical and Experimental Hypnosis, 21*, 312–323.

Council on Scientific Affairs, American Medical Association. (1985). Scientific status of refreshing recollection by the use of hypnosis. *Journal of the American Medical Association, 253*, 1918–1923.

Craik, F. I. M., & Lockhart, R. S. (1972). Levels of processing: A framework for memory research. *Journal of Verbal Learning and Verbal Behavior, 11*, 671–684.

Crawford, H. J., & Allen, S. N. (1983). Enhanced visual memory during hypnosis as mediated by hypnotic responsiveness and cognitive strategies. *Journal of Experimental Psychology: General, 112*, 662–685.

Das, J. P. (1961). Learning and recall under hypnosis and in the wake state: A comparison. *Archives of General Psychiatry, 4*, 517–521.

DePiano, F. A., & Salzberg, H. C. (1981). Hypnosis as an aid to recall of meaningful information presented under three types of arousal. *International Journal of Clinical and Experimental Hypnosis, 29*, 383–400.

Dhanens, T. P., & Lundy, R. M. (1975). Hypnotic and waking suggestions and recall. *International Journal of Clinical and Experimental Hypnosis, 23*, 68–79.

Diamond, B. L. (1980). Inherent problems in the use of pretrial hypnosis on a prospective witness. *California Law Review, 68*, 313–349.

Dinges, D. F., Orne, M. T., Whitehouse, W. G., Orne, E. C., Powell, J. W., & Erdelyi, M. H. (1987, August). *Recall in hypnosis: More memory, more confidence, or more mistakes?* Paper presented at the meeting of the American Psychological Association, New York.

Dywan, J. (1983). *Hypermnesia, hypnosis and memory: Implications for forensic investigation.* Unpublished doctoral dissertation, University of Waterloo.

Dywan, J., & Bowers, K. S. (1983). The use of hypnosis to enhance recall. *Science, 222*, 184–185.

Ellenberger, H. F. (1970). *The discovery of the unconscious: The history and evolution of dynamic psychiatry.* New York: Basic Books.

Ellis, H. C. (1985). On the importance of mood intensity and encoding demands in memory: Commentary on Hasher, Rose, Zacks, Sanft, and Doren. *Journal of Experimental Psychology: General, 114*, 392–395.

Erdelyi, M. H. (1984). The recovery of unconscious (inaccessible) memories: Laboratory studies of hypermnesia. In G. Bower (Ed.), *The psychology of learning and motivation* (Vol. 18, pp. 95–127). New York: Academic Press.

Erdelyi, M. H. (1985). *Psychoanalysis: Freud's cognitive psychology.* New York: W. H. Freeman.

Erdelyi, M. H., & Becker, J. (1974). Hypermnesia for pictures: Incremental memory for pictures but not words in multiple recall trials. *Cognitive Psychology, 6*, 159–171.

Erdelyi, M. H., Finkelstein, S., Herrell, N., Miller, B., & Thomas, J. (1976). Coding modality versus input modality in hypermnesia: Is a rose a rose a rose? *Cognition, 4*, 311–319.

Erdelyi, M. H., & Kleinbard, J. (1978). Has Ebbinghaus decayed with time? The growth of recall (hypermnesia) over days. *Journal of Experimental Psychology: Human Learning and Memory, 4*, 275–289.

Erickson, M. H. (1935). A study of an experimental neurosis hypnotically induced in a case of ejaculatio praecox. *British Journal of Medical Psychology, 15*, 34–50.

Erickson, M. H., & Rossi, E. L. (1980). The February Man: Facilitating new identity in hypnotherapy. In E. L. Rossi (Ed.), *The collected papers of Milton H. Erickson on hypnosis* (Vol. 4, pp. 525–542). New York: Irvington.

Eysenck, H. J. (1941). An experimental study of the improvement of mental and physical functions in the hypnotic state. *British Journal of Medical Psychology, 18*, 304–316.

Frankel, F. H. (1976). *Hypnosis: Trance as a coping mechanism.* New York: Plenum.

Freud, S. (1953). My views on the part played by sexuality in the aetiology of the neuroses. In J. Strachey (Ed. and Trans.), *The standard edition of the complete psychological works of Sigmund Freud* (Vol. 7, pp. 269–279). London: Hogarth Press. (Original work published 1906)

Garver, R. B., Fuselier, G. D., & Booth, T. B. (1981). The hypnotic treatment of amnesia in an Air Force basic trainee. *American Journal of Clinical Hypnosis, 24,* 3–6.

Geiselman, R. E., Fisher, R. P., Firstenberg, I., Hutton, L. A., Sullivan, S., Avetissian, I., & Prosk, A. (1984). Enhancement of eyewitness memory: An empirical evaluation of the cognitive interview. *Journal of Police Science and Administration, 12,* 74–80.

Geiselman, R. E., Fisher, R. P., MacKinnon, D. P., & Holland, H. L. (1985). Eyewitness memory enhancement in the police interview: Cognitive retrieval mnemonics versus hypnosis. *Journal of Applied Psychology, 70,* 401–412.

Gidro-Frank, L., & Bowers Buch, M. K. (1948). A study of the plantar response in hypnotic age regression. *Journal of Nervous and Mental Disease, 107,* 443–458.

Gleitman, H. (1981). *Psychology.* New York: Norton.

Green, D. M., & Swets, J. A. (1966). *Signal detection theory and psychophysics.* New York: Wiley.

Hasher, L., Rose, K. C., Zacks, R. T., Sanft, H., & Doren, B. (1985). Mood, recall, and selectivity effects in normal college students. *Journal of Experimental Psychology: General, 114,* 104–118.

Helwig, C. V. (1978). A comparison of the effectiveness of hypnotic-motivational, task-motivational, and relaxation instructions in eliciting the recall of anxiety inducing material (Doctoral dissertation, University of Toronto, 1976). *Dissertation Abstracts International, 38,* 6013A.

Hilgard, E. R. (1965). *Hypnotic susceptibility.* New York: Harcourt, Brace & World.

Hilgard, E. R. (1984). Comments on the BSECH report on the Home Office draft circular on the use of hypnosis by the police in the investigation of crimes. *British Journal of Experimental and Clinical Hypnosis, 1,* 69.

Hilgard, J. R. (1970). *Personality and hypnosis: A study of imaginative involvement.* Chicago: University of Chicago Press.

Hilgard, J. R., & LeBaron, S. (1984). *Hypnotherapy of pain in children with cancer.* Los Altos, CA: William Kaufmann.

Hodge, J. R., Wagner, E. E., & Schreiner, F. (1966). The validity of hypnotically induced emotional states: Part II. *American Journal of Clinical Hypnosis, 9,* 129–134.

Hull, C. L. (1933). *Hypnosis and suggestibility.* New York: Appleton-Century-Crofts.

Huse, B. (1930). Does the hypnotic trance favor the recall of faint memories? *Journal of Experimental Psychology, 13,* 519–529.

International Society of Hypnosis. (1979). Resolution. *International Journal of Clinical and Experimental Hypnosis, 27,* 453.

Janet, P. (1925). *Psychological healing: A historical and clinical study* (Vol. 1). London: Allen & Unwin.

Kihlstrom, J. F., & Evans, F. J. (1979). Memory retrieval processes during posthypnotic amnesia. In J. F. Kihlstrom & F. J. Evans (Eds.), *Functional disorders of memory* (pp. 179–218). Hillsdale, NJ: Erlbaum.

Klatzky, R. L., & Erdelyi, M. H. (1985). The response criterion problem in tests of hypnosis and memory. *International Journal of Clinical and Experimental Hypnosis, 33,* 246–257.

Kosslyn, S. M. (1973). Scanning visual images: Some structural implications. *Perception and Psychophysics, 14,* 90–94.

Kosslyn, S. M. (1981). The medium and the message in mental imagery: A theory. *Psychological Review, 88,* 46–66.

Kroger, W. S., & Doucé, R. G. (1979). Hypnosis in criminal investigation. *International Journal of Clinical and Experimental Hypnosis, 27,* 358–374.

Lamb, C. S. (1985). Hypnotically-induced deconditioning: Reconstruction of memories in the treatment of phobias. *American Journal of Clinical Hypnosis, 28,* 56–62.

Laurence, J.-R., & Perry, C. (1983). Hypnotically created memory among highly hypnotizable subjects. *Science, 222,* 523–524.

Lindsay, R. C. L., Wells, G. L., & Rumpel, C. M. (1981). Can people detect eyewitness-identification accuracy within and across situations? *Journal of Applied Psychology, 66,* 79–89.

Loftus, E. F. (1979). *Eyewitness testimony.* Cambridge, MA: Harvard University Press.

Loftus, E. F. (1982). Remembering recent experiences. In L. S. Cermak (Ed.), *Human memory and amnesia* (pp. 239–255). Hillsdale, NJ: Erlbaum.

Loftus, E. F., Manber, M., & Keating, J. P. (1983). Recollection of naturalistic events: Context enhancement versus negative cueing. *Human Learning, 2,* 83–92.

Loftus, E. F., Miller, D. G., & Burns, H. J. (1978). Semantic integration of verbal information into a visual memory. *Journal of Experimental Psychology: Human Learning and Memory, 4,* 19–31.

Loftus, E. F., & Zanni, G. (1975). Eyewitness testimony: The influence of the wording of a question. *Bulletin of the Psychonomic Society, 5,* 86–88.

London, P., & Fuhrer, M. (1961). Hypnosis, motivation, and performance. *Journal of Personality, 29,* 321–333.

Lytle, R. A., & Lundy, R. M. (1986, September). *Hypnosis and the recall of visually presented material: A partial replication of Stager and Lundy.* Paper presented at the meeting of the Society for Clinical and Experimental Hypnosis, Chicago.

MacHovec, F. J. (1981). Hypnosis to facilitate recall in psychogenic amnesia and fugue states: Treatment variables. *American Journal of Clinical Hypnosis, 24,* 7–13.

Malpass, R. S., & Devine, P. G. (1981). Guided memory in eyewitness identification. *Journal of Applied Psychology, 66,* 343–350.

McCloskey, M., & Zaragoza, M. (1985). Misleading postevent information and memory for events: Arguments and evidence against memory impairment hypotheses. *Journal of Experimental Psychology: General, 114,* 1–16.

McConkey, K. M., & Nogrady, H. (1984). Hypnosis, hypnotizability and story recall. *Australian Journal of Clinical and Experimental Hypnosis, 12,* 93–98.

McCranie, E. J., Crasilneck, H. B., & Teter, H. R. (1955). The electroencephalogram in hypnotic age regression. *Psychiatric Quarterly, 29,* 85–88.

Mitchell, M. B. (1932). Retroactive inhibition and hypnosis. *Journal of General Psychology, 7,* 343–359.

Moll, A. (1958). *The study of hypnosis.* New York: Institute for Research in Hypnosis Publication Society and Julian Press. (Original work published 1889)

Morgan, A. H., Johnson, D. L., & Hilgard, E. R. (1974). The stability of hypnotic susceptibility: A longitudinal study. *International Journal of Clinical and Experimental Hypnosis, 22,* 249–257.

Nace, E. P., Orne, M. T., & Hammer, A. G. (1974). Posthypnotic amnesia as an active psychic process: The reversibility of amnesia. *Archives of General Psychiatry, 31,* 257–260.

Nash, M. R., Drake, S. D., Wiley, S., Khalsa, S., & Lynn, S. J. (1986). Accuracy of recall by hypnotically age-regressed subjects. *Journal of Abnormal Psychology, 95,* 298–300.

Nash, M. R., Johnson, L. S., & Tipton, R. D. (1979). Hypnotic age regression and the occurrence of transitional object relationships. *Journal of Abnormal Psychology, 88,* 547–555.

Nash, M. R., Lynn, S. J., Stanley, S., Frauman, D., & Rhue, J. (1985). Hypnotic age regression and the importance of assessing interpersonally relevant affect. *International Journal of Clinical and Experimental Hypnosis, 33,* 224–235.

Neisser, U. (1967). *Cognitive psychology*. Englewood Cliffs, NJ: Prentice-Hall.

Neisser, U. (1982). *Memory observed: Remembering in natural contexts*. San Francisco: W. H. Freeman.

Nogrady, H., McConkey, K. M., & Perry, C. (1985). Enhancing visual memory: Trying hypnosis, trying imagination, and trying again. *Journal of Abnormal Psychology, 94,* 195–204.

O'Connell, D. N., Shor, R. E., & Orne, M. T. (1970). Hypnotic age regression: An empirical and methodological analysis. *Journal of Abnormal Psychology Monographs, 76*(3, Pt. 2).

Orne, M. T. (1951). The mechanism of hypnotic age regression: An experimental study. *Journal of Abnormal and Social Psychology, 46,* 213–225.

Orne, M. T. (1959). The nature of hypnosis: Artifact and essence. *Journal of Abnormal and Social Psychology, 58,* 277–299.

Orne, M. T. (1961). The potential uses of hypnosis in interrogation. In A. D. Biderman & H. Zimmer (Eds.), *The manipulation of human behavior* (pp. 169–215). New York: Wiley.

Orne, M. T. (1966). On the mechanisms of posthypnotic amnesia. *International Journal of Clinical and Experimental Hypnosis, 14,* 121–134.

Orne, M. T. (1977). The construct of hypnosis: Implications of the definition for research and practice. *Annals of the New York Academy of Sciences, 296,* 14–33.

Orne, M. T. (1979). The use and misuse of hypnosis in court. *International Journal of Clinical and Experimental Hypnosis, 27,* 311–341.

Orne, M. T., & Dinges, D. F. (1984). Hypnosis. In P. D. Wall & R. Melzack (Eds.), *Textbook of pain* (pp. 806–816). London: Churchill Livingstone.

Orne, M. T., Dinges, D. F., & Orne, E. C. (1984a). *The forensic use of hypnosis* (Research in Brief). Washington, DC: National Institute of Justice.

Orne, M. T., Dinges, D. F., & Orne, E. C. (1984b). On the differential diagnosis of multiple personality in the forensic context. *International Journal of Clinical and Experimental Hypnosis, 32,* 118–169.

Orne, M. T., & Hammer, A. G. (1974). Hypnosis. In *Encyclopaedia Britannica* (15th ed., pp. 133–140). Chicago: Encyclopaedia Britannica.

Orne, M. T., Soskis, D. A., Dinges, D. F., & Orne, E. C. (1984). Hypnotically induced testimony. In G. L. Wells & E. F. Loftus (Eds.), *Eyewitness testimony: Psychological perspectives* (pp. 171–213). New York: Cambridge University Press.

Orne, M. T., Soskis, D. A., Dinges, D. F., Orne, E. C., & Tonry, M. H. (1985). Hypnotically refreshed testimony: Enhanced memory or tampering with evidence? *Issues and practices in criminal justice.* Washington, DC: National Institute of Justice.

Paivio, A. (1969). Mental imagery in associative learning and memory. *Psychological Review, 76,* 241–263.

Paivio, A. (1971). *Imagery and verbal processes*. New York: Holt, Rinehart & Winston.

Paivio, A. (1975). Perceptual comparisons through the mind's eye. *Memory and Cognition, 3,* 635–647.

People v. Kempinski, No. W80CF 352 (Cir. Ct., 12th Dist., Will Co., Ill. Oct. 21, 1980).

People v. Shirley, 641 P.2d 775 (Cal. 1982), *cert. denied,* 408 U.S. (1982).

Perry, C., & Laurence, J.-R. (1983). The enhancement of memory by hypnosis in the legal investigative situation. *Canadian Psychology, 24,* 155–167.

Perry, C., & Nogrady, H. (1985). Use of hypnosis by the police in the investigation of crime: Is guided imagery a safe substitute? *British Journal of Experimental and Clinical Hypnosis, 3,* 25–31.

Popkin, S. J., & Small, M. V. (1979). Hypermnesia and the role of imagery. *Bulletin of the Psychonomic Society, 13,* 378–380.

Putnam, W. H. (1979). Hypnosis and distortions in eyewitness memory. *International Journal of Clinical and Experimental Hypnosis, 27,* 437–448.

Raginsky, B. B. (1969). Hypnotic recall of aircrash cause. *International Journal of Clinical and Experimental Hypnosis, 17,* 1–19.

Redston, M. T., & Knox, V. J. (1983, October). *Is the recognition of faces enhanced by hypnosis?* Paper presented at the meeting of the Society for Clinical and Experimental Hypnosis, Boston.

Reiff, R., & Scheerer, M. (1959). *Memory and hypnotic age regression: Developmental aspects of cognitive function explored through hypnosis.* New York: International Universities Press.

Reiser, M. (1976). Hypnosis as a tool in criminal investigation. *The Police Chief, 43,* 36, 39–40.

Reiser, M. (1985). Investigative hypnosis: Scientism, memory tricks and power plays. In J. Zeig (Ed.), *Eriksonian psychotherapy: Vol. 2. Clinical applications* (pp. 511–523). New York: Brunner/Mazel.

Reiser, M., & Nielson, M. (1980). Investigative hypnosis: A developing specialty. *American Journal of Clinical Hypnosis, 23,* 75–84.

Roediger, H. L., & Payne, D. G. (1982). Hypermnesia: The role of repeated testing. *Journal of Experimental Psychology: Learning, Memory, and Cognition, 8,* 66–72.

Roediger, H. L., & Payne, D. G. (1985). Recall criterion does not affect recall level or hypermnesia: A puzzle for generate/recognize theories. *Memory and Cognition, 13,* 1–7.

Rosenthal, B. G. (1944). Hypnotic recall of material learned under anxiety- and non-anxiety-producing conditions. *Journal of Experimental Psychology, 34,* 369–389.

Salzberg, H. C., & DePiano, F. A. (1980). Hypnotizability and task motivating suggestions: A further look at how they affect performance. *International Journal of Clinical and Experimental Hypnosis, 28,* 261–271.

Sanders, G. S., & Simmons, W. L. (1983). Use of hypnosis to enhance eyewitness accuracy: Does it work? *Journal of Applied Psychology, 68,* 70–77.

Sanders, S. (1969). The effect of hypnosis on visual imagery. *Dissertation Abstracts International, 30,* 2936B. (University Microfilms No. 69–15, 484)

Sarbin, T. R. (1950). Contributions to role-taking theory: I. Hypnotic behavior. *Psychological Review, 57,* 255–270.

Sarbin, T. R., & Coe, W. C. (1972). *Hypnosis: A social psychological analysis of influence communication.* New York: Holt, Rinehart & Winston.

Schafer, D. W., & Rubio, R. (1978). Hypnosis to aid the recall of witnesses. *International Journal of Clinical and Experimental Hypnosis, 26,* 81–91.

Shaul, R. D. (1978). Eyewitness testimony and hypnotic hypermnesia. *Dissertation Abstracts International, 39,* 2521B. (University Microfilms No. 78–21, 261)

Sheehan, P. W. (1972). A functional analysis of the role of visual imagery in unexpected recall. In P. W. Sheehan (Ed.), *The function and nature of imagery* (pp. 149–174). New York: Academic Press.

Sheehan, P. W. (1979). Hypnosis and the process of imagination. In E. Fromm & R. E. Shor (Eds.), *Hypnosis: Developments in research and new perspectives* (2nd ed., pp. 381–411). New York: Aldine.

Sheehan, P.W., Grigg, L., & McCann, T. (1984). Memory distortion following exposure to false information in hypnosis. *Journal of Abnormal Psychology, 93,* 259–265.

Sheehan, P. W., & Perry, C. W. (1976). *Methodologies of hypnosis: A critical appraisal of contemporary paradigms of hypnosis.* Hillsdale, NJ: Erlbaum.

Sheehan, P. W., & Tilden, J. (1983). Effects of suggestibility and hypnosis on accurate and distorted retrieval from memory. *Journal of Experimental Psychology: Learning, Memory, and Cognition, 9,* 283–293.

Sheehan, P. W., & Tilden, J. (1984). Real and simulated occurrences of memory distortion in hypnosis. *Journal of Abnormal Psychology, 93,* 47–57.

Shields, I. W., & Knox, V. J. (1986). Level of processing as a determinant of hypnotic hypermnesia. *Journal of Abnormal Psychology, 95,* 358–364.

Shor, R. E. (1959). Hypnosis and the concept of generalized reality-orientation. *American Journal of Psychotherapy, 13,* 582–602.

Shor, R. E., Orne, M. T., & O'Connell, D. N. (1966). Psychological correlates of plateau hypnotizability in a special volunteer sample. *Journal of Personality and Social Psychology, 3,* 80–95.

Sloane, M. C. (1981). A comparison of hypnosis versus waking state and visual versus non-visual recall instructions for witness/victim memory retrieval in actual major crimes. *Dissertation Abstracts International, 42,* 2551B. (University Microfilms No. 81-25, 873)

Smith, M. C. (1983). Hypnotic memory enhancement of witnesses: Does it work? *Psychological Bulletin, 94,* 387–407.

Smith, S. M. (1979). Remembering in and out of context. *Journal of Experimental Psychology: Human Learning and Memory, 5,* 460–471.

Society for Clinical and Experimental Hypnosis. (1979). Resolution. *International Journal of Clinical and Experimental Hypnosis, 27,* 452.

Spanos, N. P., Valois, R., Ham, M. W., & Ham, M. L. (1973). Suggestibility and vividness and control of imagery. *International Journal of Clinical and Experimental Hypnosis, 21,* 305–311.

Spence, D. P. (1982). *Narrative truth and historical truth: Meaning and interpretation in psychoanalysis.* New York: Norton.

Spiegel, H. (1980). Hypnosis and evidence: Help or hindrance? *Annals of the New York Academy of Sciences, 347,* 73–85.

Spiegel, H., & Spiegel, D. (1978). *Trance and treatment: Clinical uses of hypnosis.* New York: Basic Books.

Spiegel, H., Shor, G., & Fischman, S. (1945). An hypnotic ablation technique for the study of personality development. *Psychosomatic Medicine, 7,* 272–278.

Stager, G. L. (1974). The effect of hypnosis on the learning and recall of visually presented material. *Dissertation Abstracts International, 35,* 3075B. (University Microfilms No. 74-28, 985)

Stager, G. L., & Lundy, R. M. (1985). Hypnosis and the learning and recall of visually presented material. *International Journal of Clinical and Experimental Hypnosis, 33,* 27–39.

Stalnaker, J. M., & Riddle, E. E. (1932). The effect of hypnosis on long-delayed recall. *Journal of General Psychology, 6,* 429–440.

State v. Forney, 310 N.C. 126, 310 S.E.2d 20 (1984).

State v. Mack, Minn. 292 N.W.2d 764 (1980).

State v. McQueen, 295 N.C. 96, 244 S.E.2d 414 (1978).

Sturm, C. A. (1982). *Eyewitness memory: A comparison of guided memory and hypnotic hypermnesia techniques.* Unpublished doctoral dissertation, University of Montana.

Sutcliffe, J. P., Perry, C. W., & Sheehan, P. W. (1970). Relation of some aspects of imagery and fantasy to hypnotic susceptibility. *Journal of Abnormal Psychology, 76,* 279–287.

't Hoen, P. (1978). Effects of hypnotizability and visualizing ability on imagery-mediated learning. *International Journal of Clinical and Experimental Hypnosis, 26,* 45–54.

Tallant, B. (1984, October). *Hypnotic conditions—their effect on memory.* Paper presented at the meeting of the Society for Clinical and Experimental Hypnosis, San Antonio, TX.

Teasdale, J. D., & Fogarty, S. J. (1979). Differential effects of induced mood on retrieval of pleasant and unpleasant events from episodic memory. *Journal of Abnormal Psychology, 88,* 248–257.

Timm, H. W. (1981). The effect of forensic hypnosis techniques on eyewitness recall and recognition. *Journal of Police Science and Administration, 9,* 188–194.

Timm, H. W. (1982). *A theoretical and empirical examination of the effects of forensic hypnosis on eyewitness recall.* Paper presented at the 9th International Congress of Hypnosis and Psychosomatic Medicine, Glasgow, Scotland.

True, R. M. (1949). Experimental control in hypnotic age regression states. *Science, 110,* 583–584.

True, R. M., & Stephenson, C. W. (1951). Controlled experiments correlating electroencephalogram, pulse, and plantar reflexes with hypnotic age regression and induced emotional states. *Personality, 1,* 252–263.

Tulving, E. (1972). Episodic and semantic memory. In E. Tulving & W. Donaldson (Eds.), *Organization of memory* (pp. 381–403). New York: Academic Press.

Tulving, E., & Pearlstone, Z. (1966). Availability and accessibility of information in memory for words. *Journal of Verbal Learning and Verbal Behavior, 5,* 381–391.

Tulving, E., & Thomson, D. M. (1973). Encoding specificity and retrieval processes in episodic memory. *Psychological Review, 80,* 352–373.

Twerski, A. J., & Naar, R. (1976). Guilt clarification via age regression. *American Journal of Clinical Hypnosis, 18,* 204–206.

Velten, E. (1968). A laboratory task for induction of mood states. *Behaviour Research and Therapy, 6,* 473–482.

Wagstaff, G. F. (1982). Hypnosis and recognition of a face. *Perceptual and Motor Skills, 55,* 816–818.

Wagstaff, G. F., Traverse, J., & Milner, S. (1982). Hypnosis and eyewitness memory—two experimental analogues. *IRCS Medical Science: Psychology and Psychiatry, 10,* 894–895.

Wells, G. L., & Leippe, M. R. (1981). How do triers of fact infer the accuracy of eyewitness identifications? Memory for peripheral detail can be misleading. *Journal of Applied Psychology, 66,* 682–687.

Wells, G. L., Lindsay, R. C. L., & Ferguson, T. J. (1979). Accuracy, confidence, and juror perceptions in eyewitness identification. *Journal of Applied Psychology, 64,* 440–448.

White, R. W. (1941). A preface to the theory of hypnotism. *Journal of Abnormal and Social Psychology, 36,* 477–505.

White, R. W., Fox, G. F., & Harris, W. W. (1940). Hypnotic hypermnesia for recently learned material. *Journal of Abnormal and Social Psychology, 35,* 88–103.

Whitehouse, W. G., Dinges, D. F., Orne, E. C., & Orne, M. T. (1987, October). *Hypnotic hypermnesia assessed by forced interrogatory recall.* Paper presented at the meeting of the Society for Clinical and Experimental Hypnosis, Los Angeles.

Young, P. C. (1925). An experimental study of mental and physical functions in the normal and hypnotic states. *American Journal of Psychology, 36,* 214–232.

Young, P. C. (1926). An experimental study of mental and physical functions in the normal and hypnotic states: Additional results. *American Journal of Psychology, 37,* 345–356.

Yuille, J. C., & McEwan, H. (1985). Use of hypnosis as an aid to eyewitness memory. *Journal of Applied Psychology, 70,* 389–400.

Zelig, M., & Beidleman, W. B. (1981). The investigative use of hypnosis: A word of caution. *International Journal of Clinical and Experimental Hypnosis, 29,* 401–412.

# 3

## Hypermnesia: The Effect of Hypnosis, Fantasy, and Concentration

MATTHEW HUGH ERDELYI
*Brooklyn College and the Graduate Center*
*of the City University of New York*

### HYPNOTIC HYPERMNESIA

"Hypnotic hypermnesia," the enhancement of memory through hypnosis, is at once a classic claim and a current problem of hypnosis.

The notion that hypnosis can augment memory probably originated (in Western psychology) in the late 18th century with the work of the Marquis de Puységur on somnambulistic "lucidity" (Ellenberger, 1970), though similar claims can be found in ancient religious–psychological disciplines such as, for example, raja yoga (Mumford, 1974). The hypermnesic power of hypnosis was apparently widely assumed in the late 19th century and figured prominently in the therapeutic approaches of Janet, Breuer, and Freud, among others (Bowers & Meichenbaum, 1984; Ellenberger, 1970), though Freud, as is well known, soon abandoned hypnosis, finding concentration (retrieval effort) to be as effective (Breuer & Freud, 1895/1955; Erdelyi, 1985). Although hypnosis is not a standard instrument in traditional psychoanalytic psychotherapy, it has continued to be used by a wide spectrum of therapists for the purposes of producing recoveries of traumatic memories for abreaction (e.g., Schreiber, 1973; Spiegel & Spiegel, 1978; Thigpen & Cleckley, 1957). More recently, there has developed a surge in the practical use of hypnosis in forensic contexts, in the continued belief that hypnosis has the power to recover unconscious memories (e.g., Arons, 1967; Reiser & Nielson, 1980; Schafer & Rubio, 1978).

It is clear, then, that the assumption that hypnosis is capable of enhancing memory is widespread as well as of long standing. How well is this assumption supported by scientific evidence? Not too well, according to recent overviews of the experimental literature (e.g., Smith, 1983). The laboratory evidence, at best, is mixed. Of the three dozen or so published studies, roughly a third are positive (suggesting the existence of hypnotic hypermnesia), but the other two-thirds are null or negative (suggesting that hypnosis has no effect on memory or that it actually tends to disrupt memory). However, as my colleagues and I (Erdelyi, Dinges, Orne, Whitehouse, & Orne, 1987) have recently shown, the apparent haphazardness of the experimental literature is misleading. When outcomes are classified according to two basic factors—the *type of stimulus* being retrieved (nonsense/low-sense vs. meaningful/high-sense) and the *type of test* used to assess memory (recall vs. recognition)—the laboratory outcomes assume a striking orderliness. Figure 3-1 (adapted from Erdelyi *et al.*, 1987) demonstrates this feature of the laboratory evidence. (Table 3-1 documents the entries in Figure 3-1.)

It will be readily seen that neither recall nor recognition of nonsense/ low-sense materials is enhanced by hypnosis, nor is the recognition of meaningful/high-sense materials. The cell for recall of high-sense materials, however, in contrast to the other three, is substantially positive.

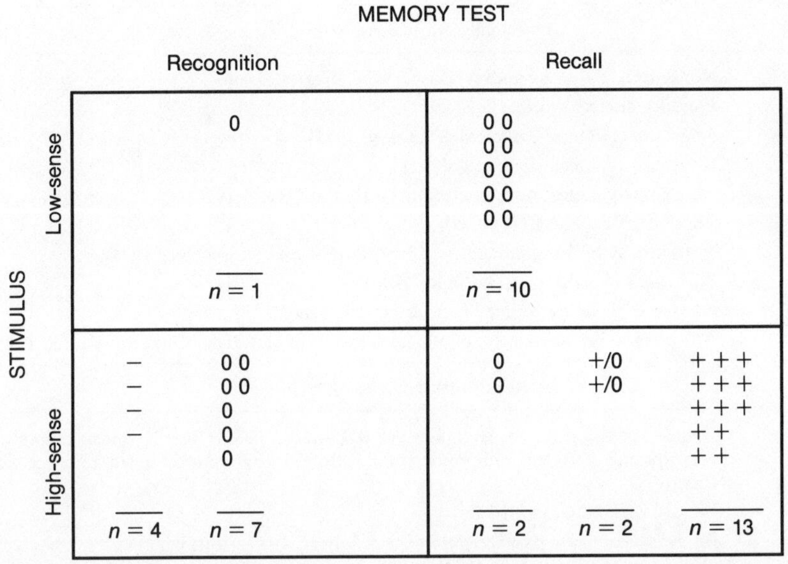

MEMORY TEST

|  |  | Recognition |  | Recall |  |  |
|---|---|---|---|---|---|---|
| **STIMULUS** | **Low-sense** | 0 | | 0 0<br>0 0<br>0 0<br>0 0<br>0 0 | | |
| | | $n = 1$ | | $n = 10$ | | |
| | **High-sense** | —<br>—<br>—<br>— | 0 0<br>0 0<br>0<br>0<br>0 | 0<br>0 | +/0<br>+/0 | + + +<br>+ + +<br>+ + +<br>+ +<br>+ + |
| | | $n = 4$ | $n = 7$ | $n = 2$ | $n = 2$ | $n = 13$ |

Figure 3-1. Effect of hypnosis on memory as a function of type of stimulus and memory test. Key to outcome symbols: +, positive (enhancement) effect; +/0, positive (enhancement) effect, but not with respect to all control conditions; 0, null outcome or nonsignificant trend; —, negative (decrement) effect. (Adapted from *The Stimulus and the Test in Hypnotic Hypermnesia* by M. H. Erdelyi, D. F. Dinges, M. T. Orne, W. G. Whitehouse, and E. C. Orne, 1987, manuscript submitted for publication.)

Table 3-1. Documentation of Figure 3-1: Outcomes by Stimulus and Test

| Out-come | Stimulus and study |
|---|---|
| | **Recognition of low-sense stimuli** |
| 0 | Inkblots (Young, 1925) |
| | **Recognition of high-sense stimuli** |
| 0 | Objective, nonleading questions about filmed accident (Putnam, 1979) |
| − | Leading questions about accident (Putnam, 1979) |
| − * | Videotape of a theft (Sanders & Simmons, 1983) |
| 0 * | Leading questions about filmed crime (Sheehan & Tilden, 1983) |
| 0 * | Leading and nonleading questions about filmed crime (Sheehan & Tilden, 1984) |
| 0 | Staged assassination (Timm, 1981) |
| 0 * | Faces (Wagstaff, 1982) |
| − * | Slides of objects, people (Wagstaff, Traverse, & Milner, 1982, Experiment 1) |
| 0 * | Staged event (Wagstaff *et al.*, 1982, Experiment 2) |
| 0 * | Objective, nonleading questions about filmed accident (Zelig & Beidleman, 1981) |
| − | Leading questions about accident (Zelig & Beidleman, 1981) |
| | **Recall of low-sense stimuli** |
| 0 | Nonsense syllables (remote) (Barber & Calverley, 1966) |
| 0 | Paired-associate words (Das, 1961) |
| 0 | Nonsense syllables (Dhanens & Lundy, 1975) |
| 0 | Nonsense syllables (Eysenck, 1941) |
| 0 | Nonsense syllables; nonsense pictorial figures (Huse, 1930) |
| 0 | Three-digit numbers (Mitchell, 1932) |
| 0 | Nonsense syllables; innocuous and profane words (Rosenthal, 1944) |
| 0 | Word lists (Salzberg & DePiano, 1980) |
| 0 | Nonsense syllables (White, Fox, & Harris, 1940) |
| 0 | Adjective–noun associates; digits; nonsense syllables; lists of names (Young, 1925) |
| | **Recall of high-sense stimuli** |
| + | Article about a rare chemical (Cooper & London, 1973) (But: Hypnosis enhanced performance only when hypnotic recall followed nonhypnotic recall, and not vice versa) |
| + | Picture details (Crawford & Allen, 1983) |
| + | Biographical prose passage (Dhanens & Lundy, 1975) (But: whereas hypnosis with motivational instructions helped those high vs. low in susceptibility [Difference Score = 4.33 vs. 1.89], motivation without hypnosis reversed the pattern [Difference Score = 2.50 vs. 4.22]) |
| + | Meaningful auditory and visual information associated with films inducing low arousal, sexual arousal, and "traumatic" arousal (DePiano & Salzberg, 1981) |
| + | Emotional events; real-life events (Dorcus, 1960) |
| + | Pictures (Dywan & Bowers, 1983) |

Table 3-1(*Continued*)

| | Recall of high-sense stimuli |
|---|---|
| +/0 | Filmed crime scenarios (Geiselman, Fisher, MacKinnon, & Holland, 1985) (Hypnotic procedure elicited more correct recalls than a standard police interview, but not more than a nonhypnotic guided-memory interview) |
| + | Pictures (Gheorghiu, 1972) |
| 0 | Story (McConkey & Nogrady, 1984) |
| 0 | Pictures (Nogrady, McConkey, & Perry, 1985) |
| + | Poetry; words associated with failure (Rosenthal, 1944) |
| + | Real-life scene (Sears, 1954) |
| + | Slide sequence of wallet snatching (Sheehan & Tilden, 1984) (But: Hypnosis increased recall only of peripheral and not of central details) |
| + | Film material (Stager & Lundy, 1985) |
| + | Poetry, structured prose (Stalnaker & Riddle, 1932) |
| +/0 | Staged assassination (Timm, 1981) (Hypnotic forensic interview yielded more correct information than free recall, but not more than a regular forensic interview) |
| + | Travel film segments, poetry (White *et al.*, 1940) |

*Note.* Adapted from *The Stimulus and the Test in Hypnotic Hypermnesia* by M. H. Erdelyi, D. F. Dinges, M. T. Orne, W. G. Whitehouse, and E. C. Orne, 1987, manuscript submitted for publication. Key to Outcome Symbols: +, positive (enhancement) effect; +/0, positive (enhancement) effect, but not with respect to all control conditions; 0, null outcome or nonsignificant trend; −, negative (decrement) effect; *, response bias was controlled or did not vary in the study. These tabulations do not include unpublished studies, PhD dissertations, clinical reports, and publications from Eastern Europe. Also not included in the tabulations are two articles (Sanders & Simmons, 1983; Yuille & McEwan, 1985) that were difficult to categorize in terms of the dimensions of interest because of the use of mixed lists (high-sense and low-sense materials combined) or mixed tests (recall and recognition combined) or both.

The role of the stimulus has been known since the ground-breaking study of White, Fox, and Harris (1940) and, except for the tabulation of outcomes in the literature, is nothing new. The importance of the memory test, however, has been largely overlooked, probably as a result of the confusion of recognition with recall in the literature on hypnotic hypermnesia. Thus, most authors whose work contributes to the uniformly null or negative cell for recognition of meaningful materials describe their studies as showing that hypnosis does not enhance "recall," when actually it is recognition that has failed to be augmented.

Except in some grey-area situations, the recall–recognition distinction is relatively straightforward. In recall, the subject must generate the sought-after information (e.g., the subject answers the question "What gifts did you receive on your last birthday?"), whereas in recognition, the subject only makes decisions about information provided by the experimenter (e.g., the subject answers "Yes" or "No" to the question "Did you get a tie?" or chooses, in the case of multiple-choice recognition tests, one of several alternatives supplied by the experimenter).

Can it be concluded from Figure 3-1 that hypnotic hypermnesia—for the case of recall of meaningful materials—has, after all, been demonstrated in the laboratory? The answer is no, though the evidence does not at least foreclose, as it does for the other three stimulus–test contingencies, a true hypermnesic effect. The problem with the existing positive studies—indeed, most of the remaining studies as well—is that none have controlled for possible shifts in response bias (cf. Klatzky & Erdelyi, 1985; Orne, 1979; Smith, 1983; but see Roediger & Payne, 1985). Thus, it is possible that the observed increases in hypnotic recall reflect not enhancements of *memory*, but merely enhancements of *responding*. Such response criterion or response bias effects would be consistent with the typical findings (e.g., Dywan & Bowers, 1983; Stalnaker & Riddle, 1932) that both hits (correct recalls) and false alarms (intrusions) increase with hypnosis. Furthermore, in view of the existence of powerful nonhypnotic hypermnesia effects (cf. Erdelyi, 1984; Erdelyi & Kleinbard, 1978), it must additionally be shown that any bona fide recall increments associated with hypnosis—if they can be demonstrated— are actually produced by hypnosis. At this juncture, we have no experimental data to help us resolve these issues. The next two sections of this chapter, dealing with nonhypnotic hypermnesia, further underscore these questions and hint at the probable answers.

To summarize the situation as it now stands, the following may be concluded from the experimental literature. First, there is no evidence that hypnosis enhances recall or recognition of nonsense materials. Second, there is no evidence that hypnosis enhances recognition memory for meaningful materials, and actually some evidence that hypnosis may slightly disrupt this type of memory. Finally, there is substantial evidence that hypnosis enhances correct responses in recall of meaningful materials, but there is no evidence one way or the other as to whether this enhancement effect is a memory or response (productivity) phenomenon, nor as to whether hypnosis adds to—or possibly subtracts from—nonhypnotic hypermnesia effects on recall.

## FANTASY AND HYPERMNESIA

This section evaluates the experimental status of the purported power of free-associative fantasy to recover inaccessible memories. The free-association technique was the major hypermnesic instrument upon which psychoanalysis finally settled (Erdelyi, 1985), supplanting the concentration procedure that

Freud briefly borrowed from Bernheim after abandoning the use of hypnosis (see the next section of this chapter).

The background of this research was the considerable experimental literature suggesting that subliminal stimuli tend to emerge in the content of a variety of fantasy-like productions, such as dreams, daydreams, free-associative fantasy, and imagery (Allers & Teler, 1924/1960; Eagle, Wolitzky, & Klein, 1966; Fisher, 1954, 1956; Fisher & Paul, 1959; Fiss, Goldberg, & Klein, 1963; Giddan, 1967; Hilgard, 1962; Pötzl, 1917/1960; Shevrin & Luborsky, 1958). If, as the preponderance of studies suggested, unconscious information can be indirectly recovered in fantasy (without, however, the subject's knowing that this information is being recovered), could it be shown that fantasy activity produces an increase in intentional recall?

## Initial Research

Haber and I (Haber & Erdelyi, 1967), following a lead from Hilgard (1962), undertook to pursue this question. We sought, specifically, to demonstrate that accessibility for the contents of a tachistoscopically flashed picture would actually increase after a period of free association, rather than decaying with time and intervening interference, as might be expected from classic memory theory (cf. Erdelyi, 1984).

We (Haber & Erdelyi, 1967) tested three groups of subjects. The experimental (free-association) group was exposed for 0.5 second to the complex stimulus shown in Figure 3-2. The subjects, all individually tested, then tried to recall as best as they could the contents of the semiliminal stimulus in the form of a labeled drawing. This first recall ($R_1$) was followed by a 40-minute period of free association that was recorded by the experimenter. Following this free-association task, the subjects were required to attempt another recall ($R_2$) of the stimulus that had been presented at the beginning of the study. One control group, the dart subjects, were treated identically except for the free-association activity; instead, these subjects engaged in a diverting sensory–motor task, dart throwing, for a comparable period of time, which was then followed by the second recall effort, $R_2$. A second control group, the yoked subjects, were tested to eliminate contextual embellishment effects that free association might engender and that could be confused with memory enhancement (for a discussion of this potential artifact, see Haber & Erdelyi, 1967; Hilgard, 1962). The yoked subjects did not see the original stimulus. Instead, each yoked subject copied an experimental counterpart's $R_1$ drawing, then free-associated for 40 minutes, and finally produced a postfantasy recall ($R_2$) of the $R_1$ they had copied prior to fantasy.

The results were unambiguous. The free-association subjects, unlike subjects in the control groups, recalled more stimulus items after the second, postfantasy recall effort than in the first, prefantasy recall effort (i.e., $R_2 >$

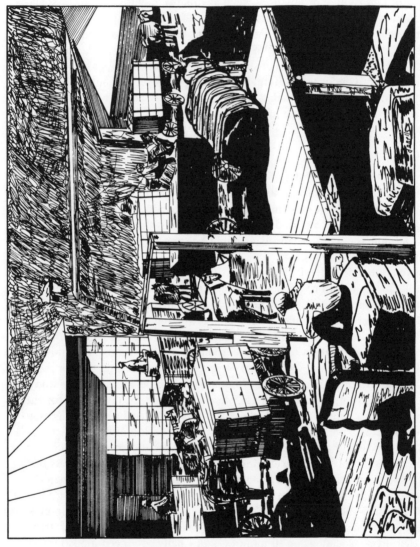

Figure 3-2. Drawing of the stimulus used by Haber and Erdelyi (1967). (From "Emergence and Recovery of Initially Unavailable Perceptual Material" by R. N. Haber and M. H. Erdelyi, 1967, *Journal of Verbal Learning and Verbal Behavior, 6,* p. 624. Copyright 1967 by Academic Press. Adapted by permission.)

$R_1$). Also, the free associations of the experimental subjects contained more stimulus-related materials than those of the yoked subjects for items never recalled in either recall trial, replicating the past findings of stimulus emergence in fantasy of subliminal input.

Figures 3-3 and 3-4 present the prefantasy and postfantasy recall efforts of two experimental subjects. It will be readily seen that postfantasy recall was superior to prefantasy recall in both these subjects. None of the control subjects (e.g., Figures 3-5 and 3-6) produced comparable results.

An evaluation of all subjects' protocols confirmed the recall-enhancing effect of fantasy. For example, a blind scorer judged all 20 $R_2$ recalls of the experimental subjects to be better than their $R_1$ recalls ($p < .000001$), but no significant trend emerged for either of the two control groups. An item-by-item content analysis of the recall protocols produced essentially the same outcome. Table 3-2 presents the number of correct stimulus elements retrieved in prefantasy and postfantasy recall for the three groups. The experimental subjects' postfantasy recalls ($R_2$) were significantly greater than their prefantasy recalls ($R_1$), and this recall enhancement was significantly greater than the small increase observed in the dart group.

Our results (Haber & Erdelyi, 1967) suggested that free-associative fantasy substantially enhances recall, and this was how we interpreted our findings at the time. If "dreams are hypermnesic" (Freud, 1900/1953, Vol. 5, p. 589), free-associative fantasy appears to be likewise.

I should pause at this point to note that the Haber and Erdelyi (1967) study leaves us essentially where the literature on hypnotic hypermnesia currently stands. The results, which are easily replicated (see below), documented that free-associative fantasy produces an enhancement in correct recalls. However, it was also the case (which may be gleaned from Figures 3-3 and 3-4) that there was a concomitant increase in intrusions or distortions in postfantasy recall. Thus, as in the case of the literature on hypnotic hypermnesia, it is not possible to determine from the Haber and Erdelyi (1967) study whether fantasy induces a true enhancement of *memory* or merely an enhancement of *reporting*.

*Response Criterion Control*

In the present case, however, an experimental answer to the response criterion question was obtained (Erdelyi, 1970, 1972a, 1972b). Since it is the same question that the area of hypnotic hypermnesia needs to resolve, the experimental strategy for dealing with the problem and the results obtained with fantasy are examined here in some detail.

For this purpose, two basic approaches were employed (Erdelyi, 1970). The first of these was to replicate the Haber and Erdelyi (1967) recall results and then to determine whether the imposition of a control over productivity

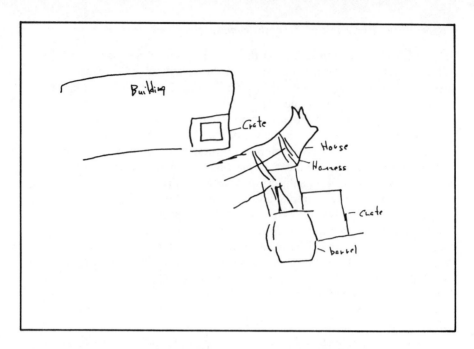

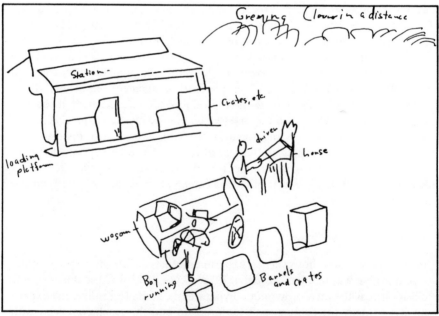

Figure 3-3. Prefantasy and postfantasy recall of subject H. J. in the Haber and Erdelyi study. (From *Psychoanalysis: Freud's Cognitive Psychology* [p. 70] by M. H. Erdelyi, 1985, New York: W. H. Freeman. Copyright 1985 by Mathew Erdelyi. Adapted by permission.)

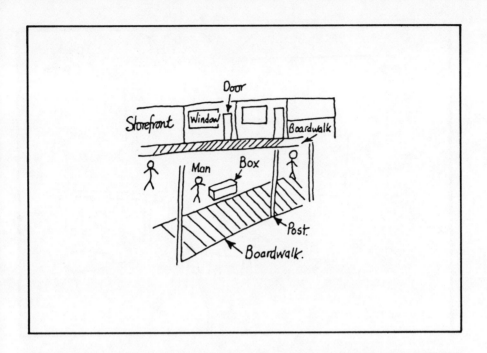

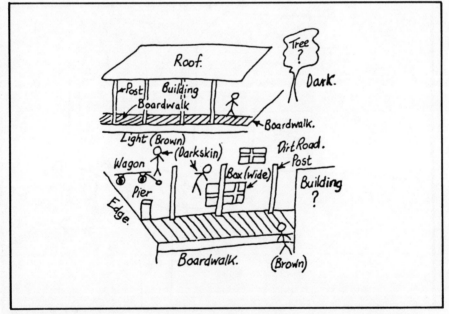

Figure 3-4. Prefantasy and postfantasy recall of subject L. B. in the Haber and Erdelyi study. (From "Emergence and Recovery of Initially Unavailable Perceptual Material" by R. N. Haber and M. H. Erdelyi, 1967, *Journal of Verbal Learning and Verbal Behavior, 6,* p. 624. Copyright 1967 by Academic Press. Adapted by permission.)

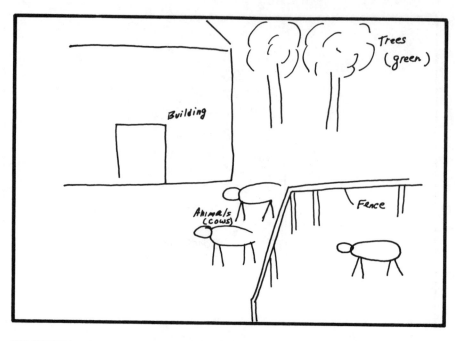

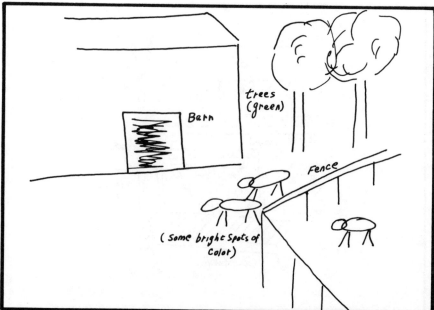

Figure 3-5. Stimulus recall before and after control task (dart playing) by subject R. L.

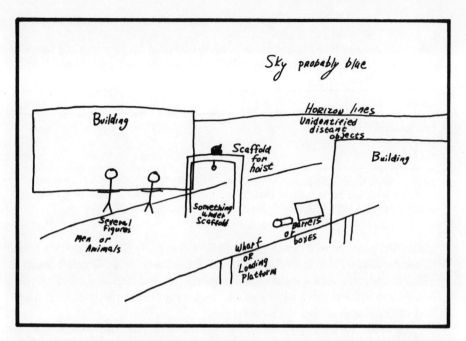

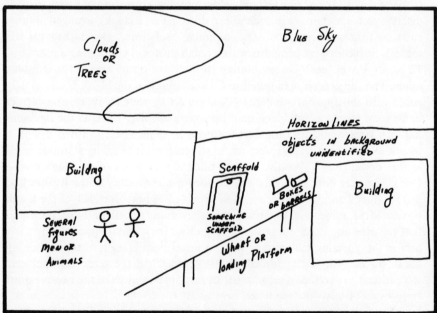

Figure 3-6. Stimulus recall before and after control task (dart playing) by subject D. S.

Table 3-2. Average Number of Correct Items Retrieved in the First ($R_1$) and Second ($R_2$) Recall Trials by the Experimental (Free-Association), Dart Control and Yoked Control Subjects

| Group | $R_1$ | $R_2$ | $R_2-R_1$ |
|---|---|---|---|
| Free association | 6.25 | 10.62 | 4.37 |
| Dart control | 6.45 | 7.70 | 1.25 |
| Yoked control | 7.20 | 7.60 | 0.40 |

*Note.* Adapted from "Emergence and Recovery of Initially Unavailable Perceptual Material" by R. N. Haber and M. H. Erdelyi, 1967, *Journal of Verbal Learning and Verbal Behavior, 6,* p. 623. Copyright 1967 by Academic Press. Adapted by permission.

would dissipate the recall enhancement effect of fantasy. The second tack was to use procedures introduced by signal detection theory (e.g., Green & Swets, 1966) to measure actual memory accessibility ($d'$) and response criterion ($\beta$) before and after fantasy with a recognition-with-ratings methodology. The first of these approaches is discussed first.

In order to gain a more ready control over response production, I (Erdelyi, 1970) shifted to a less unwieldy stimulus, consisting of a matrix of 12 discrete pictorial items (e.g., a candle, a duck, a car, a clock) arranged in three rows of four pictures each. The stimulus, as before, was flashed for 0.5 second. Subjects were provided with a recall protocol containing a matrix of 12 empty boxes, each corresponding to the position of one of the stimulus items. The subjects were required to fill in as many of the blank boxes as they could with the appropriate items. (Position errors were frequent, and correct items were scored as full hits even if they were misplaced.) After the intervening task (free association or dart throwing), subjects were provided with a second recall protocol and were asked to recall on it as many stimulus items as they could ($R_2$). Typically, subjects filled in only a few of the blank boxes. Once they were done, subjects were handed a carbon copy of the $R_2$ they had just produced and were now asked to provide a "guess" for each of the blank boxes. Most subjects complained that they could recall nothing more and that the guessing made no sense; nevertheless, they were required to do their best at the guessing task and to fill in a novel item in each of the remaining blank boxes. This latter forced recall—"forced" in the sense that subjects were forced to produce a set number of responses, unlike in the two previous "free-recall" trials—is designated here as $R_2^*$.

The first question of interest was whether the earlier finding that fantasy augments free recall could be replicated. Table 3-3 shows that it could: Experimental subjects, unlike either the dart control or yoked control subjects, evidenced a significant recall increment from $R_1$ to $R_2$. This recall increase could have resulted from either a bona fide memory enhancement or from greater response productivity as a function of free association. If it was the former, control over response productivity in $R_2^*$ should not have undermined the differential recall increments among groups. Table 3-3 shows, however, that the effect collapsed with control over response bias: $R_1$-to-$R_2^*$ increments were not different for experimental and dart control subjects. It is clear that free associations, as implemented in these studies, do not augment memory, though they do increase response productivity and therefore hits (as well as false alarms) when response bias is not controlled.

It will be of interest, of course, whether hypnotic hypermnesia effects will survive the same control over response productivity. My guess is that they will not and that hypnotic hypermnesia will turn out, like fantasy hypermnesia, to be a response bias effect.

It should be noted that the $R_1$-to-$R_2^*$ recall increases obtained by the two groups that were actually exposed to the stimulus—the free-association subjects and the dart subjects—were greater than that of the yoked subjects. The yoked subjects, it will be remembered, never saw the stimulus but instead copied the $R_1$ of an experimental counterpart; thus, the 2.54 recall increase from $R_1$ to $R_2^*$ they obtained reflects the chance guessing rate, given $R_1$. The (significantly) greater improvement of the subjects exposed to the stimulus indicates that these subjects had more information accessible than they were willing to hazard on $R_1$; for this reason, they produced, under a laxer criterion, recall increments that were greater than those associated with chance level. This is exactly what signal detection theory would predict, and it helps to account for the compelling nature of the recoveries obtained in fantasy and hypnosis. These recoveries are not mere chance guesses; they reveal accessible—but hitherto unreported—information. It is for this reason that criterion-relaxing procedures (hypnosis, fantasy) may be useful in an investigative context: Such procedures may be expected to turn up information that is accessible but that the subject is too unsure of to report under stricter-criterion conditions. (Of course, the increase in correct information will be accompanied by incorrect information in these disinhibited-criterion situa-

Table 3-3. Average Recall Performance on Pretreatment and Posttreatment Free Recall $(R_1)$ and $(R_2)$ and Posttreatment forced Recall $(R_2^*)$ for Free-Association, Dart Control and Yoked Control Subjects

| Group | $R_1$ | $R_2$ | $R_2^*$ | $R_2-R_1$ | $R_2^*-R_1$ |
|---|---|---|---|---|---|
| Free association | 3.43 | 4.48 | 7.45 | 1.05 | 4.02 |
| Dart control | 3.82 | 4.16 | 8.19 | 0.34 | 4.37 |
| Yoked control | 3.38 | 3.80 | 5.92 | 0.42 | 2.54 |

*Note.* Adapted from "The Recovery of Unavailable Perceptual Input" by M. H. Erdelyi, 1970, *Cognitive Psychology, 1,* p. 104. Copyright 1970 by Academic Press. Adapted by permission.

tions.) It does not follow, however, that all disinhibition procedures are equally effective. I (Erdelyi, 1972b) showed, for example, that free associations following a semiliminal stimulus yielded significantly fewer recoveries than guessing. Thus, it should not be assumed that hypnosis is an effective investigative procedure for turning up leads in criminal investigations (see Council of Scientific Affairs, American Medical Association, 1985) until hypnosis is shown to be superior (or, at least, not inferior) to other criterion-relaxing procedures.

The second attack upon the criterion problem that I (Erdelyi, 1970) pursued was the use of a recognition-with-ratings methodology, which allowed not just control but actual measurement of criterion ($\beta$) and sensitivity or accessibility ($d'$) effects. After the presentation of the semiliminal stimulus, subjects were given a recognition test ($R_1$), followed by either free-associative fantasy or dart throwing, followed by a second recognition test ($R_2$).

In the recognition test, which was the same for $R_1$ and $R_2$, the subjects were presented 24 pictures, 12 from the stimulus and 12 distractor items (randomly intermixed), and were required to rate on a 6-point scale how confident they were that each item had actually been one of the 12 pictures in the semiliminal stimulus. The ratings assigned permitted the experimenter to define a "yes" response on a post hoc basis according to different criterion settings. Thus, if a rating of "6" denoted a "completely confident" judgment, and the experimenter defined a "yes" as a "6" response, a very strict criterion was set, producing relatively few hits and relatively few false alarms. Defining a "yes" response a little less strictly as either a "5" ("very confident") or a "6" ("completely confident") yielded a laxer criterion setting, one that produced more hits—and more false alarms. Defining a "yes" as a "4" ("fairly confident") or "5" or "6" yielded a still laxer criterion setting and therefore even more hits and more false alarms. The laxest criterion setting defined all ratings but the least confident (a "1") as a "yes" response; that is, "yes" responses included ratings of "2," "3," "4," "5," and "6," which, of course produced very high hit and false-alarm rates. The plotting of hit rate as a function of false-alarm rate (as generated by these different criterion settings) yielded a receiver operating characteristic (ROC) curve, from which could be extracted the two parameters of interest, $\beta$ and $d'$.

Figures 3-7 and 3-8 present, for the free-association and dart control subjects, respectively, ROC curves for $R_1$ and $R_2$. These functions (from Erdelyi, 1970) are plotted on normal–normal coordinates; that is, hit rates, $P(Y/S)$, and false-alarm rates, $P(Y/N)$, are plotted as normal–deviate transforms—hence, $z_{P(Y/S)}$ and $z_{P(Y/N)}$. Without going into technical detail, it may be said that sensitivity/accessibility, $d'$, is greater the higher the ROC function is relative to the positive diagonal, and the response criteria, $\beta$, are laxer the more the criterion points are displaced rightward. (Note: An $n$-point

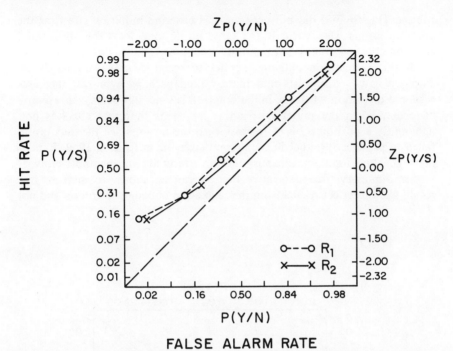

Figure 3-7. Free-association group's ROC functions for $R_1$ and $R_2$. Hit rates, P(Y/S), and false-alarm rates, P(Y/N), are plotted on normal–normal coordinates. (From "The Recovery of Unavailable Perceptual Input" by M. H. Erdelyi, 1970, *Cognitive Psychology, 1,* p. 108. Copyright 1970 by Academic Press. Reprinted by permission.)

confidence rating scale yields $n - 1$ criterion points; hence the five criterion points in the present case.)

It is immediately apparent that there was no $R_1$-to-$R_2$ improvement in recognition memory in either the free-association group (Figure 3-7) or the dart group (Figure 3-8); if anything, $R_2$ was slightly (but not significantly) lower than $R_1$ for both groups. This outcome is consistent with the recall data: There is no evidence that free-associative fantasy enhances memory. The criterion data, however, introduce an interesting wrinkle, which, if fantasy effects should generalize to hypnosis, suggests a modification in our understanding of the effects of hypnosis upon criteria. For fantasy, at any rate (see Figure 3-7), the differential shifts of the five criterion points show that there was no homogeneous criterion effect; rather, free-associative fantasy relaxed strict criteria and rendered lax criteria stricter. Note that the dart subjects (Figure 3-8) did not generate this criterion-buffering effect, as the criterion points were virtually the same for $R_1$ and $R_2$. (This differential criterion effect was obtained in another study; see Erdelyi, 1969, Experiment 4.) If this recognition outcome applies to recall memory, ultimately an empirical issue, it suggests that fantasy (and perhaps hypnosis) increases response distortion when the initial criterion is strict but decreases response distortion when the initial criterion is lax. This buffering effect is not, apparently a phenomenon of regression to the mean, since the dart group failed to produce it (either in the present study or in Erdelyi, 1969, Experiment 4). Thus, nonhomogeneous criterion effects are an open possibility.

In summary, free-associative fantasy can be shown to increase free recall, but this effect results from the relaxation of response criteria and not

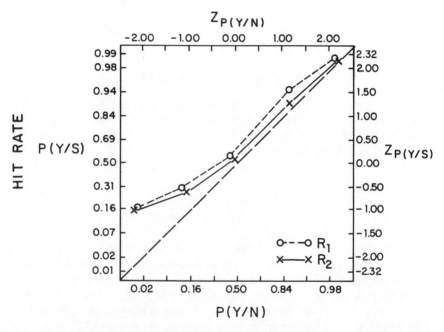

Figure 3-8. Dart control group's ROC functions for $R_1$ and $R_2$. Hit rates, P(Y/S), and false-alarm rates, P(Y/N), are plotted on normal–normal coordinates. (From "The Recovery of Unavailable Perceptual Input" by M. H. Erdelyi, 1970, *Cognitive Psychology, 1,* p. 108. Copyright 1970 by Academic Press. Reprinted by permission.)

from any enhancement of recall memory. Free-associative fantasy fails to increase recognition memory; however, fantasy appears to relax strict criterion settings while stiffening lax criterion settings.

## CONCENTRATION AND HYPERMNESIA

The studies discussed in the preceding section all involved semiliminal presentations in which the stimulus was flashed for only a fraction of a second. It may be wondered whether outcomes obtained with such stimuli generalize to clearly supraliminal materials. It is possible that not enough information is registered with semiliminal inputs for recovery and that with longer exposures hypermnesia effects may be obtained. In any case, the types of recoveries reported in the clinical literature do not involve tachistoscopic inputs, but materials that (except for the "primally repressed") were once conscious but have since become inaccessible. Thus, it is important to ascertain whether once-conscious but forgotton memories may be subject to hypermnesia.

### Fantasy Versus Concentration

Becker and I (Erdelyi & Becker, 1974) undertook to answer this question. For this purpose, we shifted away from tachistoscopic presentations to a straightforward memory procedure. Subjects were presented a supraspan memory list consisting of 80 items—40 words and 40 simply sketched pictures (e.g., a watch, a fish, a boomerang, a rat, a television), randomly intermixed. Each item was presented for 5 seconds, for a total presentation duration of about 7 minutes (5 seconds x 80 items). After the presentation of the 80 items, the subjects were administered a forced-recall trial, $R_1$, in which they were required to produce (in writing) 60 nonrepeating responses, guessing if necessary (pilot work suggested that subjects would be able to recall about 30 stimulus items from the set of 80). After this first forced recall, $R_1$, the fantasy subjects were required to generate free-associative doodles and writing (automatic writing/drawing) for 7 minutes. After this, the subjects were administered a second forced-recall test, $R_2$ (also requiring 60 responses), which was followed by a second interval of fantasy production; finally, a last forced-recall trial, $R_3$, was administered. (Since all recall trials are "forced" in this and subsequent studies, no asterisks are needed to distinguish them from free-recall trials).

Because of the disappointing effects obtained with fantasy in the previous studies, a variant of Freud's "concentration–pressure" procedure (Breuer & Freud, 1895/1955; Erdelyi, 1985) was also explored. The technique, which Freud adapted from Bernheim, and which he used after his abandonment of hypnosis but before his adoption of the free-association procedure, required patients, once they could recall nothing more, to concentrate upon the sought-after memory and to continue thinking of it until the material was recovered. When the patient complained that he or she could not remember anything more, he or she was instructed nevertheless to continue thinking of the material. In the present study, a concentration or "think" group was tested. This group was treated in exactly the same way as the fantasy subjects, except that instead of receiving the two fantasy intervals, these subjects spent the equivalent amount of time thinking (with eyes closed) of the stimulus list they had been presented.

A third group of subjects, a no-interval control group, was also tested; this group generated three consecutive forced recalls with no intervening activity between recall trials.

Table 3-4 presents the three groups' recall of pictures and words across the three forced-recall trials. The most striking effect, immediately bringing to mind the stimulus effect in studies of hypnotic hypermnesia, is the differential fate of picture versus word recall. It will be seen that every group (including the no-interval controls) produced incremental recall for pictures across trials, but that none of the groups produced significant recall increments for words.

It should be noted that the hypermnesia effects obtained with pictures cannot be attributed to shifts in response criteria, since the forced-recall procedure held subjects to a constant number of responses across trials. Thus, any increase in correct recalls was necessarily accompanied by a *decrease* in incorrect recalls. It appears, then, that true hypermnesia effects can be obtained, at least with pictures as stimuli.

What can be concluded about the effectiveness of free-associative fantasy in engendering hypermnesia for once-conscious materials? Although the free-association group produced significant increases of pictorial recall, the

Table 3-4. Average Number of Pictures and Words Recalled in Three Successive Forced-Recall Trials by the Free-Association, "Think," and No-Interval Subjects

| Group | Pictures | | | Words | | |
|---|---|---|---|---|---|---|
| | $R_1$ | $R_2$ | $R_3$ | $R_1$ | $R_2$ | $R_3$ |
| Free association | 16.65 | 18.30 | 18.59 | 14.00 | 14.17 | 14.23 |
| Think | 15.76 | 17.76 | 18.94 | 16.35 | 16.82 | 17.00 |
| No interval | 15.82 | 17.11 | 18.05 | 13.41 | 12.47 | 13.00 |
| Mean (all subjects) | 16.08 | 17.72 | 18.53 | 14.59 | 14.49 | 14.74 |

*Note.* From "Hypermnesia for Pictures: Incremental Memory For Pictures but Not Words in Multiple Recall Trials" by M. H. Erdelyi and J. Becker, 1974, *Cognitive Psychology, 6,* p. 163. Copyright 1974 by Academic Press. Reprinted by permission.

group failed to generate more picture hypermnesia than the "think" subjects or the no-interval controls; indeed, the free-association group produced the numerically lowest hypermnesia effect of the three groups, though this difference was not statistically significant. It can thus be concluded that there is not even a hint that free-associative fantasy contributes to the hypermnesia effect. This null outcome is worth underscoring because of its implications for the hypnotic hypermnesia hypothesis. It is easy to see that clinicians using hypnosis for recovering inaccessible memories may mistakenly assume that successful outcomes are the result of hypnosis. Without controls, however, it cannot be ascertained that hypnosis actually plays a role.

At the same time, the laboratory data suggest that true hypermnesias are likely to be produced in any clinical situation that requires, formally or informally, repeated efforts to recall inaccessible materials. Thus, clinicians may be right in claiming that they are able to induce hypermnesias, notwithstanding the skepticism of their experimental colleagues. Where they may be wrong, however, is in attributing their hypermnesias to a particular procedure such as hypnosis or free association. Without controls, such attributions constitute the logical error of *post hoc ergo propter hoc*.

## Further Questions about Concentration

A number of questions are prompted by the data in Table 3-4: How reliable is the hypermnesia effect? If reliable, how powerful is it? Are materials other than pictures effective? Does a concentration/"think" interval enhance the hypermnesia effect (there is a numerical trend suggesting this in Table 3-4, but it is not significant)? Will recall increase just with the passage of time, or are repeated recall efforts necessary? These and several other issues have been addressed by a growing experimental literature on hypermnesia (cf. Erdelyi, 1984; Erdelyi & Kleinbard, 1978; Payne, 1987; Roediger, Payne, Gillespie, & Lean, 1982; Roediger & Thorpe, 1978).

We pursued some of these questions in a replication study (Erdelyi & Becker, 1974, Study 2). Since the intervening free associations obviously contributed nothing to the hypermnesia effect, this group was dropped from the replication experiment. Four independent groups were tested: two "think" groups, one that attempted repeated recalls of 60 pictures, and another that attempted recalls of 60 words (the verbal counterparts of the pictures); and two parallel no-interval groups. Figure 3-9 presents the outcome of the study.

Picture recall is clearly hypermnesic, but word recall tends to remain constant across trials. In the present study, the "think" intervals were shown to enhance significantly the magnitude of the effect. However, there is nothing special about silent "think" intervals as such in enhancing hypermnesia. It appears, from further analysis, that they function as covert counterparts of

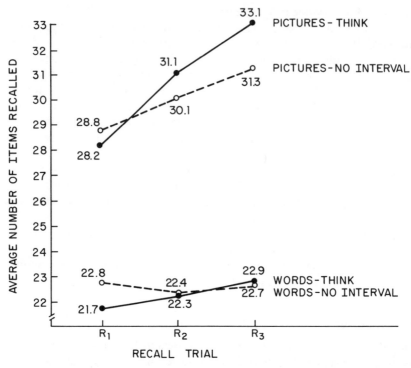

Figure 3-9. Picture and word recall with repeated recall trials with and without interpolated "think" intervals in Study 2 of Erdelyi and Becker (1974). (From "Hypermnesia for Pictures: Incremental Memory for Pictures but Not Words in Multiple Recall Trials" by M. H. Erdelyi and J. Becker, 1974, *Cognitive Psychology, 6*, p. 165. Copyright 1974 by Academic Press. Reprinted by permission.)

overt recall trials. This can be gleaned from Figure 3-10 (Erdelyi, 1977), which depicts, for Study 2 of Erdelyi and Becker (1974), recall performance as a function of retrieval time, irrespective of whether the time was spent in formal recall trials or in silent thinking. Clearly it made no difference in this study whether retrieval effort took the form of an official recall test or of silent thinking; recall of pictures, but not of words, increased with retrieval time, overt or covert (see also Erdelyi, 1984; Erdelyi & Kleinbard, 1978; Roediger & Payne, 1982; Roediger & Thorpe, 1978; Shapiro & Erdelyi, 1974).

Retrieval time should not be confused with merely the passage of time; the amount of retrieval effort (concentration, thinking, etc.) is what is crucial (Erdelyi, 1977). Roediger and Payne (1982) have shown this dramatically by demonstrating that the passage of time without retrieval effort produces no hypermnesia—or amnesia, for that matter. Nevertheless, retrieval effort is not the only factor in hypermnesia, for, obviously, the stimulus (or coding format; see below) interacts with retrieval effort.

Figures 3-9 and 3-10 suggest that the amount of hypermnesia for pictures was not exhausted in the single laboratory period used in the Erdelyi and Becker (1974) Study 2, raising the question of the limit of hypermnesia, if any, given sufficient time and retrieval effort. Kleinbard and I (Erdelyi & Kleinbard, 1978) addressed this issue, testing subjects' recall for either pictures or words for over a full week. Figure 3-11 depicts the course of recall with multiple testing over this extended time interval. It is readily seen that picture recall (but not word recall) continued to grow with retrieval effort for at least several days, increasing by some 50% over initial recall level.

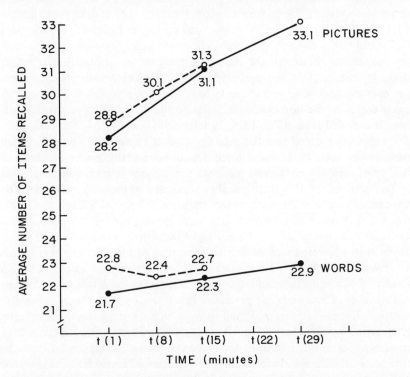

Figure 3-10. Picture and word recall as a function of retrieval time, overt or covert, in Study 2 of Erdelyi and Becker (1974). (From *Has Ebbinghaus Decayed with Time?* by M. H. Erdelyi, 1977, paper presented at the 19th Annual Meeting of the Psychonomic Society, Washington, DC.)

The hypermnesia effect with pictures is thus shown to be not only reliable, but also very powerful. If therapy sessions can be viewed as successive recall trials, a therapist can expect substantial hypermnesias to be achieved in the course of therapy. Of course, the therapist may be tempted to ascribe memory recoveries to the procedure that he or she happens to employ—hypnosis, free association, active imagination. For such ascription to be borne out, however, it will have to be demonstrated that the procedure is actually effective above and beyond the role of retrieval effort (concentration). Free association does not seem to have this property, though it does not seem to detract seriously from hypermnesia and is certainly a more enjoyable task (for both subject and experimenter) than the boring procedure of repeated recall trials. The data on hypnosis, as has been noted, are not yet in.

Even if free association or hypnosis should prove not to be hypermnesic in and of themselves, it may still be the case that they fulfill the function of inducing protracted retrieval effort (concentration) long after subjects would normally stop trying. From the complaints and the resistance to the drudgery of repeated recall trials voiced by the subjects in the Erdelyi and Kleinbard (1978) study, it is doubtful that subjects would gladly expose themselves, if they had much choice, to the pressured retrieval procedure that repeated testing represents. This was precisely Freud's experience with his concentration–pressure technique and seems to have been the impetus, following Frau Emmy von N.'s rebellion against it, for shifting to the free-association procedure (Breuer & Freud, 1895/1955; Erdelyi, 1985).

It should be noted that the data depicted in Figure 3-11 represent recall levels across successive trials. Such functions actually underestimate the number of memory recoveries achieved throughout testing, since recall on any trial reflects not only recoveries but also losses of memory over time. The appropriate measure of total item recovery would be provided by *cumulative recall* across trials, which measures the total number of correct recalls up to a particular trial, irrespective of forgetting of previously recalled items. Thus, a subject who recovered two items from one trial to the next but also forgot two items would show no net increase in recall level but would show an increase of two items in cumulative recall. The failure to distinguish between the two types of functions has produced much confusion in the experimental literature. Increases in net recall define *hypermnesia*; increases in cumulative recall define *reminiscence* (Erdelyi, 1984, 1987; Payne, 1987). Figure 3-11 provides hypermnesia functions for pictures and words. Figure 3-12, on the other hand, depicts the corresponding reminiscence functions. It is clear that subjects produced reminiscence for both pictures and words, and it is not certain whether they had reached asymptote at the end of the week of recall effort. One question that should be investigated in the hypnosis literature is whether hypnosis might have an effect on reminiscence, for it is possible for hypnotic reminiscence to exist in the absence of hypnotic hypermnesia.

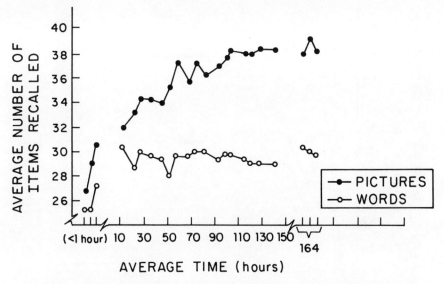

Figure 3-11. Hypermnesia for pictures and words over a week's interval: Number of items recalled in successive recall trials in Study 2 of Erdelyi and Kleinbard (1978). (From "Has Ebbinghaus Decayed with Time? The Growth of Recall (Hypermnesia) over Days" by M. H. Erdelyi and J. Kleinbard, 1978, *Journal of Experimental Psychology: Human Learning and Memory, 4,* p. 282. Copyright 1978 by the American Psychological Association. Reprinted by permission.)

*Coding Formats*

The studies examined so far all involved memory lists consisting of either pictures or words, with only pictures producing reliable hypermnesias. To what extent is the hypermnesia effect restricted to pictorial materials? In our original set of studies, we (Erdelyi & Becker, 1974) reported some hints that the mental coding of the stimulus might be more critical than the stimulus itself. Although the subjects recalling words were *on the average* nonhypermnesic, some of these subjects actually produced hefty hypermnesias (which, however, were counterbalanced by other subjects producing amnesic recall over trials). Informal querying of the subjects recalling words suggested that those who had spontaneously recoded the words into *images* produced hypermnesia, whereas those employing other mnemonic strategies, such as silent rehearsal or conceptual organization, failed to do so. This observation led to a formal test (Erdelyi, Finkelstein, Herrell, Miller, & Thomas, 1976), which replicated the flat recall functions that had been previously obtained with words but showed that if subjects were instructed to recode the word

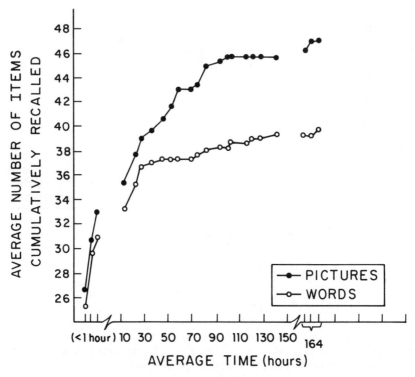

Figure 3-12. Reminiscence for pictures and words over a week's interval: Number of items cumulatively recalled in successive recall trials in Study 2 of Erdelyi and Kleinbard (1978). (From "Has Ebbinghaus Decayed with Time? The Growth of Recall (Hypermnesia) over Days" by M. H. Erdelyi and J. Kleinbard, 1978, *Journal of Experimental Psychology: Human Learning and Memory, 4,* p. 283. Copyright 1978 by the American Psychological Association. Reprinted by permission.)

inputs into images of what the words represented, hypermnesias comparable to those observed with pictures resulted. Since then, other researchers (e.g., Belmore, 1981; Erdelyi, Buschke, & Finkelstein, 1977; Roediger *et al.*, 1982) have shown that subjecting stimuli to deep processing (in the sense of Craik & Lockhart, 1972) also produces hypermnesia. Moreover, in very recent work (Erdelyi & Halberstam, 1987) substantial hypermnesias were demonstrated for a dream-like story, "The War of the Ghosts," which had been used by Bartlett (1932) to demonstrate the reconstructive–distorting nature of memory.

Thus, the literature on hypermnesia seems to parallel the literature on hypnotic hypermnesia in that effects are reliably obtained with "high-sense" stimuli (e.g., pictorial, imagistic, deeply processed, complex, and meaningful materials), but not with "low-sense" stimuli (e.g., nonsense syllables and shallowly processed lists of words). In the present case, unlike that of hypnotic hypermnesia, the effects have been shown, through the control of response bias, to be bona fide memory increments. Inasmuch as retrieval effort (in the form of overt recall or covert concentration/thinking) seems to be the critical factor with the appropriate materials, it is highly likely that the hypermnesias being produced in conjunction with hypnosis are also true hypermnesias, since concentration is inevitably involved. What needs to be shown is whether hypnosis adds anything to concentration by itself.

What of recognition hypermnesia? Is there any evidence for it, or are the data also parallel in this respect to the hypnosis literature (which, as has been seen in Figure 3-1, has produced no hint of hypnotic recognition hypermnesia)? There has been little work on this question, though it is quite clear that for lists of words, recognition hypermnesia is not readily obtained. Thus, Bernbach, Roediger, and Payne (1981), in two experiments involving words that were either imaged or semantically elaborated at the time of input, failed to find any recognition hypermnesia; actually, in one of the studies a substantial amnesia effect was obtained instead.

What of recognition hypermnesia for pictures? In this case, a peculiar methodological problem has to be faced—namely, the notoriously high recognition memory that is typically obtained with pictures (Nickerson, 1965; Shepard, 1967; Standing, Conezio, & Haber, 1970). In a pilot study I did, involving 120 pictures of the sort that have been shown to produce recall hypermnesia, virtually perfect recognition memory was obtained on an initial recognition trial (99% hits for 1% false alarms), a level that leaves no room for improvement. Except for fleeting effects that can be obtained within 90 milliseconds after input (Milner, 1968; Wallace, Coltheart, & Forster, 1970), only one experimental induction of recognition hypermnesia has been reported (Erdelyi & Stein, 1981). The trick for producing the effect was to use highly meaningful stimuli (cartoons with verbal captions) and then to test not for recognition of the whole cartoons (which yielded perfect initial recognition) but for a *component* of each cartoon—namely, the picture part without the caption. This procedure forced the subjects actively to use retrieval effort (to find the verbal complement of each picture) and resulted in significant memory improvements on repeated recognition tests (indexed by increases in $d'$ over trials) on the cartoon pictures without captions. This unusual procedure for partial stimulus testing may actually be the more ecologically valid one, since in real life one is typically obliged to recognize not the identical stimulus, but a transformed or partial version of that originally perceived. It should be added that no corresponding recognition hypermnesia was found for the cartoon captions, which may be explained by a peculiar picture–word asymmetry in these types of stimuli (Erdelyi, 1984; Erdelyi & Stein, 1981): The verbal components (i.e. captions) do not yield their pictorial complements with retrieval effort, whereas the picture components tend to do so.

In sum, there is evidence for recognition hypermnesia for pictures but none for words, and there is such hypermnesia with pictures only when retrieval plays an active role in the recognition process.

## CONCLUSION

If by "concentration" is meant retrieval effort (in the form of overt recall attempts or covert thinking of the to-be-remembered materials), there is no doubt that concentration produces reliable and powerful recall hypermnesia for pictures and imagistic/high-sense materials, but not, apparently, for low-sense materials. There is no evidence that concentration produces recognition hypermnesia for low-sense materials or for words, but there is some evidence for recognition hypermnesia for pictures when retrieval is an active component of the recognition task.

There is no evidence to date that either free association or hypnosis produces hypermnesia effects above and beyond those attributable to concentration (retrieval effort). There is much evidence, however, that in the absence of controls over response criteria, both hypnosis and free association produce increases in correct recalls—as well as accompanying increases in false recalls—for high-sense materials. For free association, it has been shown that such recall and intrusion increments are due entirely to response criterion effects, and so free association cannot be viewed as hypermnesic beyond the concentration activity that it entails. For hypnosis, the pattern of data is very similar to that obtained with free association, but since the necessary experiments to control for shifting response criteria have not yet been reported, no definitive conclusion can be reached. Thus, it remains an open question whether hypnosis contributes to the hypermnesia effects observed under hypnosis. Only the "hypermnesia" part of "hypnotic hypermnesia" has thus far been established, and it may well be shown yet that the "hypnotic" part plays no role.

## ACKNOWLEDGMENTS

This work was supported by a Public Staff Congress–City University of New York faculty research award grant (No. 6-64345) and by Grant No. 19156 from the National Institute of Mental Health, U.S. Public Health Service.

# REFERENCES

Allers, R., & Teler, J. (1960). On the utilization of unnoticed impressions in associations (J. Wolff, D. Rapaport, & S. Annin, Trans.). *Psychological Issues, 3*(Monograph 7), 121–154. (Original work published 1924)

Arons, H. (1967). *Hypnosis in criminal investigations.* Springfield, IL: Charles C Thomas.

Barber, T. X., & Calverley, D. S. (1966). Effects on recall of hypnotic induction, motivational suggestions, and suggested regression: A methodological and experimental analysis. *Journal of Abnormal Psychology, 71,* 169–180.

Bartlett, F. C. (1932). *Remembering.* Cambridge, England: Cambridge University Press.

Belmore, S. M. (1981). Imagery and semantic elaboration in hypermnesia for words. *Journal of Experimental Psychology: Human Learning and Memory, 7,* 191–203.

Bernbach, H. A., Roediger, H. L., & Payne, D. G. (1981). *Hypermnesia: Effects of encoding and retrieval manipulations.* Paper presented at the 22nd Annual Meeting of the Psychonomic Society, Boston, MA.

Bowers, K. S., & Meichenbaum, D. (Eds.). (1984). *The unconscious reconsidered.* New York: Wiley.

Breuer, J., & Freud, S. (1955). Studies on hysteria. In J. Strachey (Ed. and Trans.), *The standard edition of the complete psychological works of Sigmund Freud* (Vol. 2, pp. 1–305). London: Hogarth Press. (Original work published 1895)

Cooper, L. M., & London, P. (1973). Reactivation of memory by hypnosis and suggestion. *International Journal of Clinical and Experimental Hypnosis, 29,* 312–323.

Council of Scientific Affairs, American Medical Association. (1985). Scientific status of refreshing recollection by the use of hypnosis. *Journal of the American Medical Association, 253,* 1918–1923.

Craik, F. I. M., & Lockhart, R. S. (1972). Levels of processing: A framework for memory research. *Journal of Verbal Learning and Verbal Behavior, 11,* 671–684.

Crawford, H. J., & Allen, S. N. (1983). Enhanced visual memory during hypnosis as mediated by hypnotic responsiveness and cognitive strategies. *Journal of Experimental Psychology: General, 112,* 662–685.

Das, J. P. (1961). Learning and recall under hypnosis and in the wake state: A comparison. *Archives of General Psychiatry, 4,* 517–521.

DePiano, F. A., & Salzberg, H. C. (1981). Hypnosis as an aid to recall of meaningful information presented under three types of arousal. *International Journal of Clinical and Experimental Hypnosis, 29,* 383–400.

Dhanens, T. P., & Lundy, R. M. (1975). Hypnotic and waking suggestions and recall. *International Journal of Clinical and Experimental Hypnosis, 23,* 68–79.

Dorcus, R. M. (1960). Recall under hypnosis of amnesic events. *International Journal of Clinical and Experimental Hypnosis, 8,* 57–60.

Dywan, J., & Bowers, K. (1983). The use of hypnosis to enhance recall. *Science, 222,* 184–185.

Eagle, M. D., Wolitzky, D. L., & Klein, G. S. (1966). Imagery: Effect of a concealed figure in a stimulus. *Science, 151,* 837–839.

Ellenberger, H. F. (1970). *The discovery of the unconscious: The history and evolution of dynamic psychiatry.* New York: Basic Books.

Erdelyi, M. H. (1969). *The recovery of unavailable perceptual input.* Unpublished doctoral dissertation, Yale University.

Erdelyi, M. H. (1970). The recovery of unavailable perceptual input. *Cognitive Psychology, 1,* 99–113.

Erdelyi, M. H. (1972a). The recovery effect with a nonpictorial stimulus. *Psychological Record, 22,* 395–400.

Erdelyi, M. H. (1972b). The role of fantasy in the Poetzl (emergence) phenomenon. *Journal of Personality and Social Psychology, 24,* 186–190.

Erdelyi, M. H. (1977). *Has Ebbinghaus decayed with time?* Paper presented at the 18th Annual Meeting of the Psychonomic Society, Washington, DC.

Erdelyi, M. H. (1984). The recovery of unconscious (inaccessible) memories: Laboratory studies of hypermnesia. In G. Bower (Ed.), *The psychology of learning and motivation: Advances in research and theory* (pp. 95–127). New York: Academic Press.

Erdelyi, M. H. (1985). *Psychoanalysis: Freud's cognitive psychology.* New York: W. H. Freeman.

Erdelyi, M. H. (1987). *On the distinction between reminiscence and hypermnesia (and that between cumulative recall and recall) with some theoretical consequences.* Manuscript submitted for publication.

Erdelyi, M. H., & Becker, J. (1974). Hypermnesia for pictures: Incremental memory for pictures but not words in multiple recall trials. *Cognitive Psychology, 6,* 159–171.

Erdelyi, M. H., Buschke, H., & Finkelstein, S. (1977). Hypermnesia for Socratic stimuli: The growth of recall for an internally generated memory list abstracted from a series of riddles. *Memory and Cognition, 5,* 283–286.

Erdelyi, M. H., Dinges, D. F., Orne, M. T., Whitehouse, W. G., & Orne, E. C. (1987). *The stimulus and the test in hypnotic hypermnesia.* Manuscript submitted for publication.

Erdelyi, M. H., Finkelstein, S., Herrell, N., Miller, B., & Thomas, J. (1976). Coding modality versus input modality in hypermnesia: Is a rose a rose a rose? *Cognition, 4,* 311–319.

Erdelyi, M. H., & Halberstam, M. (1987). *Hypermnesia for "The War of the Ghosts": Preliminary report, with observations on a collapse of memory phenomenon and a Freudian Bartlett effect in a child.* Manuscript in preparation.

Erdelyi, M. H., & Kleinbard, J. (1978). Has Ebbinghaus decayed with time? The growth of recall (hypermnesia) over days. *Journal of Experimental Psychology: Human Learning and Memory, 4,* 275–289.

Erdelyi, M. H., & Stein, J. B. (1981). Recognition hypermnesia: The growth of recognition memory (*d'*) over time with repeated testing. *Cognition, 9,* 23–33.

Eysenck, H. J. (1941). An experimental study of the improvement of mental and physical functions in the hypnotic state. *British Journal of Medical Psychology, 18,* 304–316.

Fisher, C. (1954). Dreams and perception. *Journal of the American Psychoanalytic Association, 3,* 380–445.

Fisher, C. (1956). Dreams, images, and perception: A study of unconscious–preconscious relationships. *Journal of the American Psychoanalytic Association, 4,* 5–48.

Fisher, C., & Paul, I. H. (1959). The effect of subliminal visual stimulation on images and dreams: A validation study. *Journal of the American Psychoanalytic Association, 7,* 35–83.

Fiss, H., Goldberg, G., & Klein, G. (1963). Effects of subliminal stimulation on imagery and discrimination. *Perceptual and Motor Skills, 17,* 31–44.

Freud, S. (1953). The interpretation of dreams. In J. Strachey (Ed. and Trans.), *The standard edition of the complete psychological works of Sigmund Freud* (Vol. 4, pp. 1–338, and Vol. 5, pp. 339–627). London: Hogarth Press. (Work originally published 1900)

Gheorghiu, V. (1972). Experimentelle unter suchungen zur hypnotischen hypermnesie [Experimental investigation of hypnotic hypermnesia]. In D. Langen (Ed.), *Hypnose und psychosomatische medizin* (pp. 42–46). Stuttgart: Hippokrates Verlag.

Geiselman, R. E., Fisher, R. P., MacKinnon, D. P., & Holland, H. L. (1985). Eyewitness memory enhancement in the police interview: Cognitive retrieval mnemonics versus hypnosis. *Journal of Applied Psychology, 70,* 401–412.

Giddan, N. S. (1967). Recovery through images of briefly flashed stimuli. *Journal of Personality, 35,* 1–19.

Green, D. M., & Swets, J. M. (1966). *Signal detection theory and psychophysics.* New York: Wiley.

Haber, R. N., & Erdelyi, M. H. (1967). Emergence and recovery of initially unavailable perceptual material. *Journal of Verbal Learning and Verbal Behavior, 6,* 618–628.

Hilgard, E. R. (1962). What becomes of the input from the stimulus? In C. W. Eriksen (Ed.), *Behavior and awareness* (pp. 46–72). Durham, NC: Duke University Press.

Huse, B. (1930). Does the hypnotic trance favor the recall of faint memories? *Journal of Experimental Psychology, 13,* 519–529.

Klatzky, R. L., & Erdelyi, M. (1985). The response criterion problem in tests of hypnosis and memory. *International Journal of Clinical and Experimental Hypnosis, 33,* 246–257.

McConkey, K. M., & Nogrady, H. (1984). Hypnosis, hypnotizability and story recall. *Australian Journal of Clinical and Experimental Hypnosis, 12,* 93–98.

Milner, B. (1968). Visual recognition and recall after right temporal lobe excision in man. *Neuropsychologia, 6,* 191–209.

Mitchell, M. B. (1932). Retroactive inhibition and hypnosis. *Journal of General Psychology, 7,* 343–359.

Mumford, J. (1974). *Psychosomatic yoga.* New York: Samuel Weiser.

Nickerson, R. S. (1965). Short-term memory for complex meaningful configurations: A demonstration of capacity. *Canadian Journal of Psychology, 19,* 155–160.

Nogrady, H., McConkey, K. M., & Perry, C. (1985). Enhancing visual memory: Trying hypnosis, trying imagination, and trying again. *Journal of Abnormal Psychology, 94,* 195–204.

Orne, M. T. (1979). The use and misuse of hypnosis in court. *International Journal of Clinical and Experimental Hypnosis, 27,* 311–341.

Payne, D. G. (1987). Hypermnesia and reminiscence: A historical and empirical review. *Psychological Bulletin, 101,* 5–27.

Pötzl, O. (1960). The relationship between experimentally induced dream images and indirect vision (J. Wolff, D. Rapaport, & S. Annin, Trans.). *Psychological Issues, 3* (Monograph 7), 41–120. (Work originally published 1917)

Putnam, W. H. (1979). Hypnosis and distortions in eyewitness memory. *International Journal of Clinical and Experimental Hypnosis, 27,* 437–448.

Reiser, M., & Nielsen, M. (1980). Investigative hypnosis: A developing specialty. *American Journal of Clinical and Experimental Hypnosis, 23,* 75–84.

Roediger, H. L., & Payne, D. G. (1982). Hypermnesia: The role of repeated testing. *Journal of Experimental Psychology: Learning, Memory, and Cognition, 8,* 66–72.

Roediger, H. L., & Payne, D. G. (1985). Recall criterion does not affect recall level or hypermnesia: A puzzle for generate/recognize theories. *Memory and Cognition, 13,* 1–7.

Roediger, H. L., Payne, D. G., Gillespie, G. L., & Lean, D. S. (1982). Hypermnesia as determined by level of recall. *Journal of Verbal Learning and Verbal Behavior, 21,* 635–655.

Roediger, H. L., & Thorpe, L. A. (1978). The role of recall time in producing hypermnesia. *Memory and Cognition, 6,* 296–305.

Rosenthal, B. G. (1944). Hypnotic recall of material learned under anxiety- and non-anxiety-producing conditions. *Journal of Experimental Psychology, 34,* 369–389.

Salzberg, H. C., & DePiano, F. A. (1980). Hypnotizability and task motivating suggestions: A further look at how they affect performance. *International Journal of Clinical and Experimental Hypnosis, 28,* 261–271.

Sanders, G. S., & Simmons, W. L. (1983). Use of hypnosis to enhance eyewitness accuracy: Does it work? *Journal of Applied Psychology, 68,* 70–77.

Schafer, D., & Rubio, R. (1978). Hypnosis to aid the recall of witnesses. *International Journal of Clinical and Experimental Hypnosis, 26,* 81–91.

Schreiber, F. R. (1973). *Sybil.* New York: Warner Books.

Sears, A. B. (1954). A comparison of hypnotic and waking recall. *Journal of Clinical and Experimental Hypnosis, 2,* 296–304.

Shapiro, S. R., & Erdelyi, M. H. (1974). Hypermnesia for pictures but not words. *Journal of Experimental Psychology, 103,* 1218–1219.

Sheehan, P. W., & Tilden, J. (1983). Effects of suggestibility and hypnosis on accurate and distorted retrieval from memory. *Journal of Experimental Psychology: Learning, Memory, and Cognition, 9,* 283–293.

Sheehan, P. W., & Tilden, J. (1984). Real and simulated occurrences of memory distortion in hypnosis. *Journal of Abnormal Psychology, 93,* 47–57.

Shepard, R. N. (1967). Recognition memory for words, sentences, and pictures. *Journal of Verbal Learning and Verbal Behavior, 6,* 156–163.

Shevrin, H., & Luborsky, L. (1958). The measurement of preconscious perception in dreams and images: An investigation of the Pötzl phenomenon. *Journal of Abnormal and Social Psychology, 56,* 285–294.

Smith, M. C. (1983). Hypnotic memory enhancement of witnesses: Does it work? *Psychological Bulletin, 94,* 387–407.

Spiegel, H., & Spiegel, D. (1978). *Trance and treatment: Clinical uses of hypnosis.* New York: Basic Books.

Stager, G. L., & Lundy, R. M. (1985). Hypnosis and the learning and recall of visually presented material. *International Journal of Clinical and Experimental Hypnosis, 33,* 27–39.

Stalnaker, J. M., & Riddle, E. E. (1932). The effect of hypnosis on long-delayed recall. *Journal of General Psychology, 6,* 429–440.

Standing, L., Conezio, J., & Haber, R. N. (1970). Perception and memory for pictures: Single-trial learning of 2,500 visual stimuli. *Psychonomic Science, 19,* 73–74.

Thigpen, C. H., & Cleckley, H. M. (1957). *The three faces of Eve.* New York: McGraw-Hill.

Timm, H. W. (1981). The effect of forensic hypnosis techniques on eyewitness recall and recognition. *Journal of Police Science and Administration, 9,* 188–194.

Wagstaff, G. F. (1982). Hypnosis and recognition of a face. *Perceptual and Motor Skills, 55,* 816–818.

Wagstaff, G., Traverse, J., & Milner, S. (1982). Hypnosis and eyewitness memory—two experimental analogues. *IRCS Medical Science: Psychology and Psychiatry, 10,* 894–895.

Wallace, G., Coltheart, M., & Forster, K. (1970). Reminiscence in recognition memory for faces. *Psychonomic Science, 18*(6), 335–336.

White, R. W., Fox, G. F., & Harris, W. W. (1940). Hypnotic hypermnesia for recently learned material. *Journal of Abnormal and Social Psychology, 35,* 88–103.

Young, P. C. (1925). An experimental study of mental and physical functions in the normal and hypnotic state. *American Journal of Psychology, 36,* 214–232.

Yuille, J. C., & McEwan, N. H. (1985). Use of hypnosis as an aid to eyewitness memory. *Journal of Applied Psychology, 70,* 389–400.

Zelig, M., & Beidleman, W. B. (1981). The investigative use of hypnosis: A word of caution. *International Journal of Clinical and Experimental Hypnosis, 29,* 401–412.

# 4

## Confidence, Memory, and Hypnosis

PETER W. SHEEHAN
*University of Queensland, Australia*

Few would quarrel with the existence of the phenomena that deeply hypnotized subjects display so effortlessly in hypnosis. Typically, such persons can report objects that are not in fact physically present, or respond as if objects that are truly present are not—and they frequently do so with conviction. The meaning of that conviction, however, can be at issue. At a theoretical level, the expressed conviction of the hypnotic subject is taken by some (e.g., Orne & Hammer, 1974) to suggest that cognitive delusion is present and is an essential process component of hypnosis. Others, however, appeal to confidence as a dimension along which hypnotized individuals may vary according to the social-psychological characteristics of the influence communications that subjects are given by the hypnotist (Sarbin & Coe, 1972). No matter which of these contrary accounts one may support, both would predict that hypnotized subjects who suspend reality in a hallucinatory, posthypnotic, or amnesic test situation are likely to do so in ways that sustain the veracity of their response. What point would there be, for instance, for a hypnotized subject to respond as if an object present did not exist, when he or she at the same time queried whether this was really, truthfully so? The very nature of the kinds of responses that tell us diagnostically that deep hypnosis has been achieved dictates that at least some degree of conviction will accompany them.

Memory distortion is one possible facet of the suspension of reality in hypnosis. Shifts in memory may be implicated, for example, when a hypnotized subject reports something that is not true and it seems plausible to expect that such a subject will be confident about the distortion that occurs: they may especially be implicated if the degree of distortion implies a substantial suspension of reality.

To the extent that confidence in hypnotic reporting may be out of phase with the facts of memory, then the issues raised by hypnotized subjects' convictions are of considerable significance to forensic hypnosis. Hypnosis is argued by many as useful in the aid of recall (e.g., Arons, 1967; Reiser, 1980), and there are those who feel that its use should be increased (e.g., Hibbard & Worring, 1981). Considering the widespread belief among the public that hypnotized people tell the truth, then unwarranted confidence on the hypnotized person's part (as well as, of course, that of the judge and/or jury) will increase the chances of incorrect judgments occurring, and this may have damaging legal consequences. Any tendency of hypnosis to increase confidence, but not accuracy, is likely to bias the judicial process and affect the judged credibility of witnesses (for supporting evidence of this outside hypnosis, see Wells, Lindsay, & Tousignant, 1980).

## ACCURACY AND CONFIDENCE IN MEMORY

The association between accuracy and confidence has been researched in some detail in relation to eyewitnesses and earwitnesses, and the predictability of accuracy from reported confidence in the nonhypnotic setting is known to vary according to the nature of the conditions holding during memory encoding, storage, and retrieval (Deffenbacher, 1980). As Deffenbacher claims, one finds zero or even negative relationships between confidence and accuracy associated with conditions or test situations that are likely to produce errors or mistakes, but where low error rates are likely, the relationship may be positive and even quite strong. The hypothesis that Deffenbacher uses to explain this variability is expressed by him in terms of the degree of optimality of the information-processing conditions present at stimulus presentation (encoding), during the retention interval (storing), and at the time of memory test (retrieval). Under ideal processing conditions, witnesses will accurately track the adequacy of their memory performance in their confidence reports; under conditions that are not ideal or optimal, the two will covary less reliably, opening the way for other variables (such as personality characteristics) to determine the degree of confidence that is produced. Leippe (1980) recognizes this essential variability of the confidence–accuracy relationship, and importantly recasts the optimality hypothesis in terms that stress the integrative nature of subjects' memories and cognitions and the social factors that may influence confidence independently of accuracy.

According to Leippe, two characteristics of human memory and cognition—their integrative nature and their unconscious operation—may influence memory accuracy and confidence to move in different directions, especially where the test situations are highly influential. Leippe (1980) argues that as the operation of processes that alter or transform memory become more extensive, the relationship between confidence and accuracy will become smaller. Subjects have a feeling about the strength of their representations in memory, but it is unlikely that they will be conscious of the transformations that may have affected these representations during one or more of the stages of encoding, storage, and retrieval. The essential argument here is that if we are not conscious of whether and to what extent internally produced alterations of our memories have taken place, then it is likely that we will be poor judges of the accuracy of our recollections if these alterations have occurred.

Such processes as reconstruction are likely to modify accuracy independently of confidence, but other factors, such as social influence variables, may alter confidence separately from accuracy. Relevant social variables include subjects' general belief that human memory is trustworthy, and their public verbal commitment to a given position. Leippe's framework does not challenge Deffenbacher's optimality hypothesis so much as it attempts to outline more precisely what makes certain aspects of memory experience nonoptimal, and how optimality affects the accuracy–confidence relationship. It is important to note that both Deffenbacher and Leippe argue for variability in the relationship between accuracy and confidence, and that the nature of the relationship depends on the conditions of processing that hold at the moment. I return to this notion toward the end of the chapter and look further than at Deffenbacher's and Leippe's views.

The intricacies of this debate aside, there is ample evidence of the variability of the accuracy–confidence relationship as studied in the waking context, but relatively little attention has been given to systematic analysis of that same relationship in hypnosis. Yet hypnosis is one of those situations that, by its nature, can be expected to facilitate confident reporting and may easily engender the mistaken impression that accuracy should be associated closely with that conviction. This chapter directly addresses the issue of the relationship between confidence and accuracy in the hypnotic setting. It examines the evidence for possible memory distortion in hypnosis, reviews the data that bear on the association between hypnotic conviction and memory accuracy, and considers a variety of explanatory contexts that help account for effects. In particular, emphasis is placed on the question of whether observed effects can be attributed to the presence or absence of hypnosis, or whether they may be explained more appropriately by appeal to the social-contextual features of the hypnotic setting. Finally, data (both published and unpublished) are presented that help illustrate something of the nature of the influence of hypnosis and the hypnotic setting on the confidence and accuracy of hypnotic memory reports.

## MEMORY DISTORTION IN HYPNOSIS

A number of researchers in the field argue that hypnosis influences memory to make it less, not more, reliable. Timm (1983), for instance, states that hypnotic subjects seem more likely to confabulate details and are more susceptible to having their testimony distorted, while Mingay (1984) plausibly asserts that susceptible witnesses will be more influenced by subtle and unsubtle biases during interview. Orne, Soskis, Dinges, and Orne (1984) also argue that information gained prior to or during a hypnotic session is likely to be the basis for confabulation and so affect memories of events; Smith (1983) argues that the very act of recalling under hypnosis may significantly change the memory of an event, "possibly resulting in the incorporation into memory of subtle cues or suggestions provided by the hypnotist" (p. 388). These claims imply strongly that memory can be expected to be less, rather than more, accurate when assessed in the hypnotic setting, and reflections of these kinds stem from assumptions that confabulation is a regular accompaniment of mentation aroused during hypnosis. This position implies also that hypnosis induces an enhanced level of suggestibility that operates to render the hypnotized person more susceptible to being influenced. The overall picture being projected is that hypnosis creates a state of increased receptivity in which the hypnotic subject makes mistakes that ordinarily would not occur. Empirically, the phenomenon is evident in the prediction that hypnotically aided recall should be generally less reliable than normal waking memory.

The evidence supporting this hypothesis is conflicting, as it is also mixed regarding the contrary hypothesis that hypnosis reliably induces hypermnesia, or increased memory accuracy. The major issue for the distortion hypothesis is whether there is a pervasive error effect for the events under consideration that the subject attempts to remember.

Sanders and Simmons (1983) found that subjects responding under the influence of hypnosis were significantly less accurate than control subjects on tests of both recognition and structured memory. Buckhout, Eugenio, Licitra, Oliver, and Kramer (1981) have also found evidence of appreciable memory distortion effects. The study by Buckhout and his associates was unusual in that the hypnotists were misled as to who was responsible for a crime. In that research, 35 subjects who were matched for hypnotic susceptibility saw a simulated crime and were tested for their memory of events after a 48-hour retention period. Overall, there was no difference between subjects who were hypnotized or awake, but additional work showed that memory distortion effects were magnified when bias was present during hypnosis; scores for deliberately biased witnesses were lowered significantly by their having gone through hypnosis. We (Sheehan, Grigg, & McCann, 1984) found that misleading information injected into the test setting after, rather than before, hypnotic induction resulted in significantly greater acceptance of the incorrect information by actually hypnotized subjects; these subjects incorporated more misleading material into their memory than did insusceptible subjects who were simulating hypnosis. In our program of work, however, this study is distinctive in that it demonstrates an incorporation of misleading material into memory by hypnotic versus nonhypnotic subjects. The discriminating feature of the study was that subjects were exposed to false information after hypnotic induction was introduced, and not before induction was administered. When false information is given to subjects before hypnosis is introduced, hypnotic and nonhypnotic subjects generally incorporate the false information into memory to a comparable degree (Sheehan & Tilden, 1983, 1984, 1986).

Evidence on the whole has been against, rather than in support of, the hypothesis that hypnosis generally creates inherent distortion in memory reports. In a comprehensive study by Rainer (1983), for instance, which used procedures very close to those we adopted (Sheehan *et al.*, 1984), results showed no distinctive distortion effect for hypnotic subjects. The only condition across a range of memory test situations that showed a higher acceptance of false information (given to subjects who were either high or low in hypnotic susceptibility, and across both hypnotic and waking instruction) occurred where false presuppositions were given in hypnosis rather than out of it. The effect, however, was not significant. Data overall showed that acceptance of misleading information was the same under hypnotic instruction as under waking instruction and for subjects high in susceptibility as for those low in susceptibility. Rainer also did not find any distinctive effect for leading questions, where previously Putnam (1979) had demonstrated that hypnotic subjects were appreciably less accurate than waking subjects on leading questions about a car–bicycle accident; Putnam's effect has also been replicated for a stress-inducing stimulus (dealing with a crime) by Zelig and Beidleman (1981). Griffin (1980) further compared recall in hypnosis with recall in the waking state at various time intervals (2–30 days) and found that hypnotized witnesses did not confabulate more than unhypnotized witnesses.

The hypothesis that hypnosis produces general distortion in memory is further counterindicated by studies that have yielded positive evidence of hypermnesia (e.g. Augustynek, 1977; Crawford & Allen, 1983; DePiano & Salzberg, 1981; Shields & Knox, 1986; Stalnaker & Riddle, 1932) across a range of material involving, for the most part, meaningful material or stimuli processed in a deep rather than a shallow way (Shields & Knox, 1986). Stalnaker and Riddle (1932), for instance, found support for greater total information correct and greater total errors in free recall for hypnotic as opposed to waking testimony. At times, it seems, hypnosis increases the quantity of information that is remembered, and an increase in the accuracy of the testimony may be accompanied by a rise in number of errors as well. Such evidence comes from the analysis of test contexts involving both free recall and structured memory.

Using a paradigm of research geared to recognize the response criterion problem, Dywan and Bowers (1983b) asked subjects for a week to recall 60 previously presented pictures. Subjects were then either hypnotized or not and encouraged to try to remember more pictures. In the study, hypnotic subjects reported over twice as many new items, both correct and incorrect, as did subjects in a control, task-motivated condition. The evidence showed increased accuracy of recall, but at the cost of retrieving information with greater error. This study, however, does not go far enough to satisfy the conditions for optimal control of the response criterion problem as laid down by Klatzky and Erdelyi (1985) in their recent critique of studies in the area; in this respect, the results are not conclusive.

Data collected on the occurrence of pseudomemories in hypnosis also support the conclusion that hypnosis is variable in its effects on accuracy. The major study reported in this area is that by Laurence and Perry (1983c; see also, Laurence, Nadon, Nogrady, & Perry, 1986), who studied a pseudomemory of having been awakened by loud noises during the night, this event being suggested to 27 highly hypnotizable subjects during hypnosis. Results showed that 13 of 27 selected susceptible subjects reported that the suggested event had occurred. A second study from the same laboratory replicated Laurence and Perry's original findings (Labelle & Perry, 1986). The occurrence of pseudomemory can be taken to index in an indirect way a special receptivity by hypnotic subjects to misleading information that is suggested by the hypnotist: however, it is significant to note that pseudomemories do not occur among all highly susceptible subjects in hypnosis, and it is not evident that those who show the effect are markedly more susceptible to hypnosis. Individual differences in the acceptance of a pseudomemory need to be explained in terms other than the tendency of hypnosis to engender distortion.

The literature bearing on memory in hypnosis is extensive, and several reviews of pertinent studies have been published elsewhere (see Orne *et al.*, 1984; Relinger, 1984; Smith, 1983). The relevant literature is also discussed in other chapters of this volume. A brief survey of research, however, reveals support for the following set of conclusions, and they are drawn on the basis of what appear to be reasonably consistent and reliable findings in the published literature:

1. There is no general, pervasive distortion effect for hypnosis. There is evidence of greater susceptibility to misleading information when incorrect material is introduced following hypnotic induction, but the effect is not uniform or especially durable (Sheehan, 1985), and the findings are inconsistent across a range of response formats.

2. There is no general evidence of hypermnesia. The phenomenon does occur and appears to be related to the presentation of particular types of material or modes of processing (e.g., see Shields & Knox, 1986), but there appears to be much more evidence for the occurrence of memory inaccuracy in hypnosis than there is for the occurrence of increased accuracy. Klatzky and Erdelyi (1985), however, have recently suggested that the effects of

hypnosis on memory cannot be inferred entirely unambiguously from the previous work that has been conducted. They claim, for instance, that no previous study has properly tested for hypermnesia by instituting optimal control of the response criterion problem associated with hypnotic subjects' attempts to report what they remember. This problem expresses itself most clearly in the fact that hypnotic subjects' increasing response output demonstrates both increased accuracy and increased error.

3. Distortions in memory can occur outside hypnosis just as they can occur within hypnosis. Distortion in hypnosis—depending on the way it is measured—can match the degree of distortion that is evident out of hypnosis, and the degree of distortion shown by highly susceptible subjects can be matched by the extent of distortion shown by subjects low in susceptibility (Sheehan & Tilden, 1983, 1984, 1986). In these instances, memory distortion will be evident in hypnosis, but to an extent that may, at times, be comparable with the bias that can be demonstrated out of hypnosis.

The issue I now pursue in this chapter is the variability of performance accuracy in the memory test situation in hypnosis. There are strong individual differences among hypnotic subjects in the accuracy of their testimony, which may or may not be accompanied by matching conviction about what is in fact true; this variability in memory accuracy provides a fertile ground for investigating the overall relationship between confidence and accuracy in hypnosis. A preliminary analysis of the nature of the hypnotic situation is such as to suggest that, overall, confidence and accuracy are relatively independent.

## CONFIDENCE AND HYPNOSIS: THE EVIDENCE

Interesting historical data on the confidence of hypnotic subjects derive from the writings of Bernheim, Forel, and Janet, who agreed uniformly that hypnotic subjects come to believe new memories, whether confabulated or created, as real (Laurence & Perry, 1983b). This suggests, as argued previously, that confidence can be expected to be substantially out of phase with accuracy in hypnotic test situations, especially those that request a radical suspension of reality.

The empirical evidence for a poor relationship between memory accuracy and confidence in hypnosis is much more persuasive than the evidence for a positive relationship. Orne *et al.* (1984) argue, on the basis of their review of the evidence, that a disturbing consequence of the tendency of hypnotized subjects to be biased in their memory reproductions is the increased degree of confidence that hypnotized subjects develop in association with their recollections. Regardless of the accuracy of hypnotic subjects' memory reports, the conviction expressed by hypnotic subjects is frequently high. One of the impressive features of the effects found for hypnotic memory and confidence, in fact, is the consistency in the pattern of findings across different methodologies and memory test situations. Not all the data are supportive of a weak or negative relationship, but the weight of the evidence falls clearly on the side of an absence of positive correspondence.

Laurence (1982) had subjects rate their confidence for memory of stories presented dichotically both before and during hypnosis and found that subjects were significantly more confident about their recall of the stories when they were presented in hypnosis. Working with pseudomemories, the same investigator in association with Perry (Laurence & Perry, 1983c) found that when distorted memories were accepted following suggestions given by a hypnotist, subjects were typically certain that the suggested events had actually occurred. Using a Loftus-type paradigm (see Loftus, 1979a; to be explained subsequently) based on the procedure of injecting misleading information subtly into a test situation well before memory testing, we (Sheehan & Tilden, 1983) found that hypnotic instruction significantly increased subjects' confidence in their memories, especially with highly suggestible persons. This pattern of findings has been replicated across a variety of measures my colleagues and I have used in assessing subjects' convictions in the test setting (for a review, see Sheehan, 1985). In an analysis of memory in both unstructured narrative recall and forced-choice recognition testing, results have shown that hypnotic instruction yields appreciably greater confidence ratings than waking instruction for both response formats (Sheehan & Tilden, 1984, 1986). There were also indications in our program of work (albeit inconsistent ones) that acceptance of the misinformation was itself associated with especially high confidence ratings.

Using an altogether different paradigm of research, Dywan and Bowers (1983b) did not report on confidence in their original published study, but confidence was discussed in a follow-up report examining the prediction that there should be an upward shift in the confidence that subjects are willing to place in their recall as a result of hypnosis. Results in the second study confirmed predictions. Using a paradigm similar to that of the first experiment, Dywan and Bowers (1983a) found that hypnotic suggestion led to an increased production of information and increased confidence for most subjects, with no apparent increase in accuracy; this process was most in evidence for subjects who were high in hypnotic ability. The greatest confidence shift occurred for incorrect information. For highly hypnotizable subjects, even those items that were part of subject protocols before hypnosis was introduced were presented with greater confidence during hypnosis than had occurred previously.

These findings from Dywan and Bowers's research highlight a trend in the literature that appears to be a reliable one. Confidence–accuracy effects appear to be as much related to level of susceptibility as they are to the presence of hypnosis. In Dywan and Bowers's study, it was the highly susceptible group that showed the most dramatic shifts in confidence. Zelig and Beidleman (1981) also found an appreciable association between confidence and level of hypnotic susceptibility when leading questions were the source of error injected into the test situation. And in work my colleagues and I have done, highly susceptible subjects also showed significantly greater confidence in their memories than subjects low in susceptibility (see Sheehan, 1985, for a review).

One of the most comprehensive analyses of the relationship between confidence and memory accuracy has been conducted by Rainer (1983) and reported in her doctoral dissertation. Investigating a range of different sources of error (e.g., false information, leading questions), she found that for incorrect as opposed to correct responses, it was distinctively the highly susceptible subjects who were confident in hypnosis. Hypnosis altered the confidence of less suggestible subjects in the recall of correct material, but not incorrect material; and subjects high and low in suggestibility were appreciably differentiated in hypnosis, with the former subjects being more confident than the latter. Her work suggests that confidence effects differ according to the type of response being evaluated (correct or incorrect), and that both state instruction and level of suggestibility are relevant to the nature of effects that can be observed. A detailed look at Rainer's data, for example, shows that highly susceptible subjects in hypnosis were more confident of what they remembered than those low in susceptibility, irrespective of the fact that what they remembered was wrong. The less susceptible subjects, on the other hand, were more confident about accurate responses during hypnosis, but their confidence decreased when they answered incorrectly. Rainer argues that hypnosis removes hypnotized subjects' uncertainty about the accuracy of their response, but such an effect seems moderated by level of susceptibility to hypnosis. The pattern in empirical findings, however, is not always clear-cut. Consider, for example, the fact that the most dramatic increase in confidence for subjects in Rainer's study occurred for subjects low, not high, in suggestibility. This suggests that the setting of hypnosis operates to influence subjects and may do so differently for subjects who vary in their level of susceptibility to hypnosis.

It is important to note in this review that not all of the evidence supports the hypothesis that confidence increases substantially in hypnosis; however, this could be explained by the fact that the nature of effects for confidence is related to the presence or absence of error in memory, the type of measure used to test confidence, and the nature of effects of the context involved. Redston and Knox (1983), for example, tested three groups of subjects (hypnotic, relaxed, and simulating hypnosis) and presented them with material (slides of faces) that they were required to process at different levels (shallow and deep). They were predicting hypermnesia for the material that was processed deeply. No hypermnesia effect was observed, and no confidence effect was associated with hypnosis. Redston and Knox concluded that hypnotized subjects do not typically become very confident in the material that they produce in hypnosis. The absence of effects in their study, however, could have been due to the fact that there was no appreciable error effect, and the absence of error itself could be explained by the low ceiling of the material that their subjects learned. The relevance of response measures is indicated by the work of Sanders and Simmons (1983), who found that hypnotic subjects were not more appreciably confident than control subjects on the unusual measure of "willingness to testify in court." It appears that confidence effects are also related to the forensic relevance of the indices that are used to study it.

The importance, at least in some way, of setting or context characteristics is indicated by the fact that subjects who are pretending to be hypnotized display high degrees of confidence. In Redston and Knox's study, for instance, simulating subjects reported greater confidence in their confabulation than did other subjects; in our research (Sheehan & Tilden, 1984), simulating subjects actually showed more confidence than did hypnotic subjects when asked to remember details about a crime that occurred in a street, the scenes of which they had been exposed to previously. Definite demand characteristics appeared to be operating to influence role-playing subjects to report more confidently.

In conclusion, on the evidence from this review, confidence at times is related to memory accuracy in hypnosis, but the association is typically not a positive one. There seems to be a relatively reliable trend, as Rainer (1983) and Orne *et al.* (1984) have noted, for inaccurate memories in hypnosis to be confident ones. Level of susceptibility also seems to interact with hypnosis to produce significant confidence effects in hypnosis. This is perhaps not surprising, since highly hypnotizable subjects are more prone to confuse real and imagined memories than are less hypnotizable subjects, especially in the hypnotic setting. The hypnotic setting, however, may operate to influence less as well as more susceptible subjects, but not necessarily in the same way. It appears that the social influence character of the hypnotic setting will influence the less susceptible subjects to be more confident about memories that are correct, thus moving their response in the direction of a more adaptive level of performance than is evident for subjects who are highly susceptible to hypnosis. Clearly, the conditions of information processing in hypnosis appear not to be ideal, in Deffenbacher's (1980) terms, to yield a positive relationship between memory accuracy and confidence; it also appears that personality variables such as level of suggestibility operate in a more significant fashion in the hypnotic context than simple reliance on information-processing conditions would predict.

I move now to consider a sample of data that illustrates some of the effects associated with confidence assessment in the hypnotic setting. Published and unpublished data are considered that reflect a range of effects highlighting some of the different factors that may affect confidence judgments in hypnosis. All of the research is taken from work undertaken in our laboratory at the University of Queensland. Data are emphasized from the application of similar sets of procedures because this avoids to some extent the confound present when effects are compared across altogether different methods; significant results should be due to the variable of interest rather than the fact that different methodologies are involved.

## DATA ILLUSTRATING EFFECTS ON CONFIDENCE JUDGMENTS IN HYPNOSIS

### The Research Paradigm

The work reported here stems largely from the application of procedures adapted from Elizabeth Loftus's paradigm for analyzing memory distortion, which exposes subjects to incorrect information subtly introduced prior to memory test. Typically, the research forming the basis for the program of work (see Loftus, 1979a; Loftus, Miller, & Burns, 1978) presents subjects with a sequence of slides illustrating a particular series of events that is to be remembered later. One group of subjects (the experimental group) is exposed to information that contradicts what is seen, and another (the control group) is exposed to information that does not. Experimental subjects, for instance, are given false information that the man in the slide series is wearing "dark blue trousers," whereas in fact the trousers are light blue; subjects in the control condition are told simply that the trousers are blue. Experimental and control subjects are then both later asked to remember what they saw originally. Forced-choice recognition testing is the usual mode of testing for probing for acceptance of the false information into memory, and the test allows direct analysis of Loftus's distortion effect. The test typically lists true and false alternatives, where the false alternative presents the incorrect information (e.g., "dark blue trousers") that was fed incorrectly to the experimental subjects beforehand. Analysis focuses on the proportion of subjects who answer the misleading items correctly. Results from application of this set of procedures typically show that an appreciably greater proportion of experimental subjects (those exposed to the misleading information) than control subjects (those not exposed to the misleading information) report the incorrect material that was suggested. It is a matter of some controversy whether the information that was encoded originally is actually replaced by the opposing material, or whether it is simply a matter of finding the right method to retrieve it (for pursuit of this debate, see Bekerian & Bowers, 1983).

The program of work that is reported here used the same set of meaningful events as employed by Loftus and her associates (dealing with a man who steals a wallet from a woman's handbag after bumping into her in the street and knocking her handbag to the ground). It extended the testing of distortion in hypnotic memory, however, to analysis of both recognition and free recall, and employed subjects who were either hypnotized or awake and who were either high or low in hypnotic susceptibility. Furthermore, misleading information was injected either before (Sheehan & Tilden, 1983, 1984) or after (Sheehan *et al.*, 1984) hypnotic induction, and subjects' confidence and memory accuracy were recorded in detail.

## The Research Program

In the first study in the program (Sheehan & Tilden, 1983), 96 subjects preselected for hypnotic susceptibility were given either misleading or neutral information about the wallet-snatching sequence via a series of questions delivered after the stimulus sequence had been seen, but before hypnosis was introduced. In an eight-group design, independent groups of subjects high and low in susceptibility were given either waking or hypnotic instruction and received either misleading or nonmisleading information about the 24-item stimulus sequence. The misleading information introduced before hypnosis focused on three key stimulus features of the slides, and identified features such as the writing on the back of the thief's jacket and the color of the thief's clothing.

Results for the analysis of data from recognition testing conducted in hypnosis demonstrated a significant effect for presentation of the misleading information; the analysis was of the proportions of subjects in each of the eight conditions who answered the three misleading items correctly. Analysis was also conducted of the remaining 15 (objective) items on the 18-item recognition test to examine general accuracy effects. The incorrect material was incorporated appreciably into memory, but the misinformation effect did not differentiate hypnotic from waking instruction, nor subjects high in suggestibility from those low in it. Subjects' expressed conviction, however, was appreciably stronger in hypnosis than under waking instruction, especially for the highly susceptible subjects given hypnotic instruction. Hypnosis significantly increased the confidence of subjects overall, and highly suggestible subjects were the most confident of all. Table 4-1 sets out recognition results and illustrates effects pertaining to the set of 15 objective items associated overall with both confidence and accuracy.

This first study did not yield any distinctive memory distortion effect for the incorporation of misleading material into memory, and it is important to

Table 4-1. Mean Scores for Measures of Overall Accuracy and Confidence (Recognition Testing)

| Subject group | Mean number of statements "correct" (out of 15) | Mean number of statements "certain" (out of 15) | Mean confidence (scale 1–3) |
|---|---|---|---|
| Misleading condition | | | |
| Hypnotic instruction | | | |
| High suggestibility | 12.33 | 10.25 | 2.58 |
| Low suggestibility | 11.67 | 7.33 | 2.25 |
| Waking instruction | | | |
| High suggestibility | 12.33 | 7.58 | 2.28 |
| Low suggestibility | 11.42 | 8.42 | 2.30 |
| Neutral condition | | | |
| Hypnotic instruction | | | |
| High suggestibility | 11.92 | 9.67 | 2.45 |
| Low suggestibility | 11.92 | 8.58 | 2.37 |
| Waking instruction | | | |
| High suggestibility | 12.92 | 7.00 | 2.25 |
| Low suggestibility | 12.67 | 7.75 | 2.29 |
| Mean | 12.15 | 8.32 | 2.35 |

*Note.* The data are from "Effects of Suggestibility and Hypnosis on Accurate and Distorted Retrieval from Memory" by P. W. Sheehan and J. Tilden, 1983, *Journal of Experimental Psychology: Learning, Memory, and Cognition, 9,* 283–293. Copyright 1983 by the American Psychological Association. Used by permission. For each of the eight groups of subjects, $n = 12$.

note that confidence was appreciably enhanced overall in the hypnotic context, whether or not specific inaccuracy characterized the hypnotic setting. A different pattern of results emerged, however, when the misleading material was presented *after* rather than before hypnotic induction. In a later study in the program (Sheehan *et al.*, 1984), an abbreviated version of the same slide series was used in another adaptation of the Loftus methodology. In this study, subjects who were actually hypnotized and subjects who were simulating hypnosis were tested for the occurrence of memory distortion in hypnosis for both free-recall and forced-choice recognition, tested in that order; all subjects were further tested for recognition after deinduction (awakening) instructions had been delivered. The procedures of testing were as described above.

Results, as before, showed that there was a significant acceptance of the misleading material, but this time the effect emerged as distinctive for actually hypnotized subjects (vs. simulating subjects). On the same recognition-based distortion index as adopted in the earlier work (Sheehan & Tilden, 1983), actually hypnotized subjects were less accurate with respect to the misleading items than simulating subjects, and there was no appreciable difference between subject groups in the nonmisleading-information condition. Ratings of confidence taken in recognition showed that on items other than those on which subjects were misled, the memory accuracy of hypnotized subjects was comparable to that of the simulating subjects; however, as before, the hypnotic context was associated with appreciably higher confidence ratings than the waking context for hypnotized and nonhypnotized subjects alike.

Table 4-2 sets out the relevant data for recognition testing pertaining to the set of 15 objective items; the results for testing in both the hypnotic and waking states are considered. The table illustrates that confidence was greater in hypnosis than out of it, but not as great in hypnosis as the confidence expressed by simulating subjects who were pretending to be hypnotized and who were insusceptible to hypnosis. This latter finding suggests that contextual factors may determine the level of conviction expressed by subjects in hypnosis. The extent of confident reporting shown by simulating subjects tells us that the reasons why simulators expressed high confidence under hypnotic instruction may be the same as the reasons why hypnotized subjects performed in just the same way.

Table 4-2. Mean Number of Objective Questions Correctly Answered by Subjects in Hypnosis and While Awake, Together with Mean Number of Objective Questions Answered by Them as "Certain"

| | Hypnosis | | Awake | |
|---|---|---|---|---|
| Subject group | Accuracy (out of 15) | Confidence (out of 15) | Accuracy (out of 15) | Confidence (out of 15) |
| Actually hypnotized ($n = 46$) | | | | |
| Misleading information | | | | |
| $M$ | 10.39 | 9.04 | 10.43 | 8.26 |
| $SD$ | 1.50 | 1.43 | 1.65 | 2.63 |
| Nonmisleading information | | | | |
| $M$ | 10.57 | 8.61 | 10.57 | 7.13 |
| $SD$ | 1.65 | 2.73 | 1.59 | 3.09 |
| Simulating ($n = 46$) | | | | |
| Misleading information | | | | |
| $M$ | 10.30 | 10.35 | 10.69 | 8.22 |
| $SD$ | 1.69 | 2.27 | 1.36 | 2.92 |
| Nonmisleading information | | | | |
| $M$ | 10.91 | 10.00 | 10.48 | 7.86 |
| $SD$ | 1.44 | 2.28 | 1.65 | 2.78 |

*Note.* The data are from "Memory Distortion Following Exposure to False Information in Hypnosis" by P. W. Sheehan, L. Grigg, and T. McCann, 1984, *Journal of Abnormal Psychology, 93,* 259–265. Copyright 1984 by the American Psychological Association. Used by permission.

It is clear from this second study that distortion was most distinctive when incorrect material was presented following induction. Accordingly, this same procedure of presentation was preserved in a follow-up experiment that tested subjects high and low in susceptibility who were not pretending to be hypnotized at all. Here, the less susceptible group was motivated for its task by being especially instructed concerning its capacity to respond successfully. Separate groups of subjects high ($n = 22$) and low ($n = 24$) in susceptibility were given either misleading or nonmisleading information following induction; responses were examined again under tests of free recall and recognition, as adopted in the second study (Sheehan *et al.*, 1984). Accuracy and confidence were also assessed as before. The data from this study are as yet unpublished.

Results showed that the two groups of subjects were statistically differentiated in the degree to which they were influenced by the misleading material on the recognition test. The highly susceptible subjects demonstrated appreciably less accuracy on the misleading items than did the less susceptible subjects, and hypnotized subjects in this study performed comparably with the actually hypnotized subjects tested in the second study (see Table 4-2). Furthermore, there was evidence of greater certainty on the part of subjects who were misled. Overall, the groups were once again comparable with respect to general memory accuracy in recognition testing, while the two groups were again different in the degree of confidence that they expressed. Subjects high and low in susceptibility were differentiated significantly under hypnosis instructions in the confidence of their answers, with highly susceptible subjects showing the greater level of expressed conviction. Table 4-3 sets out the relevant data and illustrates the effects that were obtained overall for the objective recognition items and that enable comparison across the studies discussed up to this point. This study, as distinct from the preceding one, especially illustrates the relevance of level of susceptibility to confidence effects in the hypnotic setting. Highly susceptible subjects showed the same pattern of effects relative to less susceptible subjects in hypnosis as did hypnotized subjects relative to subjects who were awake. Such a pattern of findings suggests that person characteristics are major moderators of confidence effects in hypnosis.

In the final study reported in this series of experiments (see Doherty, 1984), 90 subjects preselected for the level of their hypnotizability were allocated to three instructional groups. One instructional set encouraged subjects to guess details of a scene they had viewed previously; another encouraged subjects to be accurate; and the third was neutral. Independent groups of subjects high and low in susceptibility were allocated to hypnotic and waking instruction, and subjects were tested for the accuracy of their narrative description of a video display of a bank robbery (Yuille, 1982). In this study, no misleading information was given; rather, the point of

Table 4-3. Mean Number of Objective Questions Correctly Answered by Subjects in Hypnosis and While Awake, Together with Mean Number of Objective Questions Answered by Them as "Certain"

| | Hypnosis | | Awake | |
|---|---|---|---|---|
| Subject group | Accuracy (out of 15) | Confidence (out of 15) | Accuracy (out of 15) | Confidence (out of 15) |
| High suggestibility (*n* = 22) | | | | |
| Misleading information | | | | |
| *M* | 11.33 | 9.42 | 10.92 | 7.42 |
| *SD* | 1.15 | 2.07 | 1.44 | 2.23 |
| Nonmisleading information | | | | |
| *M* | 10.80 | 9.00 | 10.80 | 8.50 |
| *SD* | 1.48 | 1.63 | 1.62 | 2.42 |
| Low suggestibility (*n* = 24) | | | | |
| Misleading information | | | | |
| *M* | 10.58 | 7.50 | 10.33 | 7.75 |
| *SD* | 1.16 | 1.98 | 0.98 | 2.20 |
| Nonmisleading information | | | | |
| *M* | 10.67 | 8.00 | 10.17 | 7.59 |
| *SD* | 1.50 | 2.56 | 1.53 | 3.03 |

the experiment was to examine the effect on recall of providing subjects with encouragement to shift their criterion for responding.

Figure 4-1 illustrates the data that were obtained. Groups were differentiated in terms of instructional set, with hypnotized subjects reporting far fewer correct responses in their narrative descriptions of the robbery tape. Confidence in reporting, however, was comparable across hypnotic and waking testing. This finding illustrates an important factor: Even if enhancement of confidence does not occur in hypnosis, confidence may still be out of phase with accuracy. Special note should be taken of the fact here that hypnotized subjects produced fewer total correct responses than awake subjects and yet were as confident as waking subjects. Confidence did not parallel accuracy, and the essential relationship between accuracy and confidence is expressed by the fact that confidence remained stable while accuracy shifted.

### Conclusions from the Research Program

Several conclusions are supported by the program of work that has just been outlined, and they are consistent with those drawn from the earlier review of the literature.

First, the data in Tables 4-1 through 4-3 highlight the fact that there is a substantial context effect for confidence. Regardless of accuracy (where both hypnotized and nonhypnotized subjects performed generally at the same level), confidence was frequently greater in hypnosis than in the waking state, and this effect was maintained independently of whether the conditions of testing encouraged or did not encourage memory distortion in other ways (namely, via Loftus's specific distortion effect, using misleading items). Second, it is clear that there is a substantial effect for level of susceptibility. Highly susceptible subjects tended to express more confidence than less susceptible subjects, and the level of susceptibility of subjects appeared to interact with state instruction to facilitate the enhancement of confidence. Third, there is evidence that exposure to misinformation may yield an increase in expressed confidence: A confidence effect occurred for misleading material in the third of the studies that were reported (see Table 4-3), but not in the first. It would appear that there is greater support for the hypothesis that level of confidence is associated with degree of susceptibility and presence of state instruction rather than memory distortion per se. Fourth, the absence of discrimination between simulating and actually hypnotized subjects in the level of their expressed confidence suggests that contextual cues play an important part in determining the reported conviction of subjects remembering in hypnosis. Finally, as Figure 4-1 shows, the nature of the

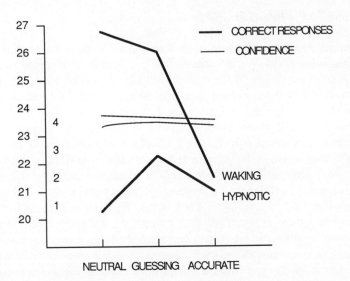

Figure 4-1. Cell means for total number of accurate and confident responses for hypnotic and waking groups in free recall. (From *The Influence of Instructional Set on Free Recall* by P. Doherty, 1984, unpublished bachelor's [honours] thesis, University of Queensland, St. Lucia, Australia. Reprinted by permission of the author.)

association between accuracy and confidence should always be examined closely, since confidence levels may take on a different interpretation when shifts in accuracy are taken into account. Confidence remained the same in the last of the studies reported, for instance, while accuracy rose substantially. The pattern of results evident in Figure 4-1 illustrates a mismatch between accuracy and confidence in the hypnotic setting that was quite distinct from the pattern of findings evident in Tables 4-1 through 4-3.

In summary, confidence effects are reliable; they may express the influence of contextual factors; and they may be out of phase with accuracy in a number of importantly different ways. A negative relationship may hold (as in the third study), where the acceptance of misleading information is accompanied by greater confidence; accuracy may be constant across state instruction while confidence varies (as reflected in Tables 4-2 and 4-3); or confidence may stay the same as accuracy varies (as reflected in Figure 4-1). The overall pattern of findings is a set of negative or null relationships.

Having presented these data and this review of the literature, I move now to consider some of the possible explanations of confidence effects in hypnosis. In considering the gap between accuracy and confidence, the important question is "What is responsible for the difference, and how does this relate to hypnosis and the hypnotic setting?"


## EXPLANATORY FRAMEWORKS

The two major explanatory frameworks that aim to account for confidence effects in hypnosis are (1) the hypothesis that confidence is enhanced by the hypnotic process itself, and (2) the hypothesis that subjects' degree of conviction is determined by the social-psychological characteristics of the context in which confidence judgments are collected. It is difficult to separate out the hypothesis that confidence in hypnosis is due to the hypnotic process from the notion that confidence reflects the effects of the hypnotic setting, but the distinctions being raised in the literature suggest that a separation of this kind is being made. Orne *et al.* (1984) argue, for instance, that hypnosis can generate misplaced confidence in memories, which can be facilitated in ways that are less likely if hypnosis has not been used. These same authors further argue that the nature of hypnosis and its effect on memory lead to the likelihood that a subject's beliefs may be changed into inaccurate memories that the subject then reports and later believes. The relevance of situational factors is appropriately acknowledged, but the ultimate appeal seems to be to the nature of hypnosis in explanation of effects.

Also consistent with the view that hypnosis creates qualitative changes in memory and confidence, relative to recollections that are nonhypnotic, Dywan and Bowers (1983a) argue that a breakdown in reality monitoring is responsible for the disruption of the accuracy–confidence relationship in hypnosis. These same authors also believe that imagery plays a role for highly susceptible subjects who are experienced with hypnosis. Little experimental evidence, however, bears on these and other viewpoints that stress the relevance of hypnosis per se to the effects associated with confidence. The data are consistent with the hypothesis that hypnosis is responsible for effects, but they do not provide a stringent test of it. This is in some part due to the fact that it is difficult to index those particular process features of hypnosis that are the characteristics responsible for confidence–accuracy effects. Reality monitoring is too elusive a process to provide the clear-cut data that are necessary to resolve the issue, and other process characteristics may be relevant as well. Rainer (1983), for instance, attributes the increase in confidence in hypnosis to the relaxing quality of the hypnotic state, which can engender a sense of well-being and thus enhance confidence.

## Process Features of Hypnosis

The two process characteristics that marshal the most supportive data for the relevance of hypnosis as distinct from the "hypnotic" setting are (1) the processes of attention and (2) motivation to respond.

The relevance of the process of attention comes from several different directions in the data. Work by Loftus and her associates (Greene, Flynn, & Loftus, 1982; Loftus, 1979b) has indicated that when new information is reviewed critically, memory distortion will be lessened. The evidence suggests that blatantly contradictory information tangibly reduces the acceptance of misleading material into memory when it is presented at the same time as other subtle information; the conflict it engenders (due to its openness) causes each piece of the new information to be scrutinized, thus rendering it less likely that other new information presented at the same time will be used to update prior recollections. As we have argued (Sheehan *et al.*, 1984), it seems plausible to assert that hypnosis increases hypnotic subjects' susceptibility to the influence of misleading information by virtue of process effects occurring at the time that material is introduced. One of those effects could be that hypnosis lowers the level of subjects' cognitive scrutiny of the postevent information that is presented. Where scrutiny of incorrect information is lowered, resistance to the influence of misleading information can be expected to be less. Such an explanation does not counter the possible influence of context effects, however. Confidence, for example, may interact with attention insofar as the hypnotic setting itself reinforces veracity, and so false information received in it may be processed less critically as a result.

The attentional hypothesis also gains additional support from the work of Crawford and Allen (1983), who found evidence of increased memory accuracy for the memory of pictorial material in hypnosis. During hypnosis, highly susceptible subjects showed a significant enhancement effect in the number of items remembered correctly. Highly susceptible subjects switched from a detailed style to a holistic style of processing the material for recall, and there were clear indications of cognitive flexibility in the way subjects processed the stimulus material. Crawford and Allen argued that highly susceptible subjects may have redistributed their attention during hypnosis, creating an accompanying freedom from distraction. Such narrowing of attention, together with an increase in absorption, may also have increased the depth of processing of events. The attentional hypothesis receives further (partial) support from evidence of greater recall for certain kinds of details in the hypnotic memory situation. We (Sheehan & Tilden, 1984), for example, found evidence of differential recall between actually hypnotized and simulating subjects in the kind of details the subjects remembered after seeing a stimulus series of events involving a wallet-snatching sequence. Sanders and Simmons (1983) have also suggested that hypnotic subjects are less aware of specific details, and Rainer (1984) argues for the validity of the notion that there are individual differences in hypnotic subjects' ability to recall central and peripheral information in the eyewitness paradigm. The differences in recall of certain kinds of details as opposed to others is compatible with the notion that attention to events is selective.

There are additional processes, however, that can lay just as strong a claim as attention to the explanation of confidence–accuracy effects in hypnosis. Timm (1983) talks of a decrease in hypnotic subjects' inhibitions about making questionable statements, and the desire of good hypnotic subjects to perform appropriately. Such concepts move close to formulating the particular relevance of subjects' "willingness to respond" as a central process accounting for effects in the hypnotic memory situation. In the study reviewed earlier by Buckhout *et al.* (1981), for example, the investigators talked of a "try harder" effect for hypnotic subjects. Hypnotic subjects appeared to exercise a "sanction to guess" even if they had no memory of certain critical details, and 90% of the hypnotized witnesses were reported as being motivated to try to recall after hypnosis, as compared with only 20% of subjects in the control group. The greater willingness to answer shown in Buckhout *et al*'s study is focused on by Mingay (1984), who stresses the importance of recognizing hypnotic subjects' willingness to guess when uncertain. Like attention, this process characteristic is not necessarily independent of the influence of contextual features. The hypnotic situation, for example, is characterized by several important stimulus features that promote or facilitate subjects' positive cooperation and willingness to respond.

The data that best fit this particular viewpoint are clearly those that provide for a looser criterion of response among hypnotic subjects in the memory test situation. Memory enhancement (indexed in terms of greater accuracy following hypnotic as opposed to waking instruction) may reflect a greater willingness on the hypnotized subjects' part to respond or to offer a memory report. Reviewing the results elsewhere, Orne *et al.* (1984) conclude generally that hypnosis produces a laxer response criterion, evidenced by the fact that subjects in hypnosis report more detail, both accurate and inaccurate. Stalnaker and Riddle (1932) found, for example, that hypnotic subjects produced more information than did nonhypnotic subjects, regardless of accuracy; the report of hypermnesia in their study fits with the hypothesis that there is a loosening of subjects' subjective criterion for responding. Dywan and Bowers (1983b), using their paradigm of research based on repeated recall, also found that the amount of both accurate and inaccurate recall was increased in hypnosis over nonhypnotic remembering, especially for hypnotizable subjects. Dywan and Bowers have further argued that the change in criterion of response can lead to a false sense of recognition, and therefore to an inflated sense of familiarity or certainty.

Not all evidence, however, is in support of these kinds of conclusions, and Klatzky and Erdelyi (1985) have catalogued the methodological pitfalls that face the researcher trying to address the response criterion problem. Stager (1974), for example, demonstrated hypermnesia for hypnotizable subjects given hypnotic instruction, but accuracy of recall was improved without any concomitant increase in the inaccuracy of recall. Working with emotionally toned material, Wagstaff and Sykes (1984) also failed to support the criterion shift hypothesis; and Shields and Knox (1986) found hypermnesia for deeply encoded material with no concomitant increase in errors, the difference between hypnotic and nonhypnotic groups occurring for accuracy scores alone. Nogrady, McConkey, and Perry (1985) also repeated many of the procedures adopted by Dywan and Bowers and failed to replicate results that favored the notion of a response criterion shift. In their study, the amount of correct and incorrect material increased over repeated testing across the recall tests, but the increase in correct material was least for highly hypnotizable subjects in the hypnosis condition. Nogrady *et al.* note that subjects in their study were not forced to generate incorrect material, as they were in the study by Dywan and Bowers.

Support for "willingness to respond" as a relevant motivational process is indicated by independent research conducted outside of the hypnotic memory test situation. In a series of studies reported in a doctoral dissertation by Ryan (1982), hypnotic, task-motivated, and simulating subjects were given sentences to hear that varied in the level of their intelligibility. Subjects listened to sentences that were high, medium, and low in intelligibility. Hypnotic subjects distinctively tried to answer questions about the most unintelligible questions, and the tendency to do this was not at all evident among task-motivated subjects or among simulating subjects motivated to respond to whatever they thought the hypnotist wanted them to do. The "willingness to respond" phenomenon was replicated across separate studies for actually hypnotized subjects but not for simulating subjects, and the presence of this difference indexes the special significance of the effect. Ryan viewed his results in terms of hypnotic subjects' being less concerned than nonhypnotic subjects with incompatibilities between objective performance and the apparent demands of the test situation, and he highlighted the relevance of test parameters to subjects' confidence judgments in hypnosis.

Few studies have actually made a direct attempt to research the relevance of "sanction to guess" to hypnotic memory testing. One such attempt, however, has been made by Doherty (1984), working within our laboratory at the University of Queensland. Doherty argued that if hypnotic subjects have a natural tendency to guess, or if they experience a lessened inhibition to respond, then the effects of specific instructions to guess should lie close in performance level to instructions that offer no specific encouragement. Accordingly, subjects high and low in susceptibility were given either waking or hypnotic instruction and allocated to one of three instructional sets: a set to sanction guessing, a set to encourage them to respond accurately, and a neutral set that did not encourage responding in any particular direction. Results showed that the guessing group in hypnosis was different in memory performance from the group that was given neutral instructions (see Figure 4-1 for the data). Results, however, were not generally supportive of the hypothesis that hypnosis specifically produces a sanction to guess that is primarily responsible for memory production in hypnosis. Clearly, further work needs to be conducted on the hypothesis that has now been proposed by many (DePiano & Salzberg, 1981; Orne *et al.*, 1984; Smith, 1983)—namely, that hypnosis encourages subjects to lower their criterion level of performance and to engage in guesswork. The special methodological difficulties raised by the response criterion problem also have yet to be addressed properly.

If hypnotized subjects feel that guessing is permissible, then the motivational relevance of this process may require especially subtle procedures to test its impact. Work outside the hypnotic memory field, for instance, has indicated that subjects' special willingness to cooperate with the hypnotist is not a process that is tapped effectively by standard hypnotic tasks, but is measured much more sensitively by specific procedures examining the impact of conflicting hypnotist demands and contextual influences (see Sheehan, 1971, 1980). Until that research is done, the possibility that increased false alarms or confabulations in hypnosis result from encouragement to guess remains an attractive process hypothesis to pursue. At the moment, however, it lacks explanatory power to cover all of the existing data, and insufficient attention has been given to its motivational relevance.

## The Relevance of Context

As Orne *et al.* (1984) argue, it is difficult to differentiate between the bona fide consequences of hypnosis and such factors as the desire of the hypnotized subject to produce responses that are consistent with the hypnotist's implicit or explicit suggestions concerning what is wanted. Yet it seems important to try to isolate the potential contribution of contextual factors to the occurrence of memory accuracy and confidence in hypnosis. Where investigators have argued that it is the experience of hypnosis that underscores the trend for memory inaccuracy (e.g., Dywan & Bowers, 1983a, 1983b), research must clearly assess the positive and negative aspects of hypnotic memory productions and try to determine what effects are due to the cognitive changes induced by hypnosis and what effects are due to those contextual influences that result when hypnosis is introduced.

Assessment of the contribution of context in this debate may be assisted by distinguishing those influences of the hypnotic setting that flow implicitly from what the hypnotist says and does, and those cues that are explicitly or actively encouraged by the hypnotist and assume the character of definite suggestions.

Addressing the former source of influence, a number of theorists in the field have drawn attention to the implicit cues for hypermnesia that exist within the hypnotic setting. Timm (1983), for instance, asserts that the hypnotist can be viewed as placing pressure on the subject to guess, and in this situation it should not be surprising that the hypnotic subject will recall additional material. Mingay (1984) also claims that prior to and during the hypnotic interview, the hypnotist is likely to build up the subject's belief that he or she will be able to remember more. The hypnotic situation is clearly one where hypnotic subjects are permitted to say things for which they are not responsible, are rarely challenged about what they report, and are hardly queried at all concerning the consistency of their reports; moreover, hypnosis is a situation where the subject feels calm and free from anxiety about whatever is being communicated (Relinger, 1984; Rosenthal, 1944). For these reasons, the hypnotic subject can be expected to report more, not fewer, ideas when asked to remember, and the output may be accurate or inaccurate.

These same cues are also consistent with the promotion of definite feelings of certainty or confidence about what is being produced. If hypnotic procedures are structured so as to engender an uncritical attitude, promote expectations of efficacy, and motivate the subject to please the hypnotist, then recall that is better is also cued as more certain. In fact, induction procedures can be said to provide the subject with a specific rationale for accepting the veridicality of what emerges during hypnosis (Laurence & Perry, 1983a, 1983b). Laurence and Perry, and Karlin (1983), also draw attention to the particular part played by the encouragement of fantasy in the hypnotic setting. Vivid and clear recall is to be expected in terms of the way the hypnotist usually structures the hypnotic situation. The role of imagery is also seen as important by Smith (1983), who argues that the occurrence of hypermnesia in procedures of memory testing based on repeated measurement creates a ritualization or formalization of performance that comes to be associated with an increase in confidence about the accuracy of the memory. It appears, then, that both confidence and accuracy fit well with cues flowing from the hypnotic induction itself, and that both are reinforced by the positive features of performance in the hypnotic setting as a whole. Whether or not these cues are enhanced in their influence because hypnosis is introduced begs a lively question. There is a widespread belief in the literature that responsiveness to cues is heightened or increased by hypnosis (Orne *et al.*, 1984), but the data sets in support of this contention are not extensive.

There are specific sets of explicit cues for accuracy and confidence that are built into the hypnotic setting, and these also need to be recognized for their potential effects. For the most part, these cues derive largely from the use in hypnosis of the "video recorder" metaphor, and the adoption of age regression procedures that encourage vivid "retelling." As Orne *et al.* (1984) indicate, informing subjects in hypnosis that they are watching events unfold contains an explicit suggestion that what the subjects will see and report is what actually took place. Use of the video recorder model (see Reiser, 1980) invariably asks subjects to remember copious details and to express the conviction that these details reflect the reality of what took place. One may well ask, in fact, what point there is in instructing subjects that they can see everything again if the hypnotist is not insisting that their reports be convincing, vivid, and detailed. What is not often acknowledged, however, is that the text of such instructions as the video recorder model cloaks powerful and often influential communications that take on the character of suggestions. And because they are suggestions that are obvious and clear-cut in their implications, they can often operate in a dramatic way. Tallant (1985), for instance, explicitly investigated the effects of instructions based on the video recorder metaphor on subjects low, medium, and high in susceptibility. Subjects were tested for recall using the Loftus accident series of slides, and the subjects recalled the slides four times during three sessions. The experimenter was also blind to subjects' susceptibility level. Tallant's analyses focused on errors of memory and ratings of confidence. Her results showed that a significant increase in error was associated with hypnosis, and a decrease in error was associated with waking recall; highly susceptible subjects also made the greatest number of errors. Increased confidence was also associated with hypnosis, and highly susceptible subjects emerged as the group that expressed most confidence in errors of memory during hypnosis. The video recorder metaphor had a dramatic effect on subjects low in susceptibility, and these instructions significantly affected the performance of highly susceptible subjects as well. Tallant's data are suggestive of a definite context effect arising from the use of instructions that are frequently employed in research on hypnotic memory.

Explicit cues of the same kind are also conveyed by age regression procedures. Such instructions usually involve an elaborate series of specific suggestions to hypnotized subjects, with the aim of convincing them that they are reliving or actually experiencing "true" events. As Relinger (1984) claims, they convey excessive demand characteristics, and it is very difficult to disentangle effects occurring because of hypnotic processes from consequences that are contextual in origin. Age regression instructions, like communications based on the video recorder metaphor, are likely to influence the hypnotic subject to report details in a way that makes for a convincing performance. In both cases, fantasy and imaginative involvement are invariably encouraged, and communications that cue subjects for truthful and accurate reporting also permit, by their nature, responses that are inaccurate and fanciful.

There is suprisingly little evidence bearing directly on the issue of context versus hypnosis as an explanation of hypnotic memory effects. In one relevant study, Timm (1981) staged a mock assassination in a lecture class and examined recognition and recall much later. Three groups were tested: One received a routine set of forensic memory assistance procedures, including hypnosis; a second group was administered the same set of memory assistance procedures, but without hypnotic induction; and a third group received neither hypnotic induction nor memory assistance. The group given forensic procedures without induction showed a near-significant enhancement effect. The low mean scores for the groups receiving the forensic procedures (with and without induction) suggested to Timm that some of the improvement in subjects' recall in hypnosis experimentation may be due to the procedures themselves, and not just to the fact that the subjects are hypnotized. The study deserves to be replicated to see whether the effect is reliable. The relative impact of context versus cognition has also been investigated by Nogrady *et al.* (1985). Here, the visual memory of subjects high and low in susceptibility for black-and-white drawings of common objects was examined under three conditions: hypnotic instructions, imagination instructions, and control (nonhypnotic) instructions. Results showed that memory performance on both accurate and inaccurate items increased appreciably across a series of multiple-recall tests, but there was no evidence of hypnotic hypermnesia. Highly hypnotizable subjects in the hypnosis condition, however, were more likely than other subjects who were tested to rate the incorrect material as correct, and they showed an appreciable confidence effect. The absence of a hypermnesia effect, as compared with the results obtained by Dywan and Bowers (1983b), suggested to Nogrady *et al.* that contextual demands rather than the experience of hypnosis was the effective variable. As stated earlier, Dywan and Bowers's subjects were forced to generate incorrect material, while in the study by Nogrady *et al.* they were not. This procedural difference suggests that hypnosis does not necessarily lead subjects to generate inaccurate material, but may lead them to embed incorrect material into their memories when they are required to produce it.

The final source of evidence bearing directly on the contextual hypothesis comes from those studies that have used simulating subjects in their design. Simulators are a group highly motivated for the task of pretense, and simulators are very efficient at isolating contextual cues that may be influencing the performance of actually hypnotized subjects. The evidence to date clearly demonstrates major parallels in the performance of simulating and hypnotized subjects. We (Sheehan *et al.*, 1984; Sheehan & Tilden, 1984) found that simulating subjects were just as confident as hypnotized subjects in their memory reports while performing the hypnotic context. Redston and Knox (1983) similarly found that simulators were enthusiastic in their belief that actually hypnotized subjects would be confident about memories expressed in hypnosis. The evidence provided by these studies does not prove in any way that hypnotic subjects are operating in their certainty levels on the basis of contextual cues, but it does indicate that the context hypothesis is tenable and that the onus of proof is on researchers in the area to demonstrate that the cue hypothesis is not sufficient to explain their data. As yet, no study has been conducted to prove that context is the crucial determinant, that memory distortion operates distinctively in hypnosis, or that hypnosis per se enhances subjects' confidence. Enhanced confidence among hypnotized subjects remains a major phenomenon and a real forensic problem. The argument is simply that we do not know yet how much influence in this effect is due to hypnosis and how much is due to situational factors explained by the social-psychological characteristics of the setting in which hypnotized subjects are typically placed. And that distinction is important.

### *The Optimality Hypothesis*

I return at this stage to reconsider the framework for conceptualizing the associations existing between memory accuracy and confidence that have been established by Deffenbacher (1980) and Leippe (1980). There is clear evidence of variability occurring in the association between memory accuracy and confidence, and it is useful to examine hypnotic data for a test of the optimality hypothesis—in particular, to examine the effects of cognitive processing and social influences as they bear on the relationship between memory accuracy and confidence. Review of the evidence described above tells us that social influence factors strongly characterize hypnosis, and it is this kind of influence that Leippe (1980) claims may affect confidence independently of accuracy and thus may reduce the association between memory accuracy and conviction. The evidence also tells us that hypnotic subjects accept misleading information that is presented to them either before or during hypnosis. The effect is not distinctive to susceptible subjects in hypnosis, but the processes of cognitive integration are clearly at work in hypnosis; they suggest the influence of factors that Leippe claims will affect accuracy independently of confidence and similarly reduce the size of the association between memory accuracy and conviction.

Tables 4-2 and 4-3 report data collected from studies that were essentially similar, except that subjects low in susceptibility were simulating hypnosis in one study (Table 4-2) and not in the other (Table 4-3). In both studies, misleading information was presented following rather than prior to hypnosis. The two experiments provided a range of memory situations in which it is possible to catalogue the associations existing between memory accuracy and confidence. Table 4-4 draws these together and summarizes the results for the significance of correlations calculated between memory accuracy and confidence in the two experiments. Results are reported separately for hypnotic and waking instruction. Essentially, three test situations are catalogued: (1) recognition testing, in which items that were not misleading ($n = 15$) were examined for subjects' overall objective accuracy; (2) free recall, in which subjects said what they remembered in their own way; and (3) testing of

Table 4-4. Correlations of Accuracy and Confidence for Different Learning Situations Considered for Hypnosis and Waking Instruction

| Test format | Nature of correlation | Hypnosis instruction | Waking instruction |
|---|---|---|---|
| Recognition testing | Positive | 1** ($r = .56$) | 1** ($r = .60$) |
|  | Zero | 3 | 2 |
|  | Negative | 0 | 1*** ($r = -.45$) |
| Free recall | Positive | 0 | 0 |
|  | Zero | 4 | 4 |
|  | Negative | 0 | 0 |
| False-information index (recognition testing)[a] | Positive | 0 | 0 |
|  | Zero | 7 | 7 |
|  | Negative | 1* ($r = -.46$) | 1* ($r = -.59$) |

*Note.* The data in this table have been computed from the results collected in the studies represented in Tables 4-2 and 4-3. Frequencies have been drawn from the sample of correlations computed separately for subjects high and low in susceptibility.

[a]Based on procedures of Loftus, as discussed in text (see also Loftus, 1979a).

*$p < .05$.

**$p < .01$.

***$p < .001$.

recognition accuracy for just the three misleading items, which provided the data for analysis of Loftus's distortion effect and which measured susceptible subjects' distinctive acceptance of incorrect information into memory. The table lists the frequency of correlations found that were positive and significant, zero (nonsignificant), and negative and significant. Positive correlations indicate that accuracy tallied with confidence, while negative correlations indicate that confidence was associated with inaccuracy rather than accuracy.

The data in Table 4-4 are revealing. There were 32 correlations calculated for hypnosis and 32 for waking instruction, and the majority of these were nonsignificant. For hypnosis, only 2 of the 32 associations were significant; 1 was positive and 1 was negative. For the waking state, a comparable pattern of results was obtained; here, only 3 of the 32 associations were significant, 1 being positive and 2 being negative. Two findings in particular are of special interest. First, the only positive associations that occurred in the studies were those associated with recognition testing, and these were not specific to hypnosis. Second, the only significant associations that were related to Loftus's distortion measure were negative; again, the results were not distinctive to hypnosis.

The incidence of significant associations was very small, and common samples were used for the difference measures; for these reasons, it is possible only to be tentative about the data. As Wells and Murray (1984) argue, however, the differences between studies are usually too numerous to permit us to discern exactly why one study finds a confidence–accuracy relationship and another study does not, so it is instructive to look at closely comparable studies to reveal something of the general patterning evident in the associations. The overall pattern of findings drawn from the results discussed here extends Wells and Murray's conclusion about the waking context to the context of hypnosis—namely, witness confidence is not a valid measure of witness accuracy—and the data give some support to the arguments of Deffenbacher (1980) concerning the optimality of hypothesis.

First, the conditions of testing in the two hypnosis experiments that have been analyzed were low in optimality. There was, for example, low familiarity with the stimuli to be remembered, and inconsistent information was presented to half the subjects during the retention interval. Furthermore, inspection time for the complex pictorial stimuli was relatively brief (5 seconds for each slide). The prevalence of nonsignificant relationships fits the hypothesis that would predict zero or negative relationships under low-optimality conditions of processing.

More specifically, there is evidence for the impact of both social influence factors and cognitive integrative factors. Consider the results for the positive associations, for example. Leippe (1980) makes the argument that some sensitivity of confidence to memory accuracy can be expected in recognition, because in this mode of testing subjects are not allowed to say "I don't know," and consequently must guess when they really do not know. It is not surprising under such conditions that low confidence ratings will accompany guesses; confidence in these responses should certainly be lower than confidence under conditions in which subjects can freely choose whether or not to respond and can make choices that they feel are the right ones. Conditions that include an option of not responding should better contribute to a high accuracy–confidence correlation. Free-recall subjects have the option of not indicating a response, but when a choice is exercised and a memory is reported, the conditions are appropriate for incorrect responses to be accompanied in memory by the confidence subjects have in making their choice. Responding in this context means that more of a commitment is made; given that a choice is exercised, both accurate and inaccurate responses are likely to have some degree of confidence associated with them. This account appeals for its justification to a variation of Bem's (1965) theory of self-persuasion. It stresses the social-contextual factors that may affect the relationship between memory accuracy and confidence, and it is significant to note that social influence factors were operating in both the hypnosis and waking contexts, not in either of them alone.

The influence of cognitive process variables is indicated also by the results for Loftus's distortion measure. The testing of the three critical items was a direct measure of the acceptance of misleading information in memory, and there was a high probability with this score that specific reconstruction processes were at work. The results in Table 4-4 show that the association between memory accuracy and confidence on this index was significantly negative, thus emphasizing the essential opposition of accuracy and confidence. The data in this respect support the findings by others as well: Loftus *et al.* (1978), for example, found that confidence was poorly related to accuracy where misinformation was studied in their design. Finally, as for social factors, the effect for cognitive influence was not distinctive to hypnosis. Processes involving unconscious integrative processes operated in an influential way, independently of the presence or absence of hypnotic or waking instruction.

*CONCLUSION*

This chapter has attempted to look in a comprehensive way at the relationship between confidence and memory accuracy in hypnosis, and it has reviewed a number of major frameworks of explanation that may help account for effects. Particular attention has been paid to the hypothesis that pervasive memory distortion occurs in hypnosis, but the evidence has been found wanting in support of this hypothesis. There appears to be no such general biasing effect of hypnosis, nor is there very consistent evidence of hypermnesia. In addition, the results from conditions that have produced greater distortion in hypnosis have not always been replicated across different memory formats or over time.

Hypnosis, however, does seem to be distinctively linked with the confidence or conviction that hypnotic subjects have in the accuracy of their reports. Regardless of the literal truth value of hypnotized subjects' memory reports, confidence is a reasonably reliable accompaniment of hypnotic testimony. As with the case of accuracy, however, level of susceptibility to hypnosis appears to play an important role in moderating its effect. In our program of research, confidence effects that have been associated with hypnosis have been most evident (across studies) for highly susceptible subjects who were in hypnosis (see also Sheehan & Grigg, 1985, and Tallant, 1985, for replication of the effect).

The sample illustration of effects demonstrated in Tables 4-1 through 4-3 and Figure 4-1 show that accuracy may stay constant across hypnosis and waking instruction while confidence varies, or that confidence may remain stable while accuracy shifts. Accuracy and confidence may also covary together, but in opposite directions. The pattern of results in Table 4-4 sustains an overall prediction of no relationship between accuracy and confidence in hypnosis. However, the usual conditions for processing events in the hypnotic situation are not optimal, and typically the conditions for information processing that hold in hypnosis lead to a test of the accuracy of hypnotic memory that establishes quite low conditions of optimality. In the hypnotic setting, therefore, one could ordinarily predict a low incidence of high positive associations between the two variables, accuracy and confidence. Significant associations do occur between accuracy and confidence in hypnosis, though, and the discussion of the data illustrated in Table 4-4 suggests that they can be explained on the basis of the hypothesized effects of cognitive integrative factors or social influence factors at work.

The explanatory frameworks for accounting for the data relating to accuracy and confidence in hypnosis are many and varied, but they can be broadly classified into those that focus on the experience of hypnosis (with attendant emphasis on process characteristics reflecting the nature of hypnosis), and those that accentuate the social or contextual features of the hypnotic setting. Hypnotic processes that appear to require further exploration in research are those of attention and motivation, the latter being reflected in the current theorizing about hypnotized subjects' "sanction to guess," which may reflect a motivated willingness on the hypnotized subjects' part to report or respond. It is difficult to separate process features of hypnotic response from contextual features, and the two are obviously intertwined. The evidence, however, points toward the definite relevance of contextual influences in determining the nature of the relationship between memory confidence and accuracy in hypnosis.

Deliberately, no attempt has been made in this chapter to draw inferences from the data on the practice of hypnosis in the law courts. The essential theme of this chapter is that good grounds can be put forward for arguing that the relationship between memory accuracy and confidence in hypnosis is poor. It would seem to help, however, to place the data within a framework of thinking that aims to order events by taking appropriate account of the variability of conditions under which information in hypnosis is gathered.

## REFERENCES

Arons, H. (1967). *Hypnosis in criminal investigation.* Springfield, IL: Charles C Thomas.

Augustynek, A. (1977). Recalling in state of awareness and under hypnosis. *Przeglad Psychologiczny, 20,* 693–705.

Bekerian, D. A., & Bowers, J. M. (1983). Eyewitness testimony: Were we misled? *Journal of Experimental Psychology: Learning, Memory, and Cognition, 9,* 139–145.

Bem, D. J. (1965). An experimental analysis of self-persuasion. *Journal of Experimental Social Psychology, 1,* 199–218.

Buckhout, R., Eugenio, P., Licitra, T., Oliver, L., & Kramer, T. H. (1981). Memory, hypnosis and evidence: Research on eyewitnesses. *Social Action and the Law, 7,* 67–72.

Crawford, H. J., & Allen, S. N. (1983). Enhanced visual memory during hypnosis as mediated by hypnotic responsiveness and cognitive strategies. *Journal of Experimental Psychology: General, 112,* 662–685.

Deffenbacher, K. A. (1980). Eyewitness accuracy and confidence: Can we infer anything about their relationship? *Law and Human Behavior, 4,* 243–260.

DePiano, F. A., & Salzberg, H. C. (1981). Hypnosis as an aid to recall of meaningful information presented under three types of arousal. *International Journal of Clinical and Experimental Hypnosis, 29,* 383–400.

Doherty, P. (1984). *The influence of instructional set on free recall.* Unpublished bachelor's (honours) thesis, University of Queensland, St. Lucia, Australia.

Dywan, J., & Bowers, K. S. (1983a, October). *Hypnosis and memory: A look at mechanisms.* Paper presented at the 35th Annual Meeting of the Society of Clinical and Experimental Hypnosis, Boston.

Dywan, J., & Bowers, K. (1983b). The use of hypnosis to enhance recall. *Science, 222,* 184–185.

Greene, E., Flynn, M. S., & Loftus, E. F. (1982). Inducing resistance to misleading information. *Journal of Verbal Learning and Verbal Behavior, 21,* 207–219.

Griffin, G. R. (1980). Hypnosis, towards a logical approach in using hypnosis in law enforcement agencies. *Journal of Police Science and Administration, 8,* 385–389.

Hibbard, W. S., & Worring, R. W. (1981). *Forensic hypnosis: The practical application of hypnosis in criminal investigations.* Springfield, IL: Charles C Thomas.

Karlin, R. A. (1983). Forensic hypnosis—two case reports. *International Journal of Clinical and Experimental Hypnosis, 31,* 227–234.

Klatzky, R. L., & Erdelyi, M. H. (1985). The response criterion problem in tests of hypnosis and memory. *International Journal of Clinical and Experimental Hypnosis, 33,* 246–257.

Labelle, L., & Perry, C. W. (1986, August). *Pseudomemory creation in hypnosis.* Paper presented at the 94th Annual Convention of the American Psychological Association, Washington, DC.

Laurence, J. R. (1982). *Memory creation in hypnosis.* Unpublished doctoral dissertation, Concordia University, Montréal.

Laurence, J. R., Nadon, R., Nogrady, M., & Perry, C. W. (1986). Duality, dissociation and memory creation in highly hypnotizable subjects. *International Journal of Clinical and Experimental Hypnosis, 34,* 295–310.

Laurence, J. R., & Perry, C. W. (1983a). The enhancement of memory by hypnosis in the legal investigative situation. *Canadian Psychology, 24,* 155–167.

Laurence, J. R., & Perry, C. W. (1983b). Forensic hypnosis in the late nineteenth century. *International Journal of Clinical and Experimental Hypnosis, 31,* 266–283.

Laurence, J. R., & Perry, C. W. (1983c). Hypnotically created memory among highly hypnotizable subjects. *Science, 222,* 523–524.

Leippe, M. R. (1980). Effects of integrative memorial and cognitive processes on the correspondence of eyewitness accuracy and confidence. *Law and Human Behavior, 4,* 261–274.

Loftus, E. F. (1979a). *Eyewitness testimony.* Cambridge, MA: Harvard University Press.

Loftus, E. F. (1979b). Reactions to blatantly contradictory information. *Memory and Cognition, 7,* 368–374.

Loftus, E. F., Miller, D. G., & Burns, H. J. (1978). Semantic integration of verbal information into a visual memory. *Journal of Experimental Psychology: Human Learning and Memory, 4,* 19–31.

Mingay, D. J. (1984). *The effect of hypnosis on a witness's memory: Reconciling forensic claims and research findings.* Unpublished manuscript, MRC Applied Psychology Unit, Cambridge, England.

Nogrady, H., McConkey, K. M., & Perry, C. W. (1985). Enhancing visual memory: Trying hypnosis, trying imagination, and trying again. *Journal of Abnormal Psychology, 94,* 195–204.

Orne, M. T., & Hammer, A. G. (1974). Hypnosis. In *Encyclopaedia Britannica* (Vol. 15, pp. 133–140). Chicago, IL: William Benton.

Orne, M. T., Soskis, D. A., Dinges, D. F., & Orne, E. C. (1984). Hypnotically induced testimony. In G. L. Wells & E. F. Loftus (Eds.), *Eyewitness testimony: Psychological perspectives* (pp. 171–215). Cambridge, England: Cambridge University Press.

Putnam, W. H. (1979). Hypnosis and distortions in eyewitness memory. *International Journal of Clinical and Experimental Hypnosis, 27,* 437–448.

Rainer, D. (1983). *Eyewitness testimony: Does hypnosis enhance accuracy, distortion, and confidence?* Unpublished doctoral dissertation, University of Wyoming.

Redston, M. T., & Knox, J. (1983, October). *Is the recognition of faces enhanced by hypnosis?* Paper presented at the 35th Annual Meeting of the Society of Clinical and Experimental Hypnosis, Boston.

Reiser, M. (1980). *Handbook of investigative hypnosis.* Los Angeles: Law Enforcement Hypnosis Institute.

Relinger, H. (1984). Hypnotic hypermnesia: A critical review. *American Journal of Clinical Hypnosis, 26,* 212–225.

Rosenthal, B. G. (1944). Hypnotic recall of material learned under anxiety and non-anxiety producing conditions. *Journal of Experimental Psychology, 34,* 369–389.

Ryan, M. (1982). *Belief, conviction, and performance in hypnosis.* Unpublished doctoral dissertation, University of Queensland, St. Lucia, Australia.

Sanders, G. S., & Simmons, W. L. (1983). Use of hypnosis to enhance eyewitness accuracy: Does it work? *Journal of Applied Psychology, 68,* 70–77.

Sarbin, T. R., & Coe, W. C. (1972). *Hypnosis: A social psychological analysis of influence communication.* New York: Holt, Rinehart & Winston.

Sheehan, P. W. (1971). Countering preconceptions about hypnosis: An objective index of involvement with the hypnotist. *Journal of Abnormal Psychology Monographs, 78,* 299–322.

Sheehan, P. W. (1980). Factors influencing rapport in hypnosis. *Journal of Abnormal Psychology, 89,* 263–281.

Sheehan, P. W. (1985, August). *Memory distortion in hypnosis.* Invited address, to the 10th International Congress of Hypnosis and Psychosomatic Medicine, Toronto.

Sheehan, P. W., & Grigg, L. (1985). Hypnosis, memory and the acceptance of an implausible cognitive set. *British Journal of Clinical and Experimental Hypnosis, 3,* 5–12.

Sheehan, P. W., Grigg, L., & McCann, T. (1984). Memory distortion following exposure to false information in hypnosis. *Journal of Abnormal Psychology, 93,* 259–265.

Sheehan, P. W., & Tilden, J. (1983). Effects of suggestibility and hypnosis on accurate and distorted retrieval from memory. *Journal of Experimental Psychology: Learning, Memory, and Cognition, 9,* 283–293.

Sheehan, P. W., & Tilden, J. (1984). Real and simulated occurrences of memory distortion in hypnosis. *Journal of Abnormal Psychology, 93,* 47–57.

Sheehan, P. W., & Tilden, J. (1986). The consistency of occurrences of memory distortion following hypnotic induction. *International Journal of Clinical and Experimental Hypnosis, 34,* 122–137.

Shields, I. W., & Knox, J. (1986). Level of processing as a determinant of hypnotic hypermnesia. *Journal of Abnormal Psychology, 95,* 358–364.

Smith, M. C. (1983). Hypnotic memory enhancement of witnesses: Does it work? *Psychological Bulletin, 94,* 387–407.

Stalnaker, J. M., & Riddle, E. E. (1932). The effect of hypnosis on long-delayed recall. *Journal of General Psychology, 6,* 429–440.

Stager, G. (1974). The effect of hypnosis on the learning and recall of visually presented material. *Dissertation Abstracts International, 35*(6), 3075-B. (University Microfilms No. 74-28, 985)

Tallant, B. K. (1985, August). *Errors of memory in hypnosis.* Paper presented at the 10th International Congress of Hypnosis and Psychosomatic Medicine, Toronto.

Timm, H. W. (1981). The effect of forensic hypnosis techniques on eyewitness recall and recognition. *Journal of Police Science and Administration, 9,* 188–194.

Timm, H. W. (1983). The factors theoretically affecting the impact of forensic hypnosis techniques on eyewitness recall. *Journal of Police Science and Administration, 11,* 442–450.

Wagstaff, G. F., & Sykes, C. T. (1984). Hypnosis and the recall of emotionally-toned material. *IRGS Medical Science, 12,* 137–138.

Wells, G. L., Lindsay, R. C. L., & Tousignant, J. P. (1980). Effects of expert psychological advice on human performance in judging the validity of eyewitness testimony. *Law and Human Behavior, 4,* 275–285.

Wells, G. L., & Murray, D. M. (1984). Eyewitness confidence. In G. L. Wells & E. Loftus (Eds), *Eyewitness testimony: Psychological perspectives* (pp. 155–170). Cambridge, England: Cambridge University Press.

Yuille, J. C. (1982). *Video as a medium for eyewitness research (1).* Unpublished manuscript, University of British Columbia.

Zelig, M., & Beidleman, W. B. (1981). The investigative use of hypnosis: A word of caution. *International Journal of Clinical and Experimental Hypnosis, 29,* 401–412.

# 5

## Hypnotic Age Regression Techniques in the Elicitation of Memories: Applied Uses and Abuses

CAMPBELL W. PERRY
JEAN-ROCH LAURENCE
JOYCE D'EON
BEVERLEA TALLANT
*Concordia University, Montréal*

Regression to an earlier age in hypnosis is often a compelling phenomenon, particularly when the regression is to childhood. It is not uncommon for the hypnotized person to manifest childlike qualities in a subjectively convincing manner, with appropriate changes in voice, gesture, and handwriting; occasionally, also, the age-regressed subject may spontaneously relive a painful and/or traumatic incident of his or her earlier life. Often, this may have such emotional accompaniments as crying, accelerated breathing, sweating, and nausea (Laurence, Nadon, Bowers, Perry, & Regher, 1985). In one case, a subject age-regressed to infancy by Erickson urinated in his trousers when frightened unexpectedly (LeCron, 1965).

As far as can be ascertained, the first report of a suggestion of age regression was published in 1883 in the *Revue Philosophique* (cited by Bernheim, 1884). The author, Charles Richet, suggested to one of his subjects that he was 6 years old again, playing with his friends outside the house. The suggestion was seen as one example of personality alterations that could be induced in hypnosis. Bernheim (1884) also reported that he used this technique with some of his patients when he wanted them to relive a past event. At the beginning of the 1890s these types of suggestions became very popular, especially because of their perceived similarity to the then-intriguing phenomenon of "double personality." Bourru and Burot (1888) and Binet (1896) devoted books to the subject of personality alterations in which hypnotized subjects assumed the characteristics of, for instance, a priest, a general, or a nun. As we shall see, some of the features demonstrated by them as intrinsic to personality alterations re-emerged subsequently within the context of age regression phenomena. This popularity rapidly led to some variations of the basic suggestion. In 1896, de Rochas published his investigation of regression not only to subjects' childhoods, but also to their alleged past lives and future lives as well.

In recent years, renewed attention has been focused on age regression as the result of attempts to apply it, particularly in clinical, investigative, and reincarnation contexts. This, in turn, has often led to brisk debate concerning the nature of regressive phenomena and the problems that emerge from utilizing them in applied settings. In order to understand these issues of definition and of application, it is helpful first to discuss the very nature of hypnosis itself, since this provides a context within which these problems are more readily identifiable.

## THE NATURE OF HYPNOSIS

The term "hypnosis" is a metaphor; it was coined by the British investigator James Braid (1843) to draw attention to the possible links between the behaviors encountered in what·Mesmer (1779/1970) had called "animal magnetism" and the behaviors of sleepwalkers. In this, Braid was following the thinking of earlier investigators who had sought to formulate animal magnetism in alternative terms. The Marquis de Puységur (Puységur, 1784–1785) had referred to Mesmeric phenomena as "artificial somnambulism," and di Faria (1819) had coined the term "lucid sleep." It is now well known that hypnosis has little to do with nocturnal sleep; indeed, the electroencephalographic (EEG) pattern for hypnosis is formally indistinguishable from that of a person when he or she is awake, alert, and relaxed with eyes closed (Barber, 1970). Nevertheless, the sleep metaphor implied by the term "hypnosis" persists, although consideration of the positions taken by current leading investigators suggests that what is involved in understanding hypnosis implies distinctly alternative mechanisms.

Despite differences in theoretical approach, there is a considerable consensus among investigators that hypnosis is a situation in which the subject is asked to set aside critical judgment without abandoning it completely, and to indulge in fantasy and make-believe (Gill & Brenman, 1959; E. R. Hilgard, 1977). This has led Orne (1980) to state that to the extent to which a person can experience the subjective phenomena of hypnosis, he or she may experience major alterations, even distortions of perception, mood, and memory. Quite stable individual differences in the ability to do this have been reported regularly. It has been found that 10–15% of individuals are highly responsive to hypnosis (i.e., are capable of suggested posthypnotic amnesia); a further 10–15% are minimally responsive; and the remaining majority of 70–80% are moderately responsive to varying degrees (E. R. Hilgard, 1965; Perry, 1977).

In recent times, considerable emphasis has been placed upon the fantasy and make-believe experienced in hypnosis, particularly by individuals who possess a high degree of hypnotic ability. Its major characteristics have been described variously as "imaginative involvement" (J. R. Hilgard, 1979) and as "believed-in imaginings" (Sarbin & Coe, 1972); indeed, these latter investigators have proposed that the central question for hypnosis research concerns identifying the conditions under which imaginings become believable. Consistent with these views, Spanos and Barber (1974) have characterized hypnosis as thinking along with, and experiencing, suggestion-related imaginings.

In addition, Sutcliffe (1961) has described the deeply hypnotized individual as "deluded" in a descriptive, nonpejorative sense. He has added that, for the highly hypnotizable person, hypnosis provides a context in which the person is able to indulge in fantasy and make-believe. He maintains that this is something that such persons enjoy doing outside of a hypnotic context, and also is an activity at which they are highly accomplished. To round off this emerging picture, S. C. Wilson and Barber (1983) have recently characterized individuals who are highly responsive to hypnosis as "fantasy addicts" (a term that may be too strong); in addition, these investigators have provided data indicating that people who are able to experience the major subjective alterations in a context defined as hypnosis also report frequent difficulty in distinguishing fact from fantasy and real from imagined events in their everyday lives.

Recent research data (see Nadon, 1983, for a review) indicate that the main characteristics that are most strongly related to hypnotizability include imagery/imagination, absorption, and possibly dissociation (as indexed by measures of selective attention). In addition, following interactionist accounts proposed by Bowers (1973) and by Sheehan and Perry (1976), it may be necessary to evaluate the degree to which the various contexts in which hypnosis is dispensed differentially affect hypnotic response. For instance, the context in which investigative police hypnosis is presented may have a much greater effect in fashioning the responses of subjects than, for instance, the experimental laboratory (Perry & Laurence, 1983).

Be this as it may, the conceptualization of hypnosis in terms of imagination—whether as "imaginative involvement" or as "believed-in imaginings"— is important for the understanding of hypnotic age regression, since it may contribute to a better understanding both of its phenomena and of the problems that can be encountered in its utilization in applied contexts.

## AGE REGRESSION AT THE DESCRIPTIVE LEVEL

The more dramatic and compelling features of age regression in hypnosis, described in the opening section of this chapter, could lead one to believe that it is confined to the highly hypnotizable individuals who constitute 10–15% of the population (E. R. Hilgard, 1965; Laurence & Perry, 1981). Reference to the norms of the Stanford Hypnotic Susceptibility Scale, Form C (SHSS:C; Weitzenhoffer & Hilgard, 1962) indicates, however, that 43% of individuals respond positively to the age regression suggestion of this standardized measure of hypnotizability.

This quite high proportion may be a direct function of the SHSS:C's scoring criterion for age regression. The age regression item of the SHSS:C is tested by having the subject write his or her name, age, and the date during hypnosis—first prior to regression, and subsequently when the subject is regressed to fifth grade and then second grade. The subject is scored as having responded to the suggestion if there is "a clear change in handwriting between the present and one of the regressed ages" (Weitzenhoffer & Hilgard, 1962, p. 25). It has since become clear that handwriting change has little relevance as a criterion of whether a subject is experiencing age regression; indeed, it can be considered as a confabulation or as behavioral compliance. This point was anticipated by Orne (1951), who characterized the drawings of age-regressed subjects as "sophisticated oversimplifications" (p. 215), which, although childlike in appearance, contain adult elements that are not present at early periods of development. Investigators have become aware that the most distinctive characteristic of age regression is the hypnotized person's report of reliving an early event, as opposed to merely imagining or thinking about it during hypnosis.

Recent data (Perry & Walsh, 1978) have shown that the subjective experience of age regression is differential. Approximately 50% of highly hypnotizable subjects who experience reliving an earlier age report duality, in which they experience being both adult and child either simultaneously or in alternation. The remaining subjects report a "quasi-literal" regression, in which they experience being the actual suggested age, and have no sense of their adult identity. The differential response had been observed earlier; Orne (M. T. Orne, personal communication to C. Perry, 1979) has indicated that subjects reporting duality in age regression were excluded from the major study of the phenomenon performed by O'Connell, Shor, and Orne (1970). A similar observation was made even earlier at the time that investigators studied personality alterations. Binet (1896) observed:

> Some authors . . . hold that in experiments of transformation of personality the subject is really playing a part, a sort of comedy, and that he may be compared to an actor who expressed sentiments which he himself does not feel.
>
> Authors who adopt this interpretation, and among them I may cite M. Delboeuf, are by no means of the opinion that the subject tries to simulate and deceive the experimenter—the old idea of simulation is no longer held. But they think that the subject obeys from a different motive. When he receives an order, like that of representing a soldier or a peasant, he performs it to the best of his ability, with no other desire than that of pleasing the person from whom

he has received the suggestion. He plays a comedy part, but with good intentions. The condition is then certainly a very complex psychological state, but yet it is easy to explain on this theory.

This position has been violently combated by other authors, notably by M. Bernheim, who holds that in every case the subject is sincere and really accepts the suggestion which he receives. A new personality is communicated to him and he accepts it, because the suggestion is for him reality itself, and because for the time being he entirely forgets his former personality.

It does not seem necessary to pass judgment upon these two diametrically opposed opinions, because they appear to me to be equally correct, only they apply to different cases. There are persons who are by no means the dupes of the suggestions given to them, but who will still carry them out because they are unable to resist the influence of the operator. This class of patients never forget who they are—their identity. If they are told to represent a priest, a general, or a nun, they will be capable of doing it as any of us might do it when requested, but they know that they are playing a part. They try to assume the characters desired, but they always retain the memory of their proper personality. Others on the contrary, are completely the victims of the suggested illusion, because the memory of their former ego is for the moment entirely obliterated.

The differences of effect result from the psychic nature of the subjects respectively, and also, perhaps, from the method employed by the suggester. It is useless, therefore, to enter into the discussion concerning the facts. Two facts, we should remember, may be different without contradicting each other. (pp. 258–260)

Bernheim (1884) also described his patients' responses to a suggestion of regression in similar differential terms. He reported:

[One subject] listens to the question of his imaginary questioner, and gives his answer without repeating the question. He grows pale and trembles when he is wounded. [Another subject], on the contrary, does not turn pale when wounded, neither does his heart beat more rapidly. It is another self that he sees and feels acting in this strange doubling of his personality of which he is not aware. He talks to me, answers me, knows that he is in the hospital sleeping, and at the same time on the battlefield; the contradiction does not surprise him. (p. 39)

This differential response to an age regression item received explicit recognition recently when Morgan and Hilgard (1978–1979) constructed the Stanford Hypnotic Clinical Scale (SHCS). On this scale, hypnotic subjects are presented with five descriptive sentences about their age regression experience and asked to select the one that most closely fits it. These sentences are as follows:

    1. I did not go back at all.
    2. I was thinking about when I was that age, but had no visual experiences.

3. Although I did not go back, I could see myself as a young child reliving an experience.

4. I know I was really my present age, but I felt in part as though I was reliving an experience.

5. I actually felt as though I was back at the suggested age, and reliving a past experience. (p. 45)

Subjects are rated as having responded to the age regression suggestion if they check either alternative 4 (the duality response) or alternative 5 (the quasi-literal age regression experience). Morgan and Hilgard (1978–1979, p. 136) report that 66% of a student normative sample of 111 subjects passed the age regression item by this criterion; this figure may be inflated, however, since it has been our own experience that some subjects are confused by the wording of the duality statement. Indeed, some subjects have sought to resolve what they perceive as an impasse by marking the response sheet for age regression as 4½. Again, in a recent study (Tallant, 1984), one subject furnished a spontaneous duality report. On being presented the response form, however, she marked alternative 5, after much hesitation.

The problem with the wording is that it places the greater emphasis upon the subject's experiencing his or her present age, whereas the experience of reliving is central to the subject, and the awareness of his or her present age is peripheral. Laurence and Perry (1981), for instance, have presented a number of subjects' verbal reports of duality. Here are two examples:

> *Subject 3*: The thing is . . . I was there, you know. It was if I was there . . . but I wasn't very long; it came and went and it didn't stay. . . . I felt like I was . . . it sort of felt like "what am I doing there" and then the next thing I'm back here, and then "what am I doing here?" It felt like that. It felt like that I was looking at myself in a sense . . . something like you would do in a dream.
>
> *Subject 22*: As soon as I began to write, I was there and I was not there. . . . It was like a merry-go-round; I was in and out of it so fast. . . . I had something like a kind of observer who was watching the class. (p. 338)

Indeed, these verbal reports suggest that duality in age regression may be more appropriately indexed by a semistructured interview than by a multiple-choice checklist, in order to capture these nuances of the experience.

The verbal reports presented in this study point also to one final characteristic of responses in age regression. Laurence and Perry (1981) reported a study in which they tested responses to age regression; at a subsequent time during the same hypnosis session, they tested subjects on E. R. Hilgard's (1977) "hidden-observer" item, in which it is suggested that cold-pressor pain that is denied by the subject at a conscious level may be registering at some other level of which he or she may not be aware. It was found that subjects reporting duality in age regression reported also having a hidden-observer experience, while subjects reporting no duality did not report such an experience. This finding has since been replicated (Laurence, Nadon, Nogrady, & Perry, 1986; Nogrady, McConkey, Laurence, & Perry, 1983). In the latter study, a group of insusceptible simulating subjects was utilized to investigate the potential artifact of demand characteristics (for a detailed rationale of this procedure, and for a critique of the inferences that can be drawn from it when actually hypnotized and simulating subjects show both similarities and differences in behavior, see Orne, 1959, 1979). Not one simulator reported either duality in age regression or the hidden-observer effect, suggesting that the hidden-observer metaphor and the experience of duality in age regression may tap a common differential dissociation response. Nogrady *et al.* (1983) also tested a group of subjects who were in medium susceptibility; not one of them reported a hidden-observer experience, although some of them manifested a duality response in age regression, suggesting that the hidden-observer effect is likely to be unique to highly hypnotizable subjects.

It should be noted, however, that a controversy exists concerning the "reality" of the hidden-observer effect. Spanos and Hewitt (1980) presented data that led them to interpret it as entirely the product of contextual cues (see Laurence, Perry, & Kihlstrom, 1983, and Spanos, 1983, for a discussion of the relevant issues). It suffices to say here that the studies performed at Concordia University and two other studies (E. R. Hilgard, Hilgard, Macdonald, Morgan, & Johnson, 1978; E. R. Hilgard, Morgan, & Macdonald, 1975) have found the incidence of the hidden-observer effect to be 40–50%, whereas Spanos and Hewitt found an almost 100% incidence of it. This suggests the hypothesis that differences in defining "hypnosis" to subjects may be in play (Kihlstrom, 1985): Spanos and his colleagues tend to define it as a willingness to cooperate, whereas E. R. Hilgard and subsequent investigators of the hidden-observer effect define it as a willingness to cooperate *and* an ability to experience subjective alterations. At the time of this writing, the controversy continues unresolved. Recently, Spanos, de Groot, Tiller, Weekes, and Bertrand (1985) were able to replicate the finding of a differential response to an age regression item; once again, however, nearly all of their subjects, both actually hypnotized and simulating, reported a hidden-observer effect. The controversy further indicates the emphasis that should be placed on the interaction between contextual demands and the behaviors and experiences of the hypnotized subjects. This complex interaction can play a major role in applied settings.

## PROBLEMS IN EVALUATING REPORTS OF AGE-REGRESSED INDIVIDUALS

Two of the most common fallacies about hypnotic age regression, which can be found even today, are (1) that it is literal and (2) that age regression techniques can enhance memory. For instance, it has been claimed that "regression has been proved beyond all doubt to be an actual reliving of the experiences, and the subject is remembering things which are beyond recall in the waking state" (Jaffe, 1980; p. 237). (For a review of the data on the literalness hypothesis, see Barber, 1970; for a review on the so-called "hypermnesia" [memory enhancement] effect, see Orne, Soskis, Dinges, & Orne, 1984.) While both are important issues, the scope and focus of the present chapter is upon the problems of unconditionally accepting as accurate the reports of hypnotically age-regressed subjects. The problems are (1) confabulation; (2) the creation of pseudomemories; (3) inadvertent cueing by the hypnotist, and the hypnotist's beliefs about hypnosis; (4) the beliefs and preconceptions of the hypnotized subject; and (5) in some cases, source amnesia (Evans & Thorn, 1966). Each of these problems is reviewed separately here and is illustrated with examples from the experimental, clinical, and field contexts (notably from the literatures of police investigative hypnosis and of reincarnation reports elicited in hypnosis).

## Confabulated Recall

Given the definition of hypnosis presented earlier, which emphasizes (1) the setting aside of critical judgment and (2) the indulgence in make-believe and fantasy (which in some subjects may become "believed-in imaginings"), it should not come as a surprise that hypnotic age regression is a fertile breeding ground for confabulation. While some authors (e.g., Reiser, 1980) equate confabulation with deliberate lying, it is actually a matter of the hypnotized person's confusing fact with fantasy.

One of the earliest examples of confabulation comes from one of the keener observers of human behavior—namely, Sigmund Freud. In his early years, Freud practiced hypnosis; he abandoned it in 1895, but by then he had made many observations that led him to propose the so-called "infantile seduction theory" of the origins of neurosis. On this view, neurosis was the product of the patient (usually female) having been sexually abused by an adult (usually her father). Freud obtained many of his observations when he utilized hypnosis, and although he abandoned the infantile seduction theory in 1897, many still take it as Biblical truth (see Malcolm, 1984, for a delightful review of this issue). It is now known from a number of studies (Dywan & Bowers, 1983; Stalnaker & Riddle, 1932) that hypnosis tends to increase "recall" of both correct and incorrect material; accordingly, it is quite likely that some of the reports of sexual molestation that Freud obtained were veridical and that others were the products of the patients' imagination, which, in some cases, may have been cued inadvertently by an overzealous pursuit of evidence for the seduction theory (Orne *et al.*, 1984).

In a classic study, Orne (1951) documented a number of instances of confabulation in the relatively benign context of the laboratory. One subject, for instance, when asked the time, looked at a hallucinated wristwatch "which he surely did not wear at the age of six" (p. 219). Another wrote, in childlike handwriting, the sentence "I am conducting an experiment that will assess my psychological capacities," and defined the word "hypochondriac" correctly. Yet another, regressed to the day of this 6th birthday, said that he was not in school because the day was a Saturday; subsequent independent evaluation indicated that his 6th birthday had fallen on a Sunday. One confabulation reported by Orne (1951) has a quite comic touch (and is discussed again below in connection with police investigative uses of hypnosis, except that it is no laughing matter that a confabulated recall can send an innocent person to prison). The German-born subject had arrived in the United States during his teenage years, and had spoken no English prior to this time. Regressed to his sixth birthday, he was asked repeatedly in English whether he understood English, and he replied, uniformly in German, that he did not—thus inadvertently demonstrating a clear understanding of English.

A number of instances of confabulation have been found in the investigative use of hypnosis in criminal cases. Whereas the laboratory is a relatively benign and neutral situation, the crime context is one where a high level of affect may be engendered. This, in itself, may heighten the propensity for confabulation to occur, especially as victims of crime in particular are usually highly motivated to assist the police in every way possible. Thus, even if the hypnotic interview is conducted in a manner low in cueing, as prescribed by Orne *et al.* (1984), the hypnotized victim/witness may be too eager to assist— to the point that in regression to the events of the crime, he or she may mistake hypnotically elicited fantasies for veridical "memory."

This problem may be compounded by at least three particular procedures that police hypnotechnicians have been taught in Reiser's (1980) 32-hour course. One concerns the use of "affectless recall," in which the subject is explicitly asked to relive the events of a crime, but not to relive the emotions. It is not as yet known whether such a procedure carries a built-in memory contaminant, over and above the mere introduction of an age regression procedure. Given, however, that recent research (Bower, 1981) indicates that individuals tend to recall happy events better when they are happy, and sad events better when they are sad, the possibility cannot be dismissed that affectless recall could be a major source of distortion for recalling potentially affect-laden material. We may hope that future research will clarify this major issue.

A second potential major contaminant concerns the practice, described by Reiser (1980), of using metaphors derived from televised sports. The hypnotized victim/witness is asked to "zoom in," "freeze-frame," and view in "slow motion" the "film" of the crime stored in the subconscious in order to obtain a better description of a relevant piece of information, such as the face of an accused, or an automobile license plate number. As has been indicated elsewhere (Perry & Laurence, 1983), "if a person is asked to 'zoom-in' on an image that, in the original experience, the retina could not resolve, there is no other source but fantasy for enhanced detail" (p. 163).

A third problem which has not been sufficiently addressed to date, is that police hypnotechnicians trained by the procedures of Reiser (1980) are encouraged to employ an apparent variation of E. R. Hilgard's (1977) hidden-observer technique. Subjects are cued strongly to refer to themselves as a separate identity, as if they were somehow observers of crimes in which they had been victims or participants. Indeed, Reiser (1980) actually describes an induction procedure in which a female victim was asked to describe an assailant, whom she had not seen, since he had held her from behind during a crime. The following interaction ensued:

> *Sub*: I can see the guy behind her. But I can't, she can't see him.
> *Hyp*: She doesn't have to see him. You can see him. You are watching the film from your chair. Now what are you seeing? *You can see more than she can.* (p. 196; italics added)

As indicated elsewhere, such an instruction, especially given to a highly hypnotizable individual, "is a free ticket to fantasy island" (Perry & Laurence, 1982, p. 447). A recent preliminary report (Tallant, 1984) suggests that such concerns about the inherent suggestiveness of Reiser's techniques are not lacking in foundation. In Tallant's study, there was a substantial augmentation of errors of memory among subjects low in susceptibility when Reiser's hypnotic induction technique was introduced, as compared to a group that received a more neutral procedure.

These preliminary considerations provide a context for understanding the confabulations that have been reliably reported in the legal investigative context. The case of *State v. Mack* (1980) in Minnesota represented a landmark in U. S. legal history: It was the first time that an American state supreme court ruled that hypnotized victims and witnesses could not testify about their hypnotically elicited reminiscence in court, although any additional material obtained in hypnosis could be used to develop investigative leads that might ultimately be presented in a court of law. No fewer than 14 American state supreme courts have followed *State v. Mack* in the ensuing years; furthermore, subsequent to *Mack*, approximately 500 additional cases involving hypnosis in Minnesota were permitted to lapse.

The details of *Mack* serve to underscore the problems that occur when hypnotic age regression techniques are inadvertently abused. A woman began to bleed during intercourse at a motel. On arrival at the hospital, the internist asked her how she had sustained the injury, and she told him that it was the result of intercourse. The internist was skeptical, and stated that it had to be the result of a sharp instrument. She was treated appropriately for her vaginal lesion and released from the hospital. The internist's statement acted, in effect, as a prehypnotic suggestion. The next day, she attempted to recall how such a knife attack could have occurred, but was unable to do so. A few days later, she phoned the police, who quite correctly informed her that there was little that could be done, given her fragmentary recall of the events. The case should have ended at this point.

Some weeks later, however, the police phoned her to ask whether she would consent to be hypnotized. An appointment was arranged. The lay hypnotist who performed the session audiotaped it, but the cassette tape was subsequently lost. In hypnosis, the woman's story was that her male partner had been extremely courteous until they entered the motel roon, whereupon he produced a knife, ordered her to strip naked, pushed her onto the bed, and stabbed her repeatedly in the vagina. The court established that she had only one vaginal lesion and that it was consistent with her gynecological history. More tellingly, there was no injury to the external labia; the court held that both of these facts were not consistent with her recall of repeated stabs. Taken in totality, the woman's hypnotically elicited recollections of the events she described are consistent with the hypothesis of confabulation; they are reminiscent of the anecdote concerning the contradictions in the responses of Orne's (1951) German-speaking subject, since in both cases the hypnotized person "recalled" information that was acquired after the time that he or she was regressed. Indeed, the hypnotically elicited "recall" of the woman in *Mack* is a classic instance of how fantasy can come to be believed as fact when an age regression procedure is used.

*People v. Kempinski* (1980), a legal proceeding that took place in Joliet, Illinois, is an additional case in point. Kempinski was charged with first-degree murder solely on the basis of the hypnotized witness's recollections. The witness testified to being 270 feet from the murder event in conditions of semidarkness, looking into some lights. The case was thrown out of court following the testimony of an ophthalmologist who testified that a positive identification would be impossible at this distance. Kempinski, meanwhile, had spent 5 months in prison awaiting trial. As in *State v. Mack*, the only evidence against Kempinski was the hypnotically elicited recall of an eyewitness. It should be added that the case could have been quite complex had the eyewitness been within the 25-foot radius that the ophthalmologist specified as the maximal outer limit for positive identification under the prevailing light conditions. Under these circumstances, a jury might have convicted Kempinski, since there would not have been any way to verify whether confabulation had occurred.

In addition, however, there were elements of confabulation in this eyewitness's hypnotically elicited "recall." At different stages of the hypnotic interview, he variously described the attacker as being "five feet ten" and "six feet one," and at different points characterized his appearance as "very ugly" and "ordinary-looking," respectively. More remarkably, perhaps, he stated with great subjective conviction, "I know him"; on another occasion, in reply to a question concerning the attacker's face, he said, "I don't forget things like that." In addition, he reported having first met Kempinski when the latter was a high school senior and he was a sophomore. It was ascertained subsequently that the accused had not progressed beyond the second year of high school. The memory elicited in hypnosis had to be confabulated (Barnes, 1982).

Finally, a number of reincarnation reports elicited in hypnosis show evidence of confabulated memory. These are not discussed here, since they better illustrate other problems that arise when hypnotic age regression techniques are utilized in an applied setting.

## Creation of Pseudomemories

The possibility of creating a pseudomemory that comes to be accepted as veridical was recognized a century ago by the two eminent French investigators Pierre Janet and Hippolyte Bernheim. Indeed, Janet (1925/1976) devoted an entire chapter of his classic two-volume treatise, *Psychological Healing* (Vol. 1, pp. 589–698) to what he called "treatment by mental liquidation." Perhaps his most celebrated case was Marie, a 19-year-old woman who suffered from "serious crises" (p. 590) every month during menstruation. These lasted several days; each time, the menstrual flow ceased and delirium began. Between crises, she suffered acute panic attacks in which she hallucinated pools of blood. She also had several hysterical symptoms, including anesthesia on the left side of the face and blindness of the left eye.

Janet removed all of these symptoms by his technique of "mental liquidation." For instance, he ascertained that the blindness had occurred at the age of 6, when she was obliged to share a bed with another child who had an outbreak of impetigo on the left side of the face. Marie developed a similar outbreak, which was treated successfully by orthodox medical means, but the blindness persisted into young adulthood. Indeed, Marie believed it to be congenital. Janet treated the blindness by regressing her to the night in question and suggesting that the other child did not have impetigo. Janet reports that there were approximately 50 other such cases where he successfully used this treatment approach; they are scattered through his writings, dating from *L'Automatisme Psychologique* (1889/1973).

Bernheim (1888/1973) was also aware of the possibility of creating a pseudomemory; he described an analogue item that he constructed, in which he suggested to a female patient that she had awakened four times during the course of a designated night in order to go to the toilet, and had slipped and fallen on her nose on the fourth occasion. After hypnosis, she stated that she had had severe diarrhea on that night, which occasioned the four visits, and that she had fallen and hurt her nose on the last occasion. She remained convinced that these events were veridical memories, despite Bernheim's insisting that the events had been dreamed.

Several decades later, in apparent unawareness of Janet's work, Erickson reported two cases that have since been taken as additional instances of memory creation (Lamb, 1985; Mott, 1986). In the first of these (Erickson, 1935), Erickson successfully treated a young man for ejaculatio praecox by giving him a fabricated story during hypnosis, containing Freudian symbolism thought to be related to the presenting problem. The story concerned the patient's placing a lighted, partially smoked cigarette in a hand-painted glass ashtray, proferred to him by a young female artist who had made it. This heated the ashtray unevenly, causing it to crack into several pieces. His feelings of guilt, anxiety, and humiliation evoked by this suggested incident appeared to become related to his feelings following premature ejaculation. It is clear, however, from Erickson's report that the patient was aware at follow-up of the suggested nature of the story. For this reason, it does not appear to be an instance of the creation of a pseudomemory as described by Janet.

The case of the "February Man" (Erickson & Rossi, 1980) also may not qualify as an instance of memory creation, but for other reasons. It involved a case of a pregnant woman who feared that she would be an inadequate mother as the result of her own childhood, which was devoid of parental love, particularly on the part of her mother. The case itself is described as a synthesis of several such cases where Erickson used this technique with certain patients, though, like Janet, Erickson did not make his reason for choosing this technique (as opposed to any other) explicit. The term "February Man" was chosen because the patient's birthday fell during that month; he was intended to be "a kindly granduncle type who became a secure friend and confidant" (p. 525). The technique was to hypnotically age-regress the patient to various childhood ages and to introduce Erickson in the avuncular role of the February Man, a close friend of her father, who visited her and discussed various painful and/or humiliating incidents of her childhood. It is not clear from the report whether the February Man, a fictitious entity, came to be seen as real rather than as imagined. The memory creation procedure, however, appears to have been a technique of altering the manner in which the patient recalled past events of her life, by emphasizing their positive as opposed to their negative features. For instance, she regarded her fall on a dance floor at the age of 17 as an entirely devastating experience; through the February Man, it was restructured as a minor and unimportant event that was perhaps even amusing. Her first adolescent jilting by a male, her entering a university against her mother's wishes, her choice of studies, her scholastic struggles, and her limited social life at the time were all similarly treated. In short, there appears to have been no creation of pseudomemories; rather, Erickson appears to have confined himself to restructuring the affect attached to pre-existing veridical memories.

In recent years, there have been four clinical reports dealing with memory creation that more closely resemble Janet's cases. Baker and Boaz (1983) successfully treated a dental phobia by suggesting in hypnotic age regression that a traumatic dental experience some years earlier was in fact not at all traumatic. This alteration of the affect attached to the memory was effected by changing actual details of the memory, and was successful to the point that, some months later, the woman was able to undergo major oral surgery without fear. Lamb (1985) presented three cases (one fear of the dark, one dental phobia, and one airplane phobia) in which memories of a traumatic event were altered in a similar fashion. For instance, the dental phobia had originated at the age of 6, when a dentist had begun drilling before the Novocain had taken effect, despite the child's screams of pain. This memory was altered to the child's demanding that her dentist give her more Novocain, or else she would hit him in the mouth and bite his fingers if he did not comply—a request to which he was now remembered as complying. After hypnosis, the patient reported that the traumatic experience with the dentist seemed never to have occurred and was no longer important, since the dentist had been obliged to give her more Novocain and the drilling had been painless. She reported no further problems with dentistry at a 3-year follow-up. Domangue (1985) reported similar successful treatment using a memory creation technique (which she called "hypnotic regression and reframing") with two cases of insect phobia. Similarly, Miller (1986) reported success with this technique in two cases of performance anxiety and one of separation anxiety.

Experimental evidence was obtained recently to indicate that the creation of a pseudomemory is possible even in the benign context of the laboratory. Laurence and Perry (1983) reported that of 27 highly hypnotizable subjects, approximately 50% accepted the relatively neutrally cued suggestion that they *might* have been awakened one night of the previous week (for which it had been ascertained previously that they had no competing memories) and *might* have heard *some* loud nosies. Subsequent analyses (Laurence *et al.*, 1986) suggested that the acceptance of a suggested pseudomemory was linked to reports of the hidden-observer experience, duality in age regression, and intrusions (i.e., fabrications) found during the performance of a difficult dichotic-listening task both before *and* during hypnosis.

This suggested pseudomemory item was modeled on one that had previously been developed by Orne, and had been used in a television demonstration of this phenomenon (Barnes, 1982). The only difference between it and Orne's item was that the latter was more highly cued deliberately for demonstration purposes; the subject was told in hypnosis that she had been awakened by three loud noises. Subsequently, she stood by her hypnotically elicited recollections, even when presented with an audiocassette of her prehypnosis recall of the night in question, in which she had maintained that she had not dreamed and had not been awakened.

The purpose of Orne's demonstration was to mimic the situation of what may occur when a well-intended hypnotist who has access to information available only to the police tries to help a victim/witness to recall the events of a crime more clearly. Recently, such a situation actually occurred *in vivo*. It involved a particularly heinous rape, torture, and murder of an 88-year-old woman. A murder suspect was hypnotized, at the request of the police, by a colleague with professional credentials. The case was described by the Honorable Justice Mr. Michael Kirby (Kirby, 1984). He wrote:

> At his trial, much play was made by the prosecution of the fact that Forney [the accused] under hypnosis, described seeing a "rake" at the scene of the crime. The prosecution pointed out that no mention had been made of the rake by any report in any of the newspapers. To know about the rake, it was suggested, Forney had to have been at the scene. The trial ended before it was discovered that Forney did not mention the rake until after the following occurred whilst he was under hypnosis:
>
> *Forney*: (describing walking home after the crime). Seems like I grabbed something and ran back to . . . I walked most of the way because I was so tired.
> *Hypn*: (handed a note by the policeman which instructed him to ask about a rake). What did you grab?
> *Forney*: Base of something. Base of something.
> *Hypn*: Was it a rake?
> *Forney*: I don't know. It could have been.
> *Hypn*: Where did you get the rake from?
> *Forney*: I think I got it from the yard of a house. I was so mad. . . .
> *Hypn*: What are you doing with the rake?
> *Forney*: Running down at them . . . seems like I was fighting them.
> *Hypn*: Did they take the rake from you?
> *Forney*: Yeah.
> *Hypn*: And what did they do with it?
> *Forney*: I don't know.                                              (p. 160)

During a subsequent posthypnosis free-recall period, Forney mentioned "spontaneously" that he had grasped a rake that was at the scene of the crime. This case demonstrates, once again, that an inadequate grasp of the clinical and experimental literature on the phenomena of age regression can lead to misapplications of the most potentially fatal kind.

## Inadvertent Cueing by the Hypnotist, and His or Her Preconceptions

Orne (1982) recounts the telling incident of True's (1949) experiment on hypnotic age regression, which was published in the journal *Science*. True reported that 92% of his subjects, regressed to the day of their 10th birthday, could correctly identify the day of the week. By contrast 84% correctly identified the day of their 7th birthday, and 62% their 4th birthday. This finding could not be replicated by a number of other investigators, who had assumed that True had followed the habitual procedure of providing suggestions to return in time to a particular age, and then asking subjects questions pertaining to such matters as age, the date, and the day of the week. It transpired that no such procedure had been adopted by True, and *Science*, without consultation with the author, had altered his manuscript so that it did not in fact reflect what he had done at the procedural level. In fact, True's procedure was quite different from what had been generally assumed. When a subject reported experiencing the suggested age level, True proceeded to ask, "Is it Monday? Is it Tuesday? Is it Wednesday?" and so on. Furthermore, he had a perpetual calendar on his desk, and was thus in a position to verify instantly the accuracy of the subject's response.

Evidence supporting the view that True was inadvertently cueing his subjects, probably as a function of his beliefs about hypnosis, was provided in an experiment by O'Connell *et al.* (1970). In a definitive study of hypnotic age regression, these investigators employed a control group of actual 4-year-old children. Not one of them knew the day of the week. Barber (1970) summarized a number of studies that failed to replicate True's findings: He noted a general tendency for age-regressed subjects to report either that they did not know the day of the week on which a specific birthday occurred, or else to give the wrong answer.

A similar state of affairs exists in the police investigative literature. For instance, in *People v. Kempinski* (1980), it may at first blush appear surprising that the police, who are trained to be hard-nosed and skeptical of verbal reports, did not notice the contradictions in the eyewitness's hypnotically elicited testimony, particularly the confabulation of his having known Kempinski as a high school senior. The reason may well lie in the fact that the accused was known to the police. He had previously been charged with entering a home and stealing two firearms. The home belonged to the chief of detectives of the Joliet, Illinois, police department, who was in charge of the homicide investigation of which Kempinski had been accused. He was in a position to convey any hypotheses he had about the case to the police hypnotechnician who conducted the hypnotic interview. In a similar vein, the Forney case (Kirby, 1984) is a classical example of inadvertent cueing. In both of these cases, police acceptance of the confabulated memories elicited in hypnosis may have been facilitated additionally by the fact that the officers involved accepted the commonly held but erroneous view that hypnosis leads to accurate recall.

In addition, the literature on hypnotically elicited reports of reincarnation is replete with examples of inadvertent cueing that appear, in turn, to be closely linked to the hypnotist's beliefs. I. Wilson (1981/1982) compared the verbal reports of a previous existence provided by the clients of two British lay hypnotists. He found that, in both cases, the clients remained British in their hypnotically elicited prior life or lives. For both of them, also, no reincarnation reports occurred for periods earlier than the 16th century; not one caveman or cavewoman was found. The two lay hypnotists differed, however, in one crucial respect. One of them elicited fresh reincarnations 9 months to the day of the death of the previous incarnation; the clients of the other often took as many as 70 years before a new persona emerged. These differential reincarnation reports were in line with the hypnotists' beliefs.

There were further differences when these two hypnoreincarnationists were compared with three others (two American and one Welsh). The clients of these latter practitioners reported prior lives in ancient Egypt and Tibet. Furthermore, there was "a distinct silence from less fashionable civilizations such as the Hittites, the Assyrians or the Scythians" (I. Wilson, 1981/1982, p. 90). As we shall see, though, reports of reincarnation elicited in hypnosis cannot be understood entirely in terms of hypnotists' beliefs about hypnosis and of their inadvertent cueing of subjects.

## Beliefs and Needs of the Hypnotized Subject

As indicated earlier, the crime victim/witness who becomes a candidate for investigative hypnosis is likely to provide additional but not necessarily accurate information during hypnosis—partly as a function of wanting to help police; partly because the mere introduction of hypnosis may create an automatic expectancy that additional information is "stored" at nonconscious levels; and partly also because in hypnosis, the criterion for a veridical memory is liable to become reduced in this context. All of this probably occurs, even if the hypnotist does not create dramatic expectations for hypnosis.

Perhaps the best illustration of how subjects' needs and beliefs may color the reports they provide in age regression is given by Kampman and Hirvenoja (1978). Two subjects were regressed to previous existences on two occasions separated by a several-year interval. The first subject located five different reincarnated identities on the first occasion, and seven different ones on the second occasion seven years later. The other subject identified eight distinct personae on the first occasion, and an additional four personae on the second occasion. The authors concluded that the current needs of the individual were reflected in the reincarnated personae that each reported, both in terms of apparent realistic needs described, and also in terms of the emotional experiences the subjects "relived."

At a broader level, a considerable volume of research has focused upon the role of motives, attitudes, and sets in fashioning responses to an hypnotic procedure. While we do not maintain that hypnotic response is entirely the product of social-psychological variables, such variables may be particularly potent in field applications of hypnotic age regression, particularly those in which fantasy is licensed to wander freely. Summaries of these research data can be found in Barber (1969) and in Barber, Spanos, and Chaves (1974).

To round off this section on subjects' beliefs and needs, we should point out that such potential influencers of verbal reports are not always amenable to conscious awareness. A particularly eloquent example of this point is provided in a case report (Mutter, 1979). A woman claimed innocence of being an accomplice to a double murder. Her boyfriend was a drug dealer who had "ripped off" his supplier. To avoid retaliation, the dealer, accompanied by the female witness, visited the supplier's home and shot him to death. He sent the woman upstairs in order to determine whether anyone else was in the house, where she found a young woman. Despite the witness's repeated pleas, the dealer shot and killed the woman. He then left town, and after some consideration of her own position, the woman sought immunity from prosecution from the state attorney's office. The state attorney indicated his willingness to permit this, provided she could pass a polygraph test, which she proceeded to fail.

Mutter used the ingenious procedure of hypnotically dissociating the woman's left hand and teaching her an ideomotor response signal with it. She was told, during hypnosis, that whenever Mutter tapped the dorsum of her left hand, the index finger and thumb would touch with a reflexive movement. Having established this reflex action, Mutter regressed her to the time of the offense, and added the suggestion that the index finger and thumb would touch whenever he tapped her hand and whenever she said anything that was untrue.

She was asked whether she had killed the woman, and she replied, "No." The polygraph indicated deception, but there was no ideomotor response. She was then asked whether she had pulled the trigger of the gun that had killed the woman; again the reply was negative. This time both the polygraph and the ideomotor response supported her verbal report of innocence. Mutter (1979) commented: "The conflicting responses suggested that Kay's unconscious mind believed she killed the girl. Further questioning revealed that Kay felt guilty when she found the female victim and felt directly responsible for her death, even though she pleaded for the victim's life" (p. 48).

Clearly, subjects' beliefs and needs, particularly in affect-laden field contexts, can be extremely complicated and can have a major bearing upon what is obtained when an age regression technique is utilized.

*Source Amnesia*

The main problem of evaluating verbal reports of reincarnation[1] experiences is that, in the majority of cases, the hypnotically elicited verbal reports of such phenomena are routinely taken at face value, and no attempt is made to verify independently the veracity of subjects' verbal reports. For example, in only three cases known to us was any attempt made to verify whether hypnotically elicited reincarnated personae ever lived, whether any of the people (e.g., spouses, friends, and parents) identified ever lived, whether places that were named actually existed, and whether events described (e.g., marriages or property transactions) ever occurred.

Two of these cases are inconclusive. Despite extensive investigation, it could not be established that Bridey Murphy (Bernstein, 1956) ever existed, nor could any of the people, places, and events she described be verified. In a Canadian case (Stearn, 1969), the reports of similar matters furnished by Joanne McIver, a teenage schoolgirl, who in hypnotically induced reincarnation became Susan Garnier, likewise could not be verified independently. These cases are inconclusive because records may still exist, but cannot be found. In the third case (Stevenson, 1976), independent evidence was found that bore upon the reports of Dolores Jay, who in hypnosis reported that she was Gretchen Gottleib. Gretchen was allegedly the daughter of the mayor of Ebeswalde, now in East Germany, at the time of Bismarck's reunification of Germany. Both church and village records dating from 1740 indicated that no Gottleib had ever lived in the village during this time span, and that no Gottleib had ever been mayor.

There was, however, a quite interesting aspect of this case that suggests an additional hypothesis for evaluating hypnotically elicited reports of reincarnation. In hypnosis, Dolores/Gretchen spoke German in answer to questions put to her in English. Unlike Orne's (1951) German-speaking subject, Dolores claimed never to have learned German, and she was born in the United States. Reports vary as to her degree of fluency in that language. Stevenson (1976), while noting errors in grammar, rated her German as "responsive"; that is, in his opinion, she could provide sensible answers to questions posed in German. By contrast, Roby (1975), a German-speaking United Press International journalist, characterized her German linguistic

---

1. Reincarnation is a spiritualist belief that meets our criterion of acceptability: Believing in it does no harm to other people. Unfortunately, since Bernstein (1956) reported on Bridey Murphy, a new publishing genre for books on reincarnation and hypnosis has emerged. The dust-jacket descriptions of these books frequently imply that science, via the utilization of hypnosis, has *proved* that reincarnation is a veridical phenomenon. As with the beliefs of many religions concerning the possibility of an afterlife, the scientific method is probably too blunt a method to confirm or disconfirm such an hypothesis. Indeed, many theologians maintain that an afterlife is entirely a matter of belief, on which scientific data cannot possibly be brought to bear.

skills as at a Berlitz level. He noted, however, that she used words that were current in German a century ago but have since become archaic, as well as contemporary words that were *not* in usage a century ago. This puzzling issue suggests that, certainly for reincarnation reports, and possibly in the police investigative context as well, the hypothesis of source amnesia needs to be entertained.

Source amnesia is one of the more fascinating of the amnesias. It was first documented by Evans and Thorn (1966); it involves the tendency of highly hypnotizable subjects to learn esoteric items of general knowledge in hypnosis, such as the color of amethyst, a blue or purple gemstone, when it is heated. Few people know that the correct answer is yellow. Questioned after hypnosis, subjects have no difficulty in providing the correct answer, almost invariably with a fast latency. When asked how they knew this, those who are capable of passing this highly difficult item are amnesic to the hypnotic context (or source) in which this information was learned. Some report that they do not know; others rationalize and reply, for instance, that they have a geologist friend with whom they have talked recently. The incidence of the phenomenon ranges across studies from 33% (Evans, 1979) to approximately 50% (Laurence *et al.*, 1986). It is also a phenomenon confined to highly hypnotizable individuals. There are at least two reports in the reincarnation and hypnosis literature in which source amnesia was demonstrated clearly to provide the only viable alternative explanation to the hypothesis of reincarnation.

E. R. Hilgard (1977) documented a case in which a college student had been subjected to hypnosis at a party, and had discovered himself apparently re-experiencing life as it was at the time of Queen Victoria. He was convinced that he was reincarnated, but had the good sense to seek expert advice and to accept the procedures Hilgard recommended. These included an initial session of nonhypnotic free recall, which, as Orne *et al.* (1984) have indicated, is mandatory in the legal investigative situation. On careful interview, Hilgard established that, years earlier, the client had studied the British royal family intensively, and had since forgotten that he had done this. In the meantime, his interests had changed from literary to scientific pursuits. It is instructive to reread Janet (1889/1973), in which he maintained that, as the result of stress, ideas could become *désagrégées* (disassociated) when they had the potential to fuel neurotic symptoms. In the case presented by Hilgard (1977), the evidence appears to be that a person can have an encapsulated idea without its being detrimental to normal, adaptive functioning. This is also almost invariably the case when laboratory subjects spontaneously relive a painful experience during an age regression item; among such subjects, psychopathology is extremely rare (Laurence *et al.*, 1985).

Another case of source amnesia was presented by Lowes Dickinson (1911) to the British Society for Psychical Research. It involved a woman who, when hypnotized by a physician, described in great detail an earlier existence during the reign of King Richard II of England toward the end of the 14th century. She showed an almost encyclopedic knowledge about members of the royal court, and of the customs and costumes of the period. While the subject was communicating with this earlier persona, using a planchette (a type of Ouija board) in Lowes Dickinson's presence, the source of this earlier incarnation became known. It transpired that a book by Emily Holt entitled *The Countess Maude*, which she had read when she was aged 12, contained all of the relevant information. Lowes Dickinson confirmed this in a subsequent hypnosis session.

These two cases are the only known ones where source amnesia provides a naturalistic explanation of otherwise highly puzzling phenomena; indeed, few proponents of reincarnation even attempt to explore a source amnesia hypothesis. This is unfortunate; careful exploration of this hypothesis in the case of Dolores Jay might have uncovered the source of her linguistic fluency in German. Furthermore, it has been reported by Gardner (1951) that Virginia Tighe, who became Bridey Murphy in hypnosis, was very devoted to Mrs. Anthony Corkell, an Irish widow who lived across the street from Ms. Tighe during the latter's childhood. It is possible that source amnesia was implicated in this case also; Mrs. Corkell's maiden name was Bridie Murphy, according to Gardner's information.

## CONCLUSION

In a recent paper, Reiser (1985) wrote:

> Assertions have been made in articles and in numerous court cases that a previously hypnotized witness automatically has tainted memory, is unable to discriminate among temporal events, becomes more certain about his recall and is impervious to cross-examination (Diamond, 1980). The evidence to support these statements consists of a few "horror stories" where hypnosis was misused or abused, most often by improperly trained health professionals. (pp. 516–517)

As the present chapter maintains, Reiser's assertion is inaccurate but beside the point. On *any* occasion that an age regression technique is used to elicit memories, what is recalled may be fact or fantasy, and is likely to be a subtle admixture of both. In the clinical situation there is usually no need to independently verify the truth or falsity of hypnotically elicited memories, given the long-standing clinical belief that it can be just as effective to treat a person's fantasies of his or her past as it is to treat documented realities of that past (Orne *et al.*, 1984). This is not the case in the legal investigative setting, where, far too often, the unverified hypnotically elicited recall of a witness is the *only* source of "evidence" against the accused person's protestations of innocence. The potential for a "horror story" exists on every occasion that a court of law permits such a practice. Such a situation constitutes the most dangerous abuse of age regression techniques at present.

Notwithstanding, hypnosis has a limited but often useful role to play in the legal system. When police investigations have dried up and the police have no leads to pursue, hypnosis, if conducted properly following the guidelines spelled out by Orne *et al.* (1984), may occasionally provide a necessary vital scintilla of evidence; this may be sufficient to build up a case that can be prosecuted independently of the victim/witness' hypnotically elicited recollections presented as testimony.

*People v. Woods et al.* (1977) is a case in point. A busload of children and their driver were abducted by some men driving vans. They were herded into the vans, driven to an abandoned quarry, and sealed inside. The bus driver was subsequently able to dig his way out. He had attempted to memorize the license plate numbers of two of the vans, but was unable to supply them during police questioning. In hypnosis he reported two seven-digit license plate numbers, one of which was correct to one digit, although he had provided three of the correct digits prior to hypnosis. This information led to the arrest and conviction of three individuals who had planned to demand a ransom. This particular case, which took place at Chowchilla, California, is often cited favorably by proponents of unrestricted use by police of hypnosis devoid of safeguards. Ironically, it is rarely pointed out that the bus driver did not have to testify in court. He did not need to, since the police were able to utilize the license plate data to develop an independent case against the defendants that stood up in court under cross-examination.

There are other potential positive applications of age regression techniques. For instance, as indicated earlier, Janet (1925/1976) reported that he obtained therapeutic success in approximately 50 cases during the years between 1889 and 1925. His work deserves a careful rereading in order to ascertain the conditions under which he attempted his "mental liquidation" technique, and, more importantly, to locate the situations where he felt that such a treatment technique was ill advised. Moreover, data suggest (Fiore, 1978) that reincarnation therapy, which depends upon a regression procedure, may benefit a percentage of patients. Sexton and Maddock's (1979) imaginative use of an age progession technique (in which patients were reunited with a deceased love one in a hypnotically elicited heaven) in the successful treatment of schizophrenia and depression appears to be the reverse side of this coin. Clinical research is clearly needed to ascertain the conditions under which treatment programs would benefit from a reincarnation or age progression technique.

The investigator charting this *terra incognita* would be wise, however, to tread carefully. The phenomena of hypnotic age regression can, at the subjective level, be highly convincing, so much so that Perry once had the experience of a female subject in a laboratory study crying during age regression and recounting a painful childhood experience; after hypnosis, in reviewing this incident, the subject stated that she was almost certain that the painful childhood experience had never occurred. When hypnotized subjects themselves cannot be certain whether their hypnotically elicited recollections are fact or fantasy, it behooves the investigator to be cautious in interpreting the age regression phenomena that he or she encounters. As the British poet Alexander Pope, in *"An Essay on Criticism"* (1711/1980), put it with much wit and elegance:

> A little learning *is a dangerous thing;*
> *Drink deep, or taste not the Pierian spring*[2];
> *There shallow draughts intoxicate the brain,*
> *And drinking largely sobers us again.*
> 　　　　　　　　　　(Pope, 1711/1980, p. 51)

While it is a historical impossibility that Pope had age regression in mind when he wrote these couplets, his caution is mandatory for *any* discussion of the applied use of age regression techniques.

## ACKNOWLEDGMENTS

This chapter was prepared while Campbell Perry was in receipt of Grant No. A6361 ("Errors of Memory in Hypnosis") from the Natural Sciences and Engineering Research Council (NSERC) of Canada, and while Jean-Roch Laurence was supported by an NSERC 5-year University Research Fellowship. NSERC's continuing support is acknowledged gratefully. Joyce D'Eon is now affiliated with the Department of Psychology, Royal Ottawa Regional Rehabilitation Centre, Ottawa, Ontario, Canada. We wish especially to thank Robert Nadon for his critical reading of the manuscript during its preparation, and Sherri Rufh and Danielle Laurence for their careful typing of it during various phases of its preparation.

## REFERENCES

Baker, S. R., & Boaz, D. (1983). The partial reformulation of a traumatic memory of a dental phobia during trance: A case study. *International Journal of Clinical and Experimental Hypnosis, 31,* 14–18.

Barber, T. X. (1969). *Hypnosis: A scientific approach.* New York: Van Nostrand Reinhold.

Barber, T. X. (1970). *LSD, marijuana, yoga and hypnosis.* Chicago: Aldine.

Barber, T. X., Spanos, N. P., & Chaves, J. F. (1974). *Hypnosis, imagination and human potentialities.* New York: Pergamon Press.

Barnes, M. (Director). (1982). *Hypnosis on trial* [Television program]. London: British Broadcasting Corporation.

Bernheim, H. (1884). *De la suggestion dans l'état hypnotique et dans l'état de veille.* Paris: Doin.

2. The Pierian spring was a spring that was held to be sacred to the Muses.

Bernheim, H. (1973). *Hypnosis and suggestion in psychotherapy.* New York: Jason Aronson. (Original work published 1888)

Bernstein, M. (1956). *The search for Bridey Murphy.* New York: Lancer.

Binet, A. (1896). *Alterations of personality* (H.G. Galdwin, Trans.). London: Chapman & Hall.

Bourru, H., & Burot, F. (1888). *Variations de la personalité.* Paris: Hachette.

Bower, G. H. (1981). Mood and memory. *American Psychologist, 36,* 129–148.

Bowers, K. S. (1973). Situationism in psychology: An analysis and a critique. *Psychological Review, 80,* 307–336.

Braid, J. (1843). *Neurypnology; or the rationale of nervous sleep considered in relation with animal magnetism.* London: J. Churchill.

de Rochas, A. (1896). *Les états profonds de l'hypnose* (3rd ed.) Paris: Charmel.

Diamond, B. L. (1980). Inherent problems in the use of pretrial hypnosis on a prospective witness. *California Law Review, 68,* 313–349.

di Faria, J. C. (1906). *De la cause du sommeil lucide; ou étude sur la nature de l'homme* (2nd ed., D. G. Dalgado, ed.) Paris: Henri Jouve. (Original work published 1819)

Domangue, B. B. (1985). Hypnotic regression and reframing in the treatment of insect phobias. *American Journal of Psychotherapy, 34,* 206–214.

Dywan, J., & Bowers, K.S. (1983). The use of hypnosis to enhance recall. *Science, 222,* 184–185.

Erickson, M. H. (1935). A study of an experimental neurosis hypnotically induced in a case of ejaculatio praecox. *British Journal of Medical Psychology, 15,* 34–50.

Erickson, M. H., & Rossi, E. L. (1980). The February Man: Facilitating new identity in hypnotherapy. In E. L. Rossi (Ed.), *The collected papers of Milton H. Erickson on hypnosis* (Vol. 4, pp. 525–542). New York: Irvington.

Evans, F. J. (1979). Contextual forgetting: Posthypnotic source amnesia. *Journal of Abnormal Psychology, 88,* 556–563.

Evans, F. J., & Thorn, W. A. F. (1966). Two types of post-hypnotic amnesia: Recall amnesia and source amnesia. *International Journal of Clinical and Experimental Hypnosis, 14,* 162–179.

Fiore, E. (1978). *You have been here before: A psychologist looks at past lives.* New York: Ballantine.

Gardner, M. (1951). *Fads and fallacies in the name of science.* New York: Dover.

Gill, M. M., & Brenman, M. (1959). *Hypnosis and related states.* New York: International Universities Press.

Hilgard, E. R. (1965). *Hypnotic susceptibility.* New York: Harcourt, Brace & World.

Hilgard, E. R. (1977). *Divided consciousness: Multiple controls in human thought and action.* New York: Wiley.

Hilgard, E. R., Hilgard, J. R., Macdonald, H., Morgan, A. H., & Johnson, L. S. (1978). Covert pain in hypnotic analgesia: Its reality as tested by the real–simulator design. *Journal of Abnormal Psychology, 87,* 655–663.

Hilgard, E. R., Morgan, A. H., & Macdonald, H. (1975). Pain and dissociation in the cold pressor test: A study of hypnotic analgesia with "hidden reports" through automatic key pressing and automatic talking. *Journal of Abnormal Psychology, 84,* 280–289.

Hilgard, J. R. (1979). *Personality and hypnosis: A study of imaginative involvement* (2nd ed.). Chicago: University of Chicago Press.

Jaffe, J. R. (1980). Hypnosis. *Police Journal, 53,* 233–237.

Janet, P. (1973). *L'automatisme psychologique.* Paris: Centre National de la Recherche Scientifique. (Original work published 1889)

Janet, P. (1976). *Psychological healing* (2 vols., E. Paul & C. Paul, Trans.). New York: Arno. (Original work published 1925)

Kampman, R., & Hirvenoja, R. (1978). Dynamic relation of the secondary personality induced by hypnosis to the present personality. In F. H. Frankel & H. S. Zammansky (Eds.), *Hypnosis at its bicentennial: Selected papers* (pp. 183–188). New York: Plenum.

Kihlstrom, J. F. (1985). Hypnosis. *Annual Review of Psychology, 36*, 385–418.

Kirby, M. D. (1984). Hypnosis and the law. *Criminal Law Journal, 8*, 152–165.

Lamb, C. S. (1985). Hypnotically-induced deconditioning: Reconstruction of memories in the treatment of phobias. *American Journal of Clinical Hypnosis, 28*, 56–62.

Laurence, J.-R., Nadon, R., Bowers, K., Perry, C., & Regher, G. (1985). *Clinical encounters in the experimental context.* Paper presented at the 93rd Annual Convention of the American Psychological Association, Los Angeles.

Laurence, J.-R., Nadon, R., Nogrady, H., & Perry, C. (1986). Duality, dissociation, and memory creation in highly hypnotizable subjects. *International Journal of Clinical and Experimental Hypnosis, 34*, 295–310.

Laurence, J.-R., & Perry, C. (1981). The "hidden observer" phenomenon in hypnosis: Some additional findings. *Journal of Abnormal Psychology, 90*, 334–344.

Laurence, J.-R., & Perry, C. (1983). Hypnotically created memory among highly hypnotizable subjects. *Science, 222*, 523–524.

Laurence, J.-R., Perry, C., & Kihlstrom, J. (1983). "Hidden observer" phenomena in hypnosis: An experimental creation? *Journal of Personality and Social Psychology, 44*, 163–169.

LeCron, L. M. (1965). A study of age regression under hypnosis. In L. M. LeCron (Ed.), *Experimental hypnosis* (pp. 155–174). New York: Citadel Press.

Lowes Dickinson, G. (1911). A case of emergence of a latent memory under hypnosis. *Proceedings of the Society for Psychical Research, 25*, 455–467.

Malcolm, J. (1984). *In the Freud archives.* New York: Knopf.

Mesmer, F. A. (1970). *Mémoire sur la découverte de magnétisme animal.* In M. M. Tinterow (Ed.), *Foundations of hypnosis: From Mesmer to Freud* (pp. 31–57). Springfield, IL: Charles C. Thomas. (Original work published 1779)

Miller, A. (1986). Brief reconstructive hypnotherapy for anxiety reactions: Three case reports. *American Journal of Clinical Hypnosis, 28*, 138–146.

Morgan, A. H., & Hilgard, J. R. (1978–1979). The Stanford Hypnotic Clinical Scale for Adults. *American Journal of Clinical Hypnosis, 21*, 134–147.

Mott, T., Jr. (1986). Editorial: Current status of hypnosis in the treatment of phobias. *American Journal of Clinical Hypnosis, 28*, 135–137.

Mutter, C. B. (1979). Regressive hypnosis and the polygraph: A case study. *American Journal of Clinical Hypnosis, 22*, 47–50.

Nadon, R. (1983). *The skills of hypnosis.* Unpublished master's thesis, Concordia University, Montréal.

Nogrady, H., McConkey, K. M., Laurence, J.-R., & Perry, C. (1983). Dissociation, duality, and demand characteristics in hypnosis. *Journal of Abnormal Psychology, 92*, 223–235.

O'Connell, D. N., Shor, R. E., & Orne, M. T. (1970). Hypnotic age regression: An empirical and methodological analysis. *Journal of Abnormal Psychology Monographs, 76* (3, Pt. 2).

Orne, M. T. (1951). The mechanisms of hypnotic age regression: An empirical study. *Journal of Abnormal and Social Psychology, 46*, 213–225.

Orne, M. T. (1959). The nature of hypnosis: Artifact and essence. *Journal of Abnormal and Social Psychology, 58*, 277–299.

Orne, M. T. (1979). On the simulating subject as a quasi-control group in hypnosis research: What, why and how. In E. Fromm & R. E. Shor (Eds.), *Hypnosis: Developments in research and new perspectives* (2nd ed., pp. 519–565). Chicago: Aldine.

Orne, M. T. (1980). On the construct of hypnosis: How its definition affects research and its clinical application. In G. D. Burrows & L. Dennerstein (Eds.), *Handbook of hypnosis and psychosomatic medicine* (pp. 29–51). Amsterdam: Elsevier/North Holland.

Orne, M. T. (1982). *Affidavit to the State Supreme Court of California on People v. Shirley.* Mimeograph.

Orne, M. T., Soskis, D. A., Dinges, D. G. & Orne, E. C. (1984). Hypnotically induced testimony and the criminal justice system. In G. L. Wells & E. F. Loftus (Eds.), *Advances in the psychology of eyewitness testimony* (pp. 171–213). New York: Cambridge University Press.

People v. Kempinski, No. W80CF 352 (Cir. Ct., 12th Dist., Will Co., Ill. Oct. 21, 1980).

People v. Woods et al., No. 63187 ABNC (Alameda Co., Cal., Dec. 15, 1977).

Perry, C. (1977). Is hypnotizability modifiable? *International Journal of Clinical and Experimental Hypnosis, 25,* 125–146.

Perry, C., & Laurence, J.-R. (1982). Review of M. Reiser, *Handbook of investigative hypnosis. International Journal of Clinical and Experimental Hypnosis, 30,* 443–448.

Perry, C., & Laurence, J.-R. (1983). The enhancement of memory by hypnosis in the legal investigative situation. *Canadian Psychology/Psychologie Canadienne, 24,* 155–167.

Perry, C., & Walsh, B. (1978). Inconsistencies and anomalies of response as a defining characteristic of hypnosis. *Journal of Abnormal Psychology, 87,* 574–577.

Pope, A. (1980). An essay on criticism. In M. Price (Ed.), *The selected poetry of Pope* (pp. 45–67). New York: Meridian. (Original work published 1711)

Puységur, A. M. J. Chastenet, Marquis de. (1784–1785). *Mémoires pour servir à l'histoire et à l'établissement du magnétisme animal* (2 vols.). Paris: Cellot.

Reiser, M. (1980). *Handbook of investigative hypnosis.* Los Angeles: Law Enforcement Hypnosis Institute.

Reiser, M. (1985). Investigative hypnosis: Scientism, memory tricks and power plays. In J. K. Zeig (Ed.), *Ericksonian psychotherapy*: Vol. I (pp. 511–523). New York: Brunner/Mazel.

Roby, E. F., (1975, February 3). Another life emerges from "Gretchen's" mysterious past. *Montréal Gazette,* section C, p. 21.

Sarbin, T. R., & Coe, W. C. (1972). *Hypnosis: A social-psychological analysis of influence communication.* New York: Holt, Rinehart & Winston.

Sexton, R. O., & Maddock, R. C. (1979). Age regression and age progression in psychotic and neurotic oppression. *American Journal of Clinical Hypnosis, 22,* 37–41.

Sheehan, P. W., & Perry, C. W. (1976). *Methodologies of hypnosis: A critical appraisal of contemporary paradigms of hypnosis.* Hillsdale, NJ: Erlbaum.

Spanos, N. P. (1983). The hidden observer as an experimental creation. *Journal of Personality and Social Psychology, 44,* 170–176.

Spanos, N. P., & Barber, T. X. (1974). Toward a convergence in hypnosis research. *American Psychologist, 29,* 500–511.

Spanos, N. P., de Groot, H. P., Tiller, D. K., Weekes, J. R., & Bertrand, L. P. (1985). Trance logic duality and hidden observer responding in hypnotic, imagination control, and simulating subjects: A social psychological analysis. *Journal of Abnormal Psychology, 94,* 611–623.

Spanos, N. P., & Hewitt, E. C. (1980). The hidden observer in hypnotic analgesia: Discovery or experimental creation? *Journal of Personality and Social Psychology, 39,* 1201–1214.

Stalnaker, J. M., & Riddle, E. E. (1932). The effect of hypnosis on long-delayed memory. *Journal of General Psychology, 6,* 429–440.

State v. Mack, Minn. 292 N.W.2d 764 (1980).

Stearn, J. (1969). *The search for the girl with the blue eyes.* New York: Bantam.

Stevenson, I. (1976). A preliminary report of a new case of responsive xenoglossy: The case of Gretchen. *Journal of the American Society for Psychical Research, 70,* 65–77.

Sutcliffe, J. P. (1961). "Credulous" and "skeptical" views of hypnotic phenomena: Experiments on esthesia, hallucination and delusion. *Journal of Abnormal and Social Psychology, 62,* 189–200.

Tallant, B. K. (1984). *Hypnotic conditions—their effect on memory.* Paper presented at the 36th Annual Meeting of the Society for Clinical and Experimental Hypnosis, San Antonio, TX.

True, R. M. (1949). Experimental control in hypnotic age regression states. *Science, 110,* 583–584.

Weitzenhoffer, A. M., & Hilgard, E. R. (1962). *Stanford Hypnotic Susceptibility Scale, Form C.* Palo Alto, CA: Consulting Psychologists Press.

Wilson, I. (1982). *Reincarnation?* Harmondsworth, England: Penguin. (Original work published as *Mind Out of Time?,* 1981)

Wilson, S. C., & Barber, T. X. (1983). The fantasy-prone personality: Implications for understanding imagery, hypnosis and parapsychological phenomena. In A. A. Sheikh (Ed.), *Imagery: Current theory, research and application* (pp. 340–387). New York: Wiley.

# INDUCED AND SPONTANEOUS MODELS OF REVERSIBLE MEMORY DISRUPTION

# 6

## Posthypnotic Amnesia: Dissociation of Content and Context

FREDERICK J. EVANS
*University of Medicine and Dentistry of*
*New Jersey–Robert Wood Johnson Medical School*

### POSTHYPNOTIC AMNESIA: OVERVIEW

#### Posthypnotic Amnesia and Memory

A review of posthypnotic amnesia may at first seem out of place in a book on hypnosis and memory. Like the claims of memory enhancement with hypnosis, memory loss is yet another suggestion that some people experience when hypnotized. The relevance of posthypnotic amnesia is clear if the use of hypnosis to manipulate recall involves cognitive mechanisms, especially so if forgetting and retrieval share similar cognitive processes. The temporary nature of the induced amnesia provides one method for studying the subsequent postamnesia retrieval process, particularly if the suggested memory loss obeys normal memory mechanisms.

Posthypnotic amnesia is dramatic because of the ease with which it can be induced in some deeply hypnotized subjects. The hypnotist casually suggests that, upon awakening from hypnosis, the subject will be unable to recall his or her hypnotic experiences, usually until an appropriate cue word is given. The deeply hypnotized subject will typically report that the hypnotic experiences seem discontinuous from normal waking life. Even if a subject recalls some of these experiences, he or she may have considerable difficulty doing so, sometimes showing confusion about the sequence of events or about such details as whether a suggestion of arm rigidity involved the left or right arm. It seems incongruous that some people can have so much difficulty describing what they have been doing during the preceding few minutes. The ease with which the amnesia can be reversed (Nace, Orne, & Hammer, 1974) indicates that any forgetting that occurs is at best a temporary phenomenon.

Because of the ease with which verbal reports can be manipulated, some investigators reject verbal reports as unreliable, and mistakenly dismiss posthypnotic amnesia as merely the result of compliance (Coe, 1978), role playing (Sarbin & Coe, 1972), strategic enactment (Spanos, 1986), or other strictly motivational influences (Barber & Calverley, 1966). These viewpoints are in contrast to those showing theoretical allegiance to a contemporary neodissociation view of hypnosis (Hilgard, 1977), which treats posthypnotic amnesia as being similar to other functional amnesias observed in the clinic (Bowers, 1976; Evans, 1980) and potentially understandable within a framework of modern cognitive psychology (Kihlstrom, 1977). From this viewpoint, the experience of posthypnotic amnesia is like forgetting where one has laid down the car keys, blocking an acquaintance's name at a cocktail party, the tip-of-the-tongue phenomenon, or difficulty in remembering nighttime dreams. In some respects, posthypnotic amnesia also parallels "state-dependent" learning (Overton, 1968), in which information processed under the influence of a drug (e.g., alcohol, sedatives, etc.) is not available for recall in the nondrugged condition. However, a recent study (Kihlstrom, Brenneman, Pistole, & Shor, 1985) points out some important empirical differences between state-specific learning and posthypnotic amnesia.

Historically, posthypnotic amnesia has been viewed as similar to the functional memory disturbances observed in clinical cases of hysteria, fugue, dissociative states, and multiple personality (Nemiah, 1979; Reed, 1979), and to the "islands of memory" often observed in Korsakoff syndrome (Talland, 1965). These involve compelling disturbances of memory for personal experiences and for material with strong autobiographical components (Kihlstrom & Evans, 1979). The essential intactness of the critical memories during the posthypnotic amnesia period is documented by their eventual recovery (Hull, 1933; Nace et al., 1974), as well as by subtle hints of their presence and availability in other cognitive operations, such as relearning or recognition (Hull, 1933; Williamsen, Johnson, & Ericksen, 1965).

Hull (1933) originally suggested that the mechanisms of posthypnotic amnesia involve either the way in which the material is *processed* in the memory store, or the way in which it is *retrieved* from the memory store. The observation that subjects high and low in hypnotizability recall the same number of experiences after amnesia has been lifted (Cooper, 1972; Kihlstrom & Evans, 1976) would seem to rule out the former hypothesis.

Much of the previous research on posthypnotic amnesia has been reviewed earlier (Cooper, 1972; Evans, 1980; Hilgard, 1965; Hull, 1933; Kihlstrom, 1985; Kihlstrom & Evans, 1979; Orne, 1966; Spanos, 1986; Weitzenhoffer, 1953). The present overview is selective, examining one specific hypothesis: Posthypnotic amnesia involves a temporary disruption of normal retrieval strategies, possibly related to dissociative processes. This hypothesis is directly relevant to the theme of this volume on hypnosis and memory. For example, using hypnosis to facilitate recall of currently unavailable experiences may well involve the same kind of cognitive restructuring that occurs when retrieval cues are temporarily disrupted during posthypnotic amnesia. The temporarily forgotten material is almost certainly dissociated from normal encoding or retrieval strategies to the extent that the experienced material is available for other cognitive processes, such as relearning, savings, and recognition (Graham & Patton, 1968; Hull, 1933; Williamsen *et al.*, 1965). The fact that reversibility occurs is itself a form of recovery of memory utilizing a hypnotic paradigm, even though the material has been forgotten only minutes before. The reversibility process is currently less understood than the temporary failure to utilize normal retrieval strategies that seems to be the central cognitive process of posthypnotic amnesia.

## Measurement and Assessment of Posthypnotic Amnesia

### Posthypnotic Amnesia and Standardized Hypnosis Scales

For the reader who is unfamiliar with research in the area, a digression is necessary to describe posthypnotic amnesia as it occurs in the laboratory setting. Research in hypnosis has been aided enormously by the development of standardized hypnosis scales, including the Stanford Hypnotic Susceptibility Scale, Forms A, B, and C (SHSS:A, SHSS:B, SHSS:C) developed by Weitzenhoffer and Hilgard (1959, 1962), and the Harvard Group Scale of Hypnotic Susceptibility, Form A (HGSHS:A), a self-scored adaptation of the SHSS:A developed for group administration by Shor and Orne (1962). These scales have been constructed with considerable care and have adequate psychometric properties (Hilgard, 1965).

Each of these scales consists of a standard hypnotic induction procedure (about 20 minutes). A series of 12 suggestions of graded difficulty is administered; each of these suggestions calls for an alteration in subjective experience that does not necessarily reflect objective reality. For example, during the HGSHS:A,[1] the subject is asked to extend his or her arms and feel the hands being drawn together as if by magnets (Suggestion 7); he or she is asked to experience a fly buzzing closely around, darting annoyingly at his or her face (Suggestion 9). Each suggested alteration of inner, subjective experience is associated with some behavioral index by which an external observer can

---

1. Most of the research reported here is based on the HGSHS:A. The HGSHS:A suggestions are as follows: (1) head nodding forward; (2) eye closure (during induction); (3) hand lowering; (4) arm immobilization; (5) finger lock; (6) arm rigidity; (7) hands moving together; (8) inability to shake head "no"; (9) fly hallucination; (10) eye catalepsy; (11) posthypnotic suggestion; (12) posthypnotic amnesia. Suggestions 1, 2, and 12 are not included in the evaluation of posthypnotic amnesia.

gauge the subject's response to the suggestion.[2] The number of suggestions "passed" yields a score ranging from 0 to 12. Subjects are traditionally classified as low (scoring 0–4), medium (5–7), or high (8–12) in hypnotic susceptibility.[3]

Toward the end of the standardized scale, a suggestion for posthypnotic amnesia is administered:

> In a moment I shall begin counting backwards from twenty to one. You will gradually wake up, but for most of the count you will still remain in the state you are now in. By the time I reach "five" you will open your eyes, but you will not be fully aroused. When I get to "one" you will be fully alert, in your normal state of wakefulness. You probably will have the impression that you have slept because you will have difficulty in remembering all the things I have told you and all the things you did or felt. In fact, you will find it to be so much of an effort to recall any of these things that you will have no wish to do so. It will be much easier simply to forget everything until I tell you that you can remember. You will remember nothing of what has happened until I say to you: "Now you can remember everything!" (Shor & Orne, 1962, p. 11)

After termination of hypnosis and testing of the posthypnotic suggestion, the subject is asked to recall his or her experience of hypnosis. On the HGSHS:A, the memory report is collected in written form in the response booklet provided, according to the following instructions:

> Now please take your Response Booklet, break the seal and turn to the *second* page of the Booklet. Do *not* turn to the *third page* until I specifically instruct you to do so later. On the *second page* please write down briefly in your own words a list of the things that happened since you began looking at the target. (Shor & Orne, 1962, p. 11)

After 3 minutes have passed, the amnesia suggestion is canceled by means of the prearranged reversibility cue. The subjects are given 2 minutes more to report any additional memories.

> All right, now listen carefully to my words. *Now you can remember everything*. Please turn to *page three* and write down a list of anything else that you remember now that you did not remember previously. (Shor & Orne, 1962, p. 11)

## Quantifying Posthypnotic Amnesia

*Initial Recall.* Posthypnotic amnesia has traditionally been assessed in terms of the number of suggested items the subject remembers after hypnosis

---

2. Because of the group setting in which the HGSHS:A is administered, the subjects make retrospective self-ratings after hypnosis (and posthypnotic amnesia) is terminated. These self-ratings are highly reliable (O'Connell, 1964).

3. For expositional clarity, data for only subjects high and low in hypnotizability are presented in most studies reviewed here.

and before the administration of the reversibility cue. Previous studies (Hilgard & Cooper, 1965; Kihlstrom & Evans, 1979) have shown that there is a tendency for the distribution of the number of items recalled on the HGSHS:A and similar scales to be bimodal, with the two modes occurring at 0, and around 5, suggestions recalled.

Amnesia has been defined as recalling 3 or fewer of the available 9 (HGSHS:A) or 11 (SHSS:C) suggestions. For example, with an HGSHS:A sample of 691 subjects (Kihlstrom & Evans, 1979), 31% of the subjects passed this criterion. The point–biserial correlation between initial amnesia and corrected hypnotizability (omitting the amnesia item) was .35 ($p < .001$). For the more difficult, individually administered SHSS:C, 32% of the sample passed the amnesia criterion, and the correlation between items recalled and adjusted total score was .52 ($p < .001$).[4]

Some of the features of the amnesia recall found in this study parallel features of the long-term recall of serially presented episodic material (Roediger & Crowder, 1976). For example, the frequency of recall of each item showed typical primacy and recency effects, even though the frequency of recall of each item was diminished for the highly hypnotizable subjects. This indicates that the initial recall deficit of the highly hypnotizable subjects was not specific to individual items.

*Initial Recall and Reversibility Recall.* The hypnotized subject's memory does not remain incomplete. When the experimenter administers a prearranged cue, the critical memories appear to flood back into awareness, and the hitherto amnesic subject is now able to remember the events and experiences of hypnosis clearly and without difficulty.

The basic recall characteristics of posthypnotic amnesia and reversibility (Kihlstrom & Evans, 1976, 1977) are summarized in Figure 6-1, which presents recall data for two samples ($n = 691$ and 372). Both groups were administered the HGSHS:A in the standard way. The results for the sample of 691 subjects (the bars labeled "Standard" in Figure 6-1) are discussed first; results for the sample of 372 (the bars labeled "Breach") are discussed in the next subsection. The shaded area of each bar shows the average number of suggestions recalled on the test of initial amnesia. The highly hypnotizable subjects recalled 3.3 of the critical suggestions, significantly fewer than the 4.9 suggestions recalled by the subjects low in hypnotizability ($p < .001$). The

---

4. At least three factors may have combined to diminish the item-to-total correlation for amnesia on the HGSHS:A: (1) There are subjects who for apparently motivational reasons fail to report items that they actually remember (Kihlstrom & Evans, 1977; Kihlstrom & Register, 1984); (2) performance on the HGSHS:A as a whole can be contaminated by social contagion and other effects inherent in the group setting (Evans & Mitchell, 1977); and (3) if the administration of the HGSHS:A is the subjects' first exposure to hypnosis (as it often is), it correlates about .60 with later scales, even though later scales have higher intercorrelation at about .85 (Hilgard, 1965).

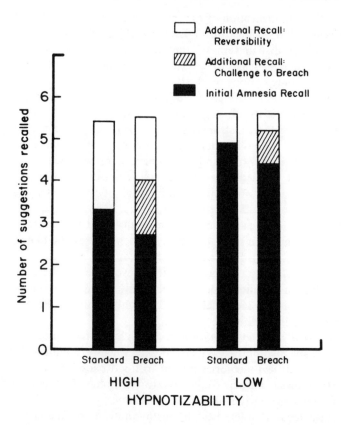

Figure 6-1. Parameters of posthypnotic amnesia in two samples ("Standard," $n = 691$, and "Breach," $n = 372$) indicating number of HGSHS:A suggestions (out of 9) recalled during amnesia ("Initial Amnesia Recall," shaded areas) and after the amnesia has been lifted ("Additional Recall: Reversibility," unshaded areas). The second sample has an additional recall during amnesia in which special instructions have been given attempting to break the amnesia ("Additional Recall: Challenge to Breach"). Recall is plotted cumulatively from amnesia trial to the reversibility trial. Subjects are classified as high (8–11) or low (0–4) in hypnotizability, based on the HGSHS:A (excluding the amnesia suggestions itself).

unshaded area of each bar represents the average number of new suggestions recalled on the final reversibility test, after the amnesia suggestion was canceled. The highly hypnotizable subjects recovered significantly more new memories than did the less hypnotizable subjects ($p < .001$), so that by the time the memory tests were concluded the subjects high and low in hypnotizability recalled, on the average, about the same total amount of critical material (5.5 suggestions). The increase in reversibility recall of about 2.1 suggestions was significant for the highly hypnotizable subjects ($p < .001$), but was inconsequential (about 0.6 suggestions) for the less hypnotizable subjects.

It was noted that even at the end of the experiment, after the amnesia was lifted, both groups combined still "forgot" about a third (31%) of the suggestions administered during hypnosis. This appeared to be normal forgetting unrelated to amnesia (Kihlstrom & Evans, 1977). Very similar findings to those described above were reported when posthypnotic amnesia was suggested for a 15-item unrelated word list (Kihlstrom, 1980).

*Breaching of Amnesia.* These data differentiating subjects high and low in hypnotizability in terms of suggested amnesic recall and its subsequent reversibility are compelling. Both initial (amnesic) recall and final (reversible) recall were lawfully related to measured hypnotizability. However, some investigators have challenged the interpretation of these data and have hypothesized that they represent nothing more than a reluctance to report on the part of the highly hypnotizable subjects (see review by Spanos, 1986). To test whether these results reflected subjects' voluntarily not reporting what they consciously knew, several studies have tried various manipulations to break down the amnesic report by exhorting subjects to recall again, being honest, open, and fully compliant, while still under the influence of the amnesia suggestion. This has become known as the "breaching" paradigm, and is derived from Bowers's (1976) "honesty" instructions as a methodological technique to improve the veracity of subjective experience in hypnosis research.

The second sample in Figure 6-1 ($n = 372$; right-hand side of each data set, labeled "Breach") presents one such attempt at breaching amnesia. This is derived from a study (Kihlstrom, Evans, Orne, & Orne, 1980; see also Kihlstrom, 1975) in which one of several instructions was used to optimize recall on a second amnesia test before amnesia was reversed. Subjects in three groups were instructed (1) to try as hard as possible to recall (challenge recall); (2) to recall items in the order in which they were administered (retrieval cue); or simply (3) to recall again (with no special instructions, as a retest control). Reversibility was tested after the second breaching test.[5] The degree of breaching of the amnesia was the same in each of the groups. The combined breaching data are indicated by the hatched area in Figure 6-1. Some subjects showed a partial recovery of hitherto unlisted material under the breaching conditions, although the extent of recovery did not account for the extent of reversibility. Reversibility occurred significantly ($p < .001$) in highly hypnotizable subjects even after considerable pressure had been exerted on them during posthypnotic amnesia encouraging them to recall fully.

5. In this study, for the reversibility test, subjects were asked to list all of the experiences they recalled instead of only additional experiences, as is standard on the HGSHS:A.

The failure to breach amnesia is disappointing to the social-contextual view of amnesia. Spanos and Coe have found similar results in several studies (Spanos, 1986; Spanos, Radtke, & Bertrand, 1985), including the use of a lie detector/polygraph paradigm to detect false and incomplete recall (Howard & Coe, 1980; Schuyler & Coe, 1981). In one study, subjects did not completely breach amnesia even after watching a videotape of themselves (McConkey & Sheehan, 1981). Some of these investigators place emphasis on the fact that some subjects *do* breach amnesia, and show sufficient additional recall so as not to show subsequent reversibility. Arguments about whether a glass is half full or half empty highlight theoretical differences but obscure the important empirical data (Evans, 1986a). However, there are clearly subjects for whom conditions have not been found to breach the amnesia, using residual reversibility as the criterion.

*Reversibility as the Criterion of Posthypnotic Amnesia.* The final point to be made about reversibility relates to the ceiling effect that could potentially mitigate against the interpretation of reversibility as indicating that amnesia is only a temporary retrieval problem. The less than perfect correlation between initial amnesia and hypnotizability introduces the possibility of artifact in the correlation between subsequent recovery of memory and hypnotizability (Nace *et al.*, 1974). Put simply, highly hypnotizable subjects may recover more new suggestions on the later test because they have a larger pool of suggestions left for recall after the first test is over, and not because of any effect of the reversibility cue as such. If a subject low in hypnotizability recalls six suggestions, compared to two for a highly hypnotizable subject, then there is a ceiling effect in that there are not as many suggestions remaining in the pool—three versus seven, respectively, on the HGSHS:A— for additional recall.

We (Kihlstrom & Evans, 1976) were able to show that the ceiling effect is not a limiting factor in using reversibility as the more important measure of amnesia. We matched subjects of high, medium, and low hypnotizability in terms of the initial number of suggestions recalled during the amnesia trial. The results are shown in Figure 6-2. Under conditions when initial recall was matched, thereby controlling for ceiling effects, the amount of reversibility for highly hypnotizable subjects was significantly greater than the amount of reversibility for subjects low in hypnotizability.[6] This was so for each level of

6. The difference between high and low subjects ($n = 691$) at any vertically plotted points (matched for level of initial amnesia recall) was significant in a one-way analysis of variance across three subgroups ($p < .02$), except for the initial recall of Suggestions 7–9, for which there was no significant difference (presumably because of ceiling effects due to the maximum of nine suggestions available for recall). The minimum $n$ was 14 for any point. Values for subjects medium in hypnotizability fell between those for high and low subjects for each vertical (amnesia recall) comparison (see Kihlstrom & Evans, 1976).

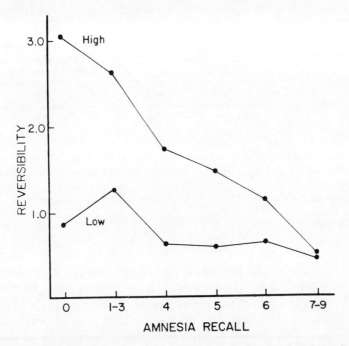

Figure 6-2. Recovery of memory after reversibility cue as a function of hypnotic susceptibility (high or low) and level of initial amnesia (number of suggestions recalled). $n = 691$; further details are given in footnote 6. Subjects medium in hypnotizability have been omitted. (Adapted from "Recovery of Memory after Posthypnotic Amnesia" by J. F. Kihlstrom and F. J. Evans, 1976, *Journal of Abnormal Psychology, 85*, p. 566. Copyright 1976 by the American Psychological Association. Adapted by permission.)

initial amnesia recall (except at levels of recall at which the ceiling effect prevented additional recall).

The mean of approximately one additional suggestion typically added by subjects low in hypnotizability during reversibility was most likely a retest or reminiscence effect. This suggests that amnesia should be defined by the reversibility of the amnesia of at least two or more suggestions, and not necessarily by initial amnesia recall (Kihlstrom & Register, 1984).

*Initial Amnesia, Reversibility, and Hypnotizability.* The reversibility data in Figure 6-2 are compelling. As testimony to the central role of reversibility, it only remains to be shown that reversible amnesia is lawfully related to hypnotic responsivity. These data are summarized in Table 6-1, which presents total scores for 691 subjects on the HGSHS:A, and scores for

Table 6-1. Hypnotizability as a Function of HGSHS:A Amnesia and Reversibility

| HGSHS:A reversibility | HGSHS:A amnesia recall | | | | | |
|---|---|---|---|---|---|---|
| | Subjects completing HGSHS:A[a] | | | Subjects completing HGSHS:A and SHSS:C[b] | | |
| | 0–3 | 4–5 | 6–9 | 0–3 | 4–5 | 6–9 |
| Pass (≥2) | 7.4 | 6.8 | 5.9 | 8.5 | 7.5 | 5.5 |
| Fail (≤2) | 5.6 | 4.9 | 5.4 | 6.6 | 5.0 | 5.0 |
| *t* | 5.5** | 6.2** | 1.1 | 4.0* | 4.6* | 0.5 |

[a]11 items on the HGSHS:A (amnesia dropped); $n = 691$. Amnesia recall based on 9 suggestions.
[b]12 items on the HGSHS:A; $n = 219$. Amnesia recall based on 11 suggestions.
*$p < .0005$.
**$p < .0001$.

the 219 subjects who also completed the SHSS:C. Data are tabulated for subjects who passed or failed the criterion for reversibility on the HGSHS:A, but for different levels of initial amnesia recall, including those who passed the traditional amnesia criterion (initially recalling three or fewer suggestions) and those who did not. Subjects who passed the criterion for amnesia or that for reversibility had higher HGSHS:A total scores (adjusted, omitting the amnesia suggestion performance), as well as higher future (SHSS:C) scores. However, subjects who passed both criteria (significant interaction effect, $p < .001$) had the highest HGSHS:A and SHSS:C scores. Those subjects who failed the initial amnesia criterion (e.g., those who recalled four or five suggestions during the amnesia test) but who still showed reversibility of the amnesia were more hypnotizable than those who did not show reversibility.

*Other Measures of Amnesia.* So far, the focus has been on the parametric data on the extent of recall during amnesia and during reversibility. Amnesia has been evaluated within the context of the episodic material experienced during administration of the hypnosis scale itself. A number of questions can be asked about the numerical parameters of amnesia recall and reversibility using different modes of testing. Many are minor variations of studies already described. For example, in the recent work on the breaching paradigm described above, the HGSHS:A reversibility procedure was usually modified so that the subjects listed afresh their total recall rather than additional recall. This procedure did not affect either the amount of material recalled or the basic parameters of posthypnotic amnesia. Studies that have examined other issues—including (1) whether it makes any difference if the amnesia suggestion is given before the remaining suggestions on the scale (incidental learning) or more traditionally at the end; and (2) dissipation of the amnesia over time (Bertrand, Spanos, & Parkinson, 1983; Dubreuil, Spanos, & Bertrand, 1982; Spanos, Tkachyk, Bertrand, & Weekes, 1984), similar to the hypermnesia over time that has occurred in normal memory studies (Erdelyi & Kleinbard, 1978; Kihlstrom, Easton, & Shor, 1983)—have not produced significant effects. Excellent discussions of these studies are available (Kihlstrom, 1977, 1978, 1985; Spanos, 1986).

Although they are not reviewed in this chapter, a number of studies have documented the basic parameters of posthypnotic amnesia and reversibility using word lists (Kihlstrom, 1980; Kihlstrom & Shor, 1978; Radtke-Bodorik, Planas, & Spanos, 1980; Spanos *et al.*, 1985; Spanos, Radtke, & Dubreuil, 1982; Spanos, Radtke-Bodorik, & Shabinsky, 1980; Spanos, Stam, D'Eon, Pawlak, & Radtke-Bodorik, 1980), or using recognition rather than recall measures (Kihlstrom & Shor, 1978; St. Jean & Coe, 1981). Although not all of the parameters of amnesia discussed above have been tested using these different paradigms, most of these studies show generally similar findings. Although measures of recognition are much more fragile as indices of posthypnotic amnesia, amnesia and reversibility can nevertheless be demonstrated (Kihlstrom & Short, 1978; St. Jean & Coe, 1981).

## The Subjective Experiences of Posthypnotic Amnesia

The mere enumeration of the number of suggestions recalled is critical for the quantification of the phenomenon, but sheds little light on the way in which subjects go about the task of trying to recall in spite of what appears to be a temporary memory block. Some of the main conclusions drawn above can be illustrated by the following verbatim transcripts obtained from subjects' HGSHS:A written amnesia reports. These transcripts also illustrate some of the important aspects of posthypnotic amnesia, to be discussed below, that are not obvious from a direct quantitative analysis.

> *Subject A*: I remember being very relaxed. My arm bothered me. Yes! The face—the clown's face. It replaced the dot on the wall. First it became colors, red and green. Then it changed into a clown's face. It was fun.

Subject A is typical of a small group of subjects who appear blithely unaware of the several events experienced during the hypnosis scale. They often show behavioral signs of puzzlement, chagrin, or embarrassed amusement during the amnesia test, and typically acknowledge a gap in memory that corresponds to a discontinuity in subjective experience, much like the similar experience following sleep. Reference to any of the targeted to-be-recalled hypnotic suggestions may be difficult to recognize (as in the present example). These subjects typically describe trivial or even confabulated aspects of the hypnotic induction procedure. Subject A gave a dramatic account of his absorption in a black fixation dot on the wall that is used during the induction procedure. The perceptual distortions occurring during the fixation were transformed into a reported experience that well served the task of filling in the memory gap that the subject appeared to have. This inability to recall is typically followed by a reasonably complete recall upon the lifting of the amnesia.

The reports from Subjects B and C are, however, more typical transcripts. Although both subjects initially recalled five suggestions during the amnesia test, the two reports are strikingly different, and they provide examples of several of the characteristics of posthypnotic amnesia described in subsequent sections.[7]

> *Subject B:* We were told we were getting tired and drowsy. Our eyelids were heavy [2]. Then we were told to raise our left arm palm downward [3], then to interlock our hands [5], then to hold them straight in front of us palms toward each other—12 inches apart [7]. Then we were told to touch our left ankle when we heard a tapping sound [11].
>
> *Subject C:* Became very tired. Eyes shut soon afterward [2]. Feel like I was floating. I made my arm stiff [6] and tried to hold out my left arm [4]. I felt a fly on my head [9]. I remember counting 1 to 20. Also holding out both of my arms [7].

Subject B was low in hypnotizability, passing only 3 of the 12 suggestions on the HGSHS:A. He recalled 4 of the 9 suggestions that are available for recall on the HGSHS:A amnesia suggestion, and added nothing new during the reversibility test. This response should be compared to that of Subject C, who also recalled 4 of the 9 suggestions. Subject C was highly hypnotizable, passing 8 out of 12 suggestions on the HGSHS:A. (Suggestion 2, eye closure, is part of the induction procedure and is not included in the amnesia test, although both subjects recalled it.) Both subjects failed the objective HGSHS:A amnesia criterion (recall of three or fewer suggestions). Several characteristics of Subject C's recall, however, suggest that he was experiencing at least a partial amnesia and was influenced by the HGSHS:A amnesia suggestion. Part of the reason for this judgment is apparent from a consideration of the transcript below, which is the transcript of Subject C's recall *after* the amnesia was lifted (reversibility). Five suggestions were recalled, although one of them (7) is a clarification of a vaguely recalled experience during the amnesia test. The contrast between the amnesia and the reversibility transcripts helps demonstrate an impressive partial amnesia, based on several criteria other than the amount of initial recall.

> *Subject C* (after amnesia was lifted):
> My left arm was forced down [3].

7. Numbers in brackets in these transcripts refer to the specific suggestions of HGSHS:A, listed in footnote 1.

> I made a fist with my left arm [6].
> I held my arms out with palms facing each
> other and then they went together [7].
> My head was very heavy [8].
> I clenched my hands together and was
> unable to undo [5].

Further comments are made on these typical transcripts later. The richness of these reports helps reinforce the decision to limit the present overview of measures of retrieval during posthypnotic amnesia to personal experiences, rather than laboratory-based word-list information. There has been controversy about whether the same memory mechanisms are involved in episodic events as are involved in less meaningful material such as word lists. (Tulving, 1972; Underwood, 1977). This review ignores this issue and focuses on aspects of hypnotic amnesia within the confines of the episodic suggestions given during a scale such as the HGSHS:A.

The remainder of this chapter turns from the basic descriptive accounts of recall and reversibility, and explores some of the data that have been obtained in my colleagues' and my own research, with some confirmation from other centers, covering a number of unique features of posthypnotic amnesia. Source amnesia, generic recall, and the disorganization of retrieval strategies during posthypnotic amnesia are discussed.

## THE AMNESIA PROCESS: DISSOCIATION OF CONTEXT AND CONTENT

### Posthypnotic Source Amnesia

A search for appropriate explanatory variables has led to a consideration of both normal and pathological memory processes. In cases of clinical amnesia and in fugue states, the patients typically do not know who they are, where they are, or what has happened over time. Nevertheless, other verbal, cognitive, motor, and sensory skills remain intact. Clinically, memories may remain functionally intact except for the *context* in which certain events occurred. Normal memory examples come to mind: A novelist may have been inspired by a personal insight into the perfect plot, or a scientist may have designed a brilliant experiment. Unfortunately, the budding novel was recently on the bestseller list, or, even worse, the potential Nobel Prize-winning experiment has already been published! Unconscious plagiarism seems to involve amnesia for the original context in which the insight occurred. Most of us probably do not remember the process of learning to walk, writing our names for the first time, or even which shoe we put on first this morning. More commonly, we have all had the experience of meeting somebody whose name or face is hauntingly familiar, but being unable to remember where we have met this particular person before—sometimes with disastrous social consequences. In these examples, the skill or information has been dissociated from the context in which it occurred. Content is recalled, but the context is forgotten.

In experimentally induced posthypnotic "recall amnesia," content is temporarily forgotten, while the context itself (the hypnosis session) is obvious. In contrast, posthypnotic "source amnesia" (Cooper, 1966; Evans & Thorn, 1966; Gheorghiu, 1967; Thorn, 1960) provides an experimental paradigm in which information is retained and reproduced, but cannot be placed in the context in which it was learned.

In an experimental session, hypnotized subjects (usually college students) are given a test of general knowledge. They are asked several questions, the answers to which they do not usually know (e.g., "An amethyst is a blue or purple gemstone. What color does it turn when exposed to heat?"). The subjects are then told the correct answers to these difficult questions. Posthypnotic amnesia is usually suggested for the content of the session in the standard way. After the subjects are tested for their memory of the content of the hypnosis session (standard recall amnesia), the same questions are asked again. For example, when asked "An amethyst is a blue or purple gemstone. What color does it turn when it is exposed to heat?", subjects with source amnesia will quickly answer, correctly, "Yellow." When they are asked how they know the answer, they typically look rather puzzled and are unable to specify how they know. They may even rationalize their inability to specify how they acquired the information ("My girlfriend must have told me," or "I guess I read it somewhere," or "I must have learned it in a geology course," or "I saw a flash of yellow light").

Now this is a surprising response. The casualness of this "Aha!"-like experience seems to be the antithesis of the clear expectations that are conveyed by the procedure. If the subjects are "role-playing" amnesia for what has transpired, it would seem to require little intelligence to realize that, when asked the color of a heated amethyst, they should respond, "I don't know." Indeed, when asked the color of a heated amethyst, subjects simulating hypnosis[8] (Orne, 1979) unhesitatingly reply, "I don't know." Simulators

---

8. In the simulator quasi-design, subjects known to be unresponsive to hypnosis are told that they will be working with an experimenter whose task it is to determine which subjects are faking and which ones are really hypnotized. They are told that intelligent subjects can fake hypnosis successfully, but that if the examiner discovers the faking the experiment will stop immediately. A blind experimenter cannot discriminate between hypnotized and simulating subjects at a level better than chance (Orne, 1959, 1979). Thus, since the blind experimenter will treat all subjects alike, the behavior of the simulators provides an objective measure of the implicit cues in the total situation, and indicates behaviorally how subjects might perceive the

apparently believe that a hypnotized subject would respond to the suggested blanket amnesia for the whole hypnosis procedure and would remember nothing posthypnotically. They give the "common-sense" answer. The behavior of the simulators indicates that the predominant cues in the situation signify that everything should be forgotten by the hypnotized subject (Coe, 1978; Evans, 1979a; Evans & Thorn, 1966). Thus the source amnesia response is not concordant with the cues in the situation; in this sense, source amnesia, when it occurs (in about one out of three deeply hypnotized subjects), is counterexpectational (Evans, 1979a).[9]

In summary, the subjects readily provide the information they were taught in hypnosis, in spite of their conviction that they remember nothing about how they acquired the information. When challenged, they have no idea that their newly found knowledge about amethysts was just acquired in hypnosis. The similarities between source amnesia and the examples given above of clinical amnesia and unconscious plagiarism should be noted. In these phenomena, memory for the content or information is intact, but memory for the context in which the information was acquired is lost. Although content is recalled, the context in which the experience occurred is for the moment inaccessible.

In two related studies by Kihlstrom (1980), subjects were asked to give either word associations or category instances during the period of posthypnotic amnesia for word lists learned before the suggestion of amnesia. The amnesia for the word-list items did not prevent their association with the target items during the posthypnotic memory tasks. Moreover, production of the critical items did not facilitate their "recall" as target amnesia items. Kihlstrom concluded that posthypnotic amnesia represents a temporary dissociation of episodic features from memory traces, so that the amnesic subjects have difficulty in reconstructing the context in which target events occur. Interpretation of studies using word-list approaches to posthypnotic

---

experiment. Any behavior elicited by simulating subjects could presumably be elicited from hypnotized ones who have the same cues available to them. Similarities in behavior between hypnotized and simulating subjects do not guarantee that the behavior came about in the same way—only that it could have. Differences between these groups obviously require further confirmation using other control strategies. The behavior of simulating and hypnotized subjects differs on several of the aspects of amnesia described below (Bowers, 1976; McConkey & Sheehan, 1981; Spanos, Radtke, Bertrand, Addie, & Drummond, 1982; Spanos, Radtke-Bodorik, & Stam, 1980; Williamsen *et al.*, 1965).

9. Elsewhere (Evans, 1979a), I have reported statistically significant differences between hypnotized and simulating subjects in the occurrence of source amnesia. Spanos (1986) reports a failure to replicate these source amnesia results, but it is unclear from his report whether his procedures were adequate to document its occurrence. A critique of the Evans and Thorn (1966) study by Coe (1978) does not appear to have correctly summarized the scoring procedures that were used.

recall amnesia may be more complex, because the recall of component parts of the word list may be special instances of the source amnesia process.[10] Words, whether meaningful or meaningless, may be recalled without awareness of the contextual features of the recall process, much as in the tip-of-the-tongue phenomenon. Elsewhere (Evans, 1979b), I have presented an experimental analogue of the tip-of-the-tongue phenomenon by tracing the consequences on an arithmetic test of a successful versus an unsuccessful suggestion that the number "six" disappears from the hypnotized subjects' counting system.

One implication of the data on source amnesia is that there may be a temporary dissociation of the hypnotic events, one at a time, as they are experienced. Perhaps they are temporarily held in some kind of intermediate memory buffer without being organized in the usual efficient way until given "permission" to do so by the retrieval cue itself. The reversibility cue may well be the dominant organizational "hook" that allows the experiential (or possibly semantic) events to have an organizational structure, but only when reversibility is invoked. Until the "future" encoding is legitimized, the events remain only loosely organized during hypnosis and during the initial amnesia recall, with only sufficient structure to prevent their permanent loss. In Kihlstrom's (1980) second study above, the categorical instances provided a similar dissociated channel or "hook" to interact with the targeted material, which was semantically unavailable but accessible (Tulving & Pearlstone, 1966). Such a dissociated channel or intermediate storage capacity may occasionally breach itself by temporal proximity, but the breaching might well be partial or even transient. In the transcript given above of Subject A's report, the statement "My arm bothered me" could be a fleeting reference to any one of several HGSHS:A suggestions (hand lowering, arm immobilization, finger lock, arm rigidity, hands moving together). It may well be that the attempts to retrieve the currently unintegrated or unorganized material may lead to the recall of peripheral or incidental material not related to target suggestions (partial confabulation), to the recall of unrecognizable events (generic recall, described below), or to difficulty in verbally reporting the almost-to-be-recalled material. My colleagues and I have found qualitative differences between the transcript reports of amnesic, partially amnesic, and nonamnesic subjects that suggest confirmation of these temporary retrieval failures.

In summary, source amnesia implies a dissociation of the recall (content)

---

10. Kihlstrom (1985) has suggested that source amnesia may reflect a dissociation of episodic and semantic components of the to-be-remembered material. Source amnesia may be closely related to other aspects of amnesia, such as the difficulty some subjects have in sequencing remembered hypnotic events (discussed later); even older studies showing similar processes using olfactory and visual stimuli (Banister & Zangwill, 1941) are also relevant.

and the contextual attributes of recall (e.g., temporal integration and retrieval). The work on generic recall during posthypnotic amnesia, described next, appears to confirm the one-instance-at-a-time struggle to retrieve temporarily unorganized material and events.

## Generic (Vague) Recall

Occasionally, a subject remembers some portion of one or more of the relevant suggestions, without remembering the important details. The specific referent experience may be fairly clear, in that it is the only scale suggestion related to the memory fragment (e.g., "something about a fly"). At other times the referent is not so clear. For example, a subject who reports merely "My arm bothered me" (see Subject A's transcript) could be referring to any one of five separate and distinct suggestions concerned with movements of the hands and/or arms (see the preceding section and footnote 1). We (Kihlstrom & Evans, 1978) have referred to this phenomenon as "generic recall" (following a similar usage by Brown & McNeil, 1966). There is a vague, general idea of the to-be-remembered material (it involved the arm), but the act of recall is not completely successful because of lack of clarity about specific details (e.g., feelings of heaviness, stiffness, or arm movement).

In a blind analysis of two samples totaling 725 subjects, generic recall was found to occur significantly more often ($p < .05$ in both samples) in the memory reports of the highly hypnotizable than in those of the less hypnotizable (23% vs. 6%, respectively). Within the group of highly hypnotizable subjects, generic recall was most often found in those who were most completely amnesic. Moreover, there was a marked shift from generic to particular (or detailed) recall following cancellation of the amnesia suggestion. During reversibility testing, the subjects high and low in hypnotizability did not differ in the rare incidence (about 2%) of generic recall. The relative poverty of the memory reports of highly hypnotizable subjects, including their vague, fragmentary, and generic qualities, appears to mark the partial influence of suggestions for posthypnotic amnesia as these subjects struggle to recall material that they cannot readily access during their efforts at retrieval. Indeed, they seem to be focusing on an experience as an isolated event that is not integrated into the ongoing stream of events during hypnosis.

Further evidence of the struggle to recall can be seen in detailed analyses of the verbal transcripts of amnesic and nonamnesic subjects (Evans, Kihlstrom, & Orne, 1973). Blind raters evaluated typed transcripts and could successfully distinguish those transcripts that were produced by amnesic subjects who reversed their amnesia from those subjects who showed no objective sign of amnesia. This could be done successfully even when the transcripts of subjects high and low in hypnotizability were matched for the initial number of items actually recalled in the amnesia testing (Pettinati & Evans, 1980). Table 6-2 presents data indicating that the recall of the amnesic subjects was identifiable using several word-count and rating criteria.

Several findings in Table 6-2 (Pettinati & Evans, 1980) support the hypothesis that the process of recalling is qualitatively different for highly hypnotizable subjects compared to subjects low in hypnotizability:

1. Even subjects who did not recall any of the suggestions wrote several comments during the amnesia test. The mean word production of highly hypnotizable subjects recalling no suggestions did not differ significantly from the mean productivity of all other highly hypnotizable subjects.

2. Subjects low in hypnotizability used more total words to list their recall than did highly hypnotizable subjects, but, of course, they also recalled more suggestions. However, highly hypnotizable subjects used a smaller proportion of their written transcripts to describe the suggestions than did the less hypnotizable subjects. Thus, the less hypnotizable subjects tended to spend most of their efforts directly listing the suggested events, while the highly hypnotizable subjects spent more than half of their less productive output describing experiences not directly relevant to enumerating the test suggestions.

3. Highly hypnotizable subjects not only recalled fewer suggestions; they used fewer suggestion-relevant words to describe each item and wrote

Table 6-2. Generic and Vague Recall: Blind comparisons of Written Amnesia Transcripts Showing Differences between Subjects of High and Low Hypnotizability in the Clarity of Recalling HGSHS:A Suggestions during Posthypnotic Amnesia

| Transcript variable | HGSHS:A hypnotizability[a] | |
| --- | --- | --- |
| | High (n = 55) | Low (n = 41) |
| Number of items recalled | 2.7 | 5.4 |
| Total number of words written | 41.1 | 61.4 |
| Percentage of words describing items | 47% | 67% |
| Item-relevant words used | 18.8 | 40.0 |
| Relevant words per item | 5.1 | 7.7 |
| Percentage of words before any item | 53% | 34% |

*Note.* The data are from *Qualitative Analysis of the Memory Reports of Amnesic and Nonamnesic Subjects* by H. M. Pettinati and F. J. Evans, 1980, October, paper presented at the 32nd Annual Meeting of the Society for Clinical and Experimental Hypnosis, Chicago.

[a]All comparisons between high and low subjects were significant at $p < .05$ (two-tailed).

more words before describing the first relevant suggestion. Highly hypnotizable subjects did not describe their memories in as great detail, perhaps because they had greater difficulty in recalling their experiences. The transcripts of Subjects B and C, above, illustrate the findings summarized in the preceding paragraph and this one.

4. Each of these variables was significantly correlated with the objective amnesia score. Thus, the proportion of irrelevant words that highly hypnotizable subjects used to describe their hypnosis experiences correlated .71 with the number of suggestions forgotten. The more amnesia that was experienced, the more likely it was that subjects had written about aspects of their experience that were unrelated to the suggestions they were trying to recall.

The question arises as to precisely what highly hypnotizable subjects with amnesia wrote about if they were writing copiously about material that was not related to the task of recalling test suggestions. Several subjects commented on either of two cognitive changes they experienced during the hypnotic induction procedure. These related to changes in the visual field (e.g., color and size changes or autokinesis of the target, blurred periphery), particularly with the fixation spot used in the induction (such as the clown's face in Subject A's transcript), and to changes in bodily sensations (e.g., feelings of floating, as in Subject C's transcript; falling; inflated limbs). Such changes were primarily obtained from the highly hypnotizable subjects with amnesia (Evans *et al.*, 1973; Pettinati & Evans, 1980).

In general, highly hypnotizable subjects with amnesia tended to spend time describing events not related to the suggested items. Instead, they wrote about some of their more compelling subjective experiences during hypnosis, or showed signs of confabulation in their responses. These results support the hypothesis that a suggestion for posthypnotic amnesia has demonstrable effects other than merely reducing the number of experiences recalled posthypnotically. Such changes are consistent with the hypothesis of a struggle to retrieve during amnesia.

## Disruption of Retrieval Processes during Posthypnotic Amnesia

In most instances, amnesic subjects appear to be actively trying to recall.[11] They are limited in their success because of some inefficiency, inaccessibility,

---

11. This is not to deny the role of motivational factors, demand characteristics, deliberate withholding of recalled information, and other factors described by several authors (Coe, 1978; Coe & Sarbin, 1977; Gregg, 1979; Kihlstrom, 1977, 1978, 1983; Spanos, 1986; Spanos, Stam *et al.*, 1980; Wagstaff, 1977). It is precisely the methodological sophistication with which many investigators have tried to circumvent these problems that has helped provide as much conceptual clarity as has now been developed.

or disruption of those mechanisms that would otherwise produce easy and efficient retrieval of target experiences. The data on generic recall and the studies of written transcripts indicate that most subjects affected by the amnesia suggestion are struggling to retrieve temporarily inaccessible memories, and that they may well get caught up in a single experience (real or imagined) as they attempt to fill in the time—memory gap they experience. The nature of this struggle to recall appears to suggest that relevant content is sometimes available, with little availability of the learning context. The hypnosis experiences are being temporarily processed one at a time, as in source amnesia, and not as an organized stream of experience that would normally facilitate ongoing recall. This suggests that temporal references to ongoing experiences (suggestions) are at least suspended, or are not integrated within the usual consolidation processes for the time being (i.e., until amnesia is lifted).

Research on normal waking memory (reviewed by Bower, 1972; Tulving & Thomson, 1973) has shown that remembering, particularly episodic memory (Tulving, 1972), is greatly facilitated by many cognitive organizational principles or contextual tags (primacy, recency, similarity, affect, meaning, temporal order, etc.). The process of searching through memory storage is guided by various organizational cues and strategies by which the retrieval mechanisms function. Without a sufficiently rich associational network, and without an adequate plan for searching through memory and sufficient cues to guide retrieval, the person will not be able to gain access to material that is available in memory (Tulving & Pearlstone, 1966). This produces either a complete failure of memory, or, in less severe instances, incomplete, vague, and fragmentary or generic recall. These organizational cues usually make recall as easy, efficient, and productive as it is for most of us most of the time. It follows, then, that when recall is difficult, inefficient, and unproductive, the impairment in memory is likely to reflect the disorganization of the search processes in retrieval. This is especially the case if the memory deficit proves to be reversible and if recognition memory is mostly intact. Posthypnotic amnesia seems to fit this description nicely.

Accordingly, it has been proposed (Evans & Kihlstrom, 1973; Kihlstrom & Evans, 1979) that posthypnotic amnesia reflects a disruption of memory retrieval stemming from a disorganization of the process of memory search. Unfortunately, it is difficult to study the retrieval process in those completely amnesic subjects who have forgotten everything. It is thus necessary to focus attention on subjects who are able to remember at least some of the critical material. Fortunately, the studies of the recovery of memory after posthypnotic amnesia (Kihlstrom & Evans, 1976) and the subjective quality of memory reports taken during amnesia (Evans, 1980; Evans et al., 1973; Pettinati & Evans, 1980) have documented the partial effects of suggestions for posthypnotic amnesia. Thus, in the studies reported below, the general research strategy has been as follows: Exclude from consideration those subjects who recall virtually nothing during the test for posthypnotic amnesia, and compare the remaining subjects, grouped according to their degree of hypnotizability (high or low), in terms of the organization of recall and other aspects of retrieval.[12] We have examined some general aspects of the organization of recall and have investigated two particular organizational principles typically involved in memory organization: temporal sequence and the recall of success and failed experiences.

## Temporal Disorganization During Posthypnotic Amnesia

A number of considerations suggest that of all the cues and strategies that may be used in organizing recall of a series of personal experiences, temporal relations among the to-be-remembered items may be the most salient and important (Neisser, 1967; Underwood, 1977). If you were asked to list exactly what you have done today, chances are you would begin at the beginning: You awakened, dressed, ate breakfast, went to work, and so on. You would make use of the available contextual tags (primarily temporal ones for episodic events) to organize your activities into a reasonably complete and coherent account. The facts of amnesia—temporary failure to recall content; dissociation, or at least blurring, of context; the difficulty and confusion shown by some subjects as they go about the task of trying to recall—suggest that those highly hypnotizable subjects who have partial posthypnotic amnesia may retrieve the few experiences that they can recall in a more random manner than the organized and sequential remembering of subjects low in hypnotizability.

*Recalling the First Item First?* Initial support for this hypothesis was obtained by examining whether the first item recalled by partially amnesic subjects was indeed among the first of the suggestions administered. In a sample of 112 subjects (Evans & Kihlstrom, 1973), the first item recalled by 85% of the subjects low in hypnotizability was the first available one administered during the scale, whereas highly hypnotizable subjects tended to place the first available scale item later in their recall list—only 34% of them recalled the first item first ($\chi^2 = 6.41$, $p < .001$). This result has been replicated with 107 and 488 subjects using the HGSHS:A (Kihlstrom & Evans,

---

12. Some comparisons of partial and complete amnesia have been made, and these are referred to where possible. In general, such comparisons show a continuity between complete and partial amnesia.

Table 6-3. Frequency of Ordered and Random Recall during HGSHS:A Posthypnotic Amnesia

|  | Temporal sequence of recall[a] | |
| --- | --- | --- |
| HGSHS:A hypnotizability | Ordered | Random |
| High | 45 | 87 |
| Low | 79 | 45 |

*Note.* The data are from three combined samples ($n$'s $= 112, 107,$ and $488$) reported separately in "Memory Retrieval Processes in Posthypnotic Amnesia" by J. F. Kihlstrom and F. J. Evans, 1979, in J. F. Kihlstrom and F. J. Evans (Eds.), *Functional Disorders of Memory* (pp. 179–215), Hillsdale, NJ: Erlbaum. Copyright 1979 by Lawrence Erlbaum Associates. Used by permission.

$\chi^2 = 21.29$, $p > .001$; contingency coefficient $= .45$.

[a]Temporal sequence of recall based on significant (ordered) or insignificant (random) rank-order correlation between order of recall of the suggestions recalled and order of suggestions administered.

1979).[13] Highly hypnotizable subjects did not necessarily give primacy in their partially recalled list to the recall of the earliest (easiest) suggestions on the scale. This observation led to the hypothesis that the temporal order of recall would be impaired in partially amnesic subjects.

*Recalling Items in Order?* The temporal sequence of recall during hypnotic amnesia was initially investigated (Evans & Kihlstrom, 1973) by calculating the rank-order correlation (rho) between the order in which the subjects recalled any suggestions and the order in which those suggestions recalled had been administered during the scale. Table 6-3 presents the frequency for three combined samples (Kihlstrom & Evans, 1979) of subjects with statistically significant versus insignificant rho values as a function of hypnotizability. Highly hypnotizable subjects were more likely to recall in a random sequence; subjects low in hypnotizability were more likely to recall in a temporally accurate sequence.

Stated in a different way (Table 6-4), the mean rho scores of highly hypnotizable subjects were significantly lower than the mean rho scores of the less hypnotizable subjects (HGSHS:A mean *rho* of .67 and .80, respectively, *t*

---

13. There are two possible ways of analyzing these data. The method used here (and in Radtke and Spanos's [1981] failure to replicate) tabulates whether or not the first scale item was recalled first. On the HGSHS:A, Suggestion 3 is the first item after the induction procedure; subjects who do not recall Suggestion 3 are eliminated from the analysis. A second approach allows for the possibility that a subject does not recall, for example, any of the first five suggestions on the HGSHS:A (including Suggestion 3). For this subject, Suggestion 6 would be the first available for recall; the data tabulated would indicate whether this suggestion is the initial one recalled, or whether it is later in the limited recall list (e.g., Suggestion 9 may have been recalled first). The results hold for both methods.

Table 6-4. Organization of Recall during Amnesia for Subjects of Low, Medium, and High Susceptibility to Hypnosis (Evans & Kihlstrom, 1973)

| Scale | Mean rho score[a] | | | Analysis of variance | | | High and low subjects compared | | |
|---|---|---|---|---|---|---|---|---|---|
| | Low | Medium | High | $F$ | $df$ | $p<$ | $t$ | $df$ | $p<$ |
| HGSHS:A | .80 | .70 | .67 | 1.44 | 2, 84 | n.s. | 1.94 | 62 | .05 |
| SHSS:B | .58 | .17 | .39 | 3.69 | 2, 77 | .05 | 1.47 | 58 | .10 |
| SHSS:C | .55 | .31 | .08 | 5.38 | 2, 87 | .01 | 3.34 | 61 | .001 |
| $n^b$ | 40 | 27 | 23 | — | — | — | — | — | — |

*Note.* From "Phenomena of Hypnosis: 2. Posthypnotic Amnesia" by F. J. Evans, 1980, in G. D. Burrows and L. Dennerstein (Eds.), *Handbook of Hypnosis and Psychosomatic Medicine* (p. 93), Amsterdam: Elsevier/North-Holland. Copyright 1980 by Elsevier/North-Holland Biomedical Press. Reprinted by permission.

[a]Rho is the rank-order correlation, calculated for each subject who recalls at least three items during amnesia, between the order in which the items were recalled and the order in which these items were administered during hypnosis.

[b]Based on the SHSS:C. As some subjects recalled less than three items on one or two of the scales, $n$'s for the HGSHS: A and the SHSS:B varied slightly (see $df$ columns).

$= 1.94$, $df = 62$, $p < .05$; SHSS:C mean *rho* of .08 and .55, respectively, $t = 3.34$, $df = 61$, $p < .001$). On each of the hypnosis scales the highly hypnotizable subjects remembered events out of correct order, whereas the less hypnotizable subjects retrieved events in relatively sequential order. To return to the transcripts given earlier, the subject low in hypnotizability (Subject B) recalled the four suggestions (3, 5, 7, 11) in the order in which they were administered. The highly hypnotizable subject (Subject C) recalled in a more scattered order (6, 4, 9, 7; a Spearman *rho* of .60).

*Robustness of Disordered Retrieval.* Attempts have been made to replicate the disordered-retrieval results in several samples in our own laboratory (Kihlstrom & Evans, 1979), as well as by several other groups of investigators using similar and modified procedures (Bertrand & Spanos, 1985; Crawford, 1974; Geiselman *et al.*, 1983; Kihlstrom & Wilson, 1984; Lavoie & Sabourin, 1980; Lieberman, Brisson, & Lavoie, 1978; Radtke & Spanos, 1981; Radtke, Spanos, Della Malva, & Stam, 1986; Schwartz, 1978, 1980; Spanos & Bodorik, 1977; Spanos & D'Eon, 1980; Spanos, Radtke-Bodorik, & Stam, 1980; St. Jean & Coe, 1981; Staats & Evans, 1983). Some of the conditions under which disrupted retrieval occurred, based on samples of subjects who completed standard or appropriately modified versions of the HGSHS:A, are summarized in Table 6-5. The disruption of retrieval order in highly hypnotizable subjects has been replicated in most of the different samples studied by different investigators. The effect was typically small, though statistically significant even in small samples.

Table 6-5. Mean Temporal Organization of Recall (Rho) during Posthypnotic Amnesia for Subjects of High and Low Hypnotizability: Summary of Several Studies Testing Partial Amnesia

| Study | Scale[a] | n | Mean rho[b] High | Mean rho[b] Low |
|---|---|---|---|---|
| Crawford (1974) | HGSHS:A | 20 | .60 | .99 |
| Evans & Kihlstrom (1973) | HGSHS:A | 112 | .67 | .80 |
| | SHSS:B | 112 | .39 | .58 |
| | SHSS:C | 112 | .08 | .55 |
| Kihlstrom & Evans (1979) | HGSHS:A | 107 | .61 | .81 |
| | SHSS:C | 107 | .16 | .68 |
| Kihlstrom, Evans, Orne, & Orne (1980) | HGSHS:A | 488 | .68 | .85 |
| | HGSHS:A | 139[c] | .74 | .87 |
| Radtke & Spanos (1981) | HGSHS:A | 149 | .71 | .75[d] |
| Radtke, Spanos, Della Malva, & Stam (1986) | HGSHS:A | 318 | .54 | .77 |
| Staats & Evans (1983) | SHSS:B | 132[e] | .56 | .77 |
| St. Jean & Coe (1981) | SHSS:B | 141 | .75 | .72[f] |
| | SHSS:C | 141 | .58 | .73 |
| | SHSS:B[g] | 141 | .72 | .75[f] |
| | SHSS:C[g] | 141 | .58 | .73 |

[a]Hypnosis scale on which amnesia suggestion was analyzed.

[b]Rho is the Spearman rank-order correlation between the order in which subjects recalled at least three of the suggestions during posthypnotic amnesia and the sequence in which those suggestions were administered.

[c]Subset of sample above, in which subjects were asked to recall again during amnesia, but to make a special effort to list the suggestions in chronological sequence.

[d]Statistical significance not reported.

[e]Psychiatric inpatients.

[f]Mean rho difference between subjects high and low in hypnotizability was not statistically significant. All other pairs of mean rho scores in table differed significantly on $t$ tests ($p < .05$).

[g]Second recall test during amnesia for the same sample, but subjects were given a list of suggestions to recognize.

The conditions under which no differences have been found in retrieval order (rho) between subjects high and low in hypnotizability are also especially important (Table 6-6); they highlight the specificity of disrupted retrieval to posthypnotic amnesia. When amnesia was *not* suggested during the HGSHS:A, highly hypnotizable subjects did *not* recall in random order, but recalled in the same almost perfect temporal sequence as did the less hypnotizable subjects (Kihlstrom & Evans, 1979; $n = 72$). In addition, when amnesia was lifted, highly hypnotizable subjects no longer recalled in random sequence: The order of recall during reversibility (modified so that subjects listed all suggestions remembered) was the same for completely amnesic,

Table 6-6. Temporal Organization of Recall in Subjects of High and Low Hypnotizability under Conditions Where Posthypnotic Amnesia Suggestions Were Not in Effect

| Study | Special condition | Amnesia scale/ condition | n | Mean rho High | Low |
|---|---|---|---|---|---|
| Evans (1980) | Reversibility | HGSHS:A[a] | 76 | .86 | .87[b] |
| Kihlstrom (1975) | Reversibility | HGSHS:A[a] | 110 | .77 | .83[b] |
| Kihlstrom & Evans (1979) | No amnesia suggestion (but initial posthypnosis recall) | HGSHS:A[c] | 72 | .88 | .89[b] |
| Evans (1972) | Itinerary recall (related travel story) | Waking Memory[d] | 76 | .67 | .59[b] |

*Note.* This is a continuation of Table 6-5, in which results are presented for amnesia testing only. This table presents comparable mean rho values when no amnesia suggestion was in effect. Rho is the Spearman rank-order correlation between the order in which subjects recalled some of the suggestions during posthypnotic amnesia and the sequence in which those suggestions were administered.

[a]Testing was done with HGSHS:A suggestions; reversibility (postamnesia) was modified to give complete relisting of recall (instead of additional recall).

[b]No significant differences between subjects high and low in hypnotizability.

[c]Posthypnotic amnesia suggestion was omitted, but recall was tested as usual.

[d]A separate waking-recall task of a story about traveling to nine European cities, each associated with a tourist activity (e.g., ". . . and you saw the Eiffel Tower in Paris . . ."), parallel to nine suggestions on the HGSHS:A. Subjects were later asked to recall the cities.

partially amnesic, and nonamnesic subjects (Evans, 1980, and Kihlstrom, 1975; total $n = 186$).

It is possible that the differences in rho scores could be related to the number of suggestions recalled during the amnesia test, particularly as the highly hypnotizable in general are more amnesic and hence have less total amnesia recall. The rho statistic itself is a fragile one, particularly with lower recall. As with reversibility (discussed above; see Figure 6-2), it is possible to capitalize on the fact that total HGSHS:A scores are only moderately correlated with the amount recalled during the amnesia test, and to match subjects high and low in hypnotizability on the number of suggestions recalled during the amnesia test. Mean rho scores for subjects high and low in hypnotizability who were matched for initial amnesic recall are provided in Figure 6-3. (No point in the figure represents fewer than seven subjects.) Even when the high and low subjects recalled the *same* number of suggestions during the amnesia test, the highly hypnotizable subjects consistently had significantly *lower* rho scores (more disrupted recall) than the less hypnotizable subjects.

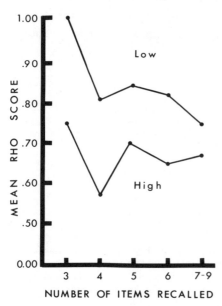

NUMBER OF ITEMS RECALLED

Figure 6-3. Mean rho index measuring temporal sequencing for subjects high (lower rho values) and low (higher rho values) in hypnotizability during HGSHS:A posthypnotic amnesia test. High and low subjects were matched for the number of suggestions recalled during the amnesia test (subjects recalling less than three items were dropped because rho could not be calculated). Vertical differences (i.e., for any level of initial recall) were statistically significant. No point is represented by fewer than seven subjects (total sample size was 691 subjects). (From "Phenomena of Hypnosis: 2. Posthypnotic Amnesia" by F. J. Evans, 1980, in G. D. Burrows and L. Dennerstein [Eds.], *Handbook of Hypnosis and Psychosomatic Medicine* [p. 96], Amsterdam: Elsevier/North-Holland. Copyright 1980 by Elsevier/North-Holland Biomedical Press. Reprinted by permission.)

This demonstrates that, like reversibility, the disrupted-recall effect is independent of the amount of recall during the amnesia test, but reflects qualitative aspects of the way in which amnesic subjects go about the task of trying to recall.[14]

*Disorganized Partial Recall and Complete Amnesia.* The data for primary recall indicate that amnesia is characterized by a partial disorganization of retrieval strategies, and that at least temporal sequencing is interfered with during posthypnotic amnesia. The dissociation between the contextual aspects of recall and the content of the recall may lead to a temporary suspension of the ability, or to the inability, to organize the ongoing episodic experiences into the normal kinds of temporal sequences that typically facilitate good recall. This temporary disruption appears to lie on a continuum of amnesic experience.

In the retrieval strategy analyses presented, it has not been possible to use the data of the more completely amnesic subjects who have had virtually no

---

14. Although highly hypnotizable subjects with partial amnesia do not seem to use temporal order as a principal organizational strategy to aid retrieval during amnesia, it is possible that they use other retrieval strategies. However, we have not yet isolated any consistent strategy used by highly hypnotizable amnesic subjects, either by adopting gross methods of analyzing overall clustering (Tulving, 1972) or by testing specific hypotheses such as the serial-position curve (Kihlstrom & Evans, 1979).

recall during amnesia, because of the inadequate methods of analyzing the data The analysis has been restricted to those who have had only a partial experience of amnesia—that is, those who have recalled some experiences—even though the more completely amnesic subjects have subsequently shown more reversibility. Table 6-7 shows that disorganized recall is on a continuum of hypnotizability with complete amnesia. Mean hypnotizability scores are presented for subjects who successfully experienced a complete amnesia and recalled virtually nothing during the amnesia test; those who had partial recall, but nevertheless showed disorganized temporal sequencing; and those who had partial initial recall and did not show disorganized temporal sequencing. The significant continuum of hypnotizibility observed in Table 6-7 indicates that the disorganized retrieval is a partial manifestation of a more generalized experience occurring in more highly hypnotized subjects.

## Failure to Recall Successful Experiences

Another major organizing principle that has been discussed in the previous literature is the experience of success and failure (Butterfield, 1964; Rosenzweig, 1938; von Restorff, 1933). It seems plausible to hypothesize that the recall data reflect not so much temporal disorganization as the differential recall of success and failure with the hypnotic suggestions that were targeted for recall during amnesia. There is a tendency on the hypnosis scales to move from easier suggestions to harder suggestions (particularly on the SHSS:C). Thus, highly hypnotizable subjects do not experience failure until later in the scales. Pettinati (1979; Pettinati & Evans, 1978; Pettinati, Evans, Orne, & Orne, 1981) has extended some of the earlier work by Hilgard and Hommel (1961) and O'Connell (1966) and has demonstrated that subjects who are low in hypnotizability and nonamnesic subjects do, as predicted, have a significant tendency to recall successful rather than failed experiences. However, there is *no* tendency for those subjects who have reversible amnesia to show a differential preference for successful or unsuccessful experiences, even when the number of suggestions failed and the number passed are taken into account.[15]

## Disorganized Retrieval and Amnesia: Summary

It has been documented that during posthypnotic amnesia there is a loss of temporal sequencing as a retrieval strategy, and there is no evidence that the experience of success and failure is used as a retrieval strategy. In addition, there is an extensive literature (reviewed elsewhere by Kihlstrom, 1985, and Spanos,

15. Coe, Baugher, Krimm, and Smith (1976) failed to replicate this finding; their failure was based in part on their use of a method of scoring relative recall that is statistically unsatisfactory (Pettinati, 1979).

Table 6-7. Prediction of Total Scores, Amnesia, and Reversibility Performance in HGSHS:A and SHSS:C from the Occurrence of Complete Amnesia or Disordered (Random) versus Ordered Recall on HGSHS:A ($n = 219$)

| Criterion | Complete amnesia ($n = 52$) | Random rho ($n = 89$) | Ordered rho ($n = 78$) | $F^a$ | $t^b$ |
|---|---|---|---|---|---|
| HGSHS: A performance | | | | | |
| Total score[c] | 7.08 | 5.83 | 5.15 | 8.6** | 1.70* |
| Amnesia recall[d] | 0.83 | 4.55 | 5.30 | 211.3*** | 3.62*** |
| Reversibility recall[e] | 2.52 | 1.17 | 0.73 | 29.1*** | 2.56* |
| SHSS:C performance | | | | | |
| Total score[c] | 7.27 | 5.98 | 4.76 | 12.8*** | 2.79** |
| Amnesia recall[d] | 3.10 | 5.30 | 6.60 | 25.1*** | 3.07** |
| Reversibility recall[e] | 3.62 | 2.30 | 1.78 | 8.5** | 1.50 |

*Note.* From "Phenomena of Hypnosis: 2. Posthypnotic Amneisa" by F. J. Evans, 1980, in G. D. Burrows and L. Dennerstein (Eds.), *Handbook of Hypnosis and Psychosomatic Medicine* (p. 93), Amsterdam: Elsevier/North-Holland. Copyright 1980 by Elsevier/North-Holland Biomedical Press. Reprinted by permission.

[a]For three groups based on HGSHS:A amnesia recall.
[b]Comparing random-recall versus ordered-recall subgroups.
[c]Based on 11 items, excluding amnesia.
[d]Number of items recalled on initial amnesia test.
[e]Number of items recalled on subsequent reversibility test.
*$p < .05$.
**$p < .005$.
***$p < .001$. (All $p$'s one-tailed.)

1986) showing a diminution in organizational strategies and categorization in word-list paradigms. It can be concluded that a primary mechanism of posthypnotic amnesia is a temporary disruption of those retrieval strategies that normally lead to efficient recall. Although not documented as extensively, the evidence also indicates that these retrieval functions return to normal with the lifting of the amnesia. There is no indication that the recall of amnesic and nonamnesic subjects is different in any situation other than during the amnesic recall. Temporary disruption of these retrieval strategies that normally aid efficient recall is a hallmark of posthypnotic amnesia.

## POSTHYPNOTIC AMNESIA: A BRIEF SYNTHESIS

The research described in this chapter not only provides heuristic hypotheses about the nature of posthypnotic amnesia, but contributes insights into the nature of normal memory processes. Posthypnotic amnesia apparently involves a temporary disruption of normal retrieval strategies, particularly those involving temporal sequencing, which is usually pre-eminent in the recall of episodic experiences. Disrupted retrieval is also observed when other paradigms are used, including word-list clustering and seriation. The disrupted retrieval during amnesia is not a function of basic differences in waking-recall styles between subjects who are high and low in hypnotizability.[16] The disruption of retrieval strategies is a robust phenomenon, even when subjects are challenged to overcome their failure to recall. The disruption is temporary because it is removed by lifting the amnesia, and it does not occur unless amnesia is specifically suggested.

Using rho as an unobtrusive measure of disrupted retrieval has limited us to the study of subjects with partial amnesia rather than those with complete amnesia. However, some deeply hypnotized subjects have experienced source amnesia, which seems to be a manifestation of the same process limited to a single experience. The source-amnesic subject remembers some content, but is unable to locate it in the temporal context of his or her hypnosis experience, just as those subjects who recall a few more items are unable to list these events in the ongoing temporal context of the hypnotic period.

The hypnotized subject has difficulty recalling his or her experiences because of a temporary disruption of the retrieval process induced by the amnesia suggestion. Obviously, the subject cannot report experiences that he or she cannot remember, even though, at another level, the experiences remain available to be used in other cognitive operations (recognition, re-learning) that make use of different access routes to memory.

The apparent paradox of the simultaneous availability and inaccessibility of memories is not unique to hypnosis. In everyday life, the inability to remember material that is present in memory occurs with the tip-of-the-tongue phenomenon, as well as in other all-too-familiar quirks of memory. When material is recalled in one form but not in another, whether in normal memory or in posthypnotic amnesia, a paradox exists only if the emphasis is placed on the forgotten material. If the nature of the retrieval process becomes the focus of investigation, the same material may seem to be both

---

16. Only limited data are available to reject the hypothesis that waking-recall style is related to posthypnotic amnesia. Retrieval disorganization occurs only in relation to suggested amnesia; it does not occur in these hypnotizable subjects during reversibility or if amnesia is not suggested nor does it occur in normal memory tests (see Table 6-6). Although subjects high and low in hypnotizability recall the same quantity of material after the reversal of any amnesia, there is at least a hint that highly hypnotizable subjects have better recall of remote world events at least 4 years old (Evans, 1980). Personal recall style may affect quantity of recall without eliminating all evidence of some amnesia. For example, we (Staats & Evans, 1983) found that anorexia nervosa patients recalled more HGSHS:A suggestions during the amnesia test than any other normal or patient group, but still showed evidence of disorganized temporal sequencing and reversibility (see Table 6-5).

"remembered" and "forgotten"—not in terms of what measure of recall is used, but rather in terms of the organizational tags available to the hypnotized amnesic subject who is actively attempting to retrieve information. The easy reversibility of the amnesia suggests that the experienced events may be stored with minimal organization in a temporary memory buffer, in which the retrieval cue itself is the primary organizational strategy that is to be used when it is appropriate to retrieve the material.

The disrupted-retrieval hypothesis has unresolved problems (Kihlstrom, 1977, 1978), but it has fared better than other hypotheses that have been offered to account for posthypnotic amnesia (Coe & Sarbin, 1977; Spanos, 1986). There are other, more general questions as well. What is the mechanism by which access to memories is blocked? The amnesia suggestion may function in a manner analogous to the cue in studies of the instructed-forgetting paradigm (Bjork, 1970; Epstein, 1972) or of state-specificity paradigms. How does the reversibility signal function to restore effective retrieval? The signal may be simply another retrieval cue, more effective than temporal sequence (and other cues) because of the manner in which the critical memories have been encoded or dissociated.[17]

The dissociation of content and context seen in source amnesia, and implicitly in generic recall, may provide some clues as to the nature of the confabulation often seen when hypnosis is used to uncover memories or refresh memory. If a specific event is stored in isolation from the context in which it has occurred, the struggle to recall will lead to a "search" to facilitate retrieval, but may involve "hooking" contextless experiences that have also become dissociated from the mainstream of memory processing. The distinction between a fixation dot and a clown face fantasy (see Subject A's transcript) is temporarily irrelevant, and so becomes generically and contextually fused or reintegrated into a false or elaborated recall. Similarly, in clinical settings, the process of focusing on a specified "tag" can facilitate the

---

17. Hypnotizable subjects experience dissociative memory effects in addition to posthypnotic amnesia. Highly hypnotizable subjects respond to suggestions administered while they remain asleep (Evans, 1981; Evans, Gustafson, O'Connell, Orne & Shor, 1966). For example, during rapid eye movement (REM) sleep subjects were given the suggestion, "Whenever I say the word 'itch' your nose will itch until you scratch it." Later, hypnotizable subjects responded appropriately to the cue word "itch" while remaining asleep (defined by electroencephalographic criteria). When they awakened the following morning, they did not remember either the suggestions or the fact that they respond (measured by free recall, word association latency, and electrodermal responses to the cue words and other control words). However, these same subjects were able to respond during sleep the next night, or even 6 months later, to the cue word "itch." Retention had clearly occurred across the intervening period in spite of total waking amnesia. It has not yet been determined whether there is an appropriate set of retrieval strategies to make the material available to the waking state. The "tag" or cue that is the primary retrieval "hook" remains dissociated from the sleep system, but is available for cognitive processes during sleep, though, paradoxically, not during normal waking conditions.

production of a hypnotic amnesia. The suggestion to "try as hard as possible to remember the hypnotic dream, even if it means you will have difficulty in recalling the beach and the boat and the rigid arm" will facilitate an amnesia for the suggestions defined as irrelevant, while helping to assure the recall of only the targeted dream. Some of these clinical applications have been discussed elsewhere (Evans, 1986b).

The retrieval failure approach advocated here is tied to ongoing attempts to develop a comprehensive view of both normal and abnormal memory disturbances within the general scope of contemporary cognitive psychology (Kihlstrom & Evans, 1979). These studies seem to provide clues about the mechanisms used by amnesic subjects as they go about the task of trying to remember. Posthypnotic amnesia seems to involve a blurring of the context, resulting in cognitions that are for a time only tenuously linked with waking experience and memory. Phenomenologically, the hypnotized subject knows, but does not know how, why, or even what he or she knows.

## ACKNOWLEDGMENTS

The research reported in this chapter was supported in part by the Carrier Foundation, and in part by Grant No. NH19156 from the National Institute of Mental Health. The influence of John F. Kihlstrom and Helen M. Pettinati is all too apparent, but they, too, may prefer to dissociate content from context. The helpful comments of Kenneth S. Mathisen and Julie Wade during the preparation of the chapter are gratefully acknowledged. Nevertheless, it would not have been completed without the technical help of Jean Balcom, as well as Marie Brown, Mary Anne Hinz, and Christine Makin.

## REFERENCES

Banister, H., & Zangwill, O. L. (1941). Experimentally induced olfactory paramnesias. *British Journal of Psychology, 32*, 153–175.

Barber, T. X., & Calverley, D. S. (1966). Toward a theory of "hypnotic" behavior: Experimental analysis of suggested amnesia. *Journal of Abnormal Psychology, 71*, 95–106.

Bertrand, L. D., & Spanos, N. P. (1985). The organization of recall during hypnotic suggestions for complete and selective amnesia. *Imagination, Cognition and Personality, 4*, 249–261.

Bertrand, L. D., Spanos, N. P., & Parkinson, B. (1983). Test of the dissipation hypothesis of hypnotic amnesia. *Psychological Reports, 52*, 667–671.

Bjork, R. A. (1970). Positive forgetting: The noninterference of items intentionally forgotten. *Journal of Verbal Learning and Verbal Behavior, 9*, 255–268.

Bower, G. H. (1972). A selective review of organizational factors in memory. In E. Tulving & W. Donaldson (Eds.), *Organization of memory* (pp. 93–137). New York: Academic Press.

Bowers, K. S. (1976). *Hypnosis for the seriously curious.* Monterey, CA: Brooks/Cole.

Brown, R., & McNeil, D. (1966). The "tip of the tongue" phenomenon. *Journal of Verbal Learning and Verbal Behavior, 5*, 325–337.

Butterfield, E. C. (1964). The interruption of tasks: Methodological, factual, and theoretical issues. *Psychological Bulletin, 62*, 309–322.

Coe, W. C. (1978). The credibility of posthypnotic amnesia: A contextualist's view. *International Journal of Clinical and Experimental Hypnosis, 26*, 218–245.

Coe, W. C., Baugher, R. J., Krimm, W. R., & Smith, J. A. (1976). A further examination of selective recall following hypnosis. *International Journal of Clinical and Experimental Hypnosis, 22*, 13–21.

Coe, W. C., & Sarbin, T. R. (1977). Hypnosis from the standpoint of a contextualist. *Annals of the New York Academy of Sciences, 296*, 2–13.

Cooper, L. M. (1966). Spontaneous and suggested posthypnotic source amnesia. *International Journal of Clinical and Experimental Hypnosis, 14*, 180–193.

Cooper, L. M. (1972). Hypnotic amnesia. In E. Fromm & R. E. Shor (Eds.), *Hypnosis: Research developments and perspectives* (pp. 217–252). Chicago: Aldine-Atherton.

Crawford, H. J. (1974). The effects of marijuana on primary suggestibility. *Dissertation Abstracts International, 35*, p. 3055.

Dubreuil, D. L., Spanos, N. P., & Bertrand, L. D. (1982). Does hypnotic amnesia dissipate with time? *Imagination, Cognition and Personality, 2*, 103–113.

Epstein, W. (1972). Mechanisms of directed forgetting. In G. H. Bower (Ed.), *The psychology of learning and motivation: Advances in research and theory* (pp. 147–191). New York: Academic Press.

Erdelyi, M. H., & Kleinbard, J. (1978). Has Ebbinghaus decayed with time? The growth of recall (hypermnesia) over days. *Journal of Experimental Psychology: Human Learning and Memory, 4*, 275–289.

Evans, F. J. (1972, September). Posthypnotic amnesia and the temporary disruption of retrieval processes. In H. W. Leibowitz (Chair), *On the nature of posthypnotic amnesia*. Symposium conducted at the 80th Annual Convention of the American Psychological Association, Honolulu.

Evans, F. J. (1979a). Contextual forgetting: Posthypnotic source amnesia. *Journal of Abnormal Psychology, 88*, 556–563.

Evans, F. J. (1979b). Hot amethysts, eleven fingers and the Orient Express. In G. D. Burrows, D. R. Collison & L. Dennerstein (Eds.), *Hypnosis, 1979* (pp. 47–53). Amsterdam: Elsevier/North-Holland.

Evans, F. J. (1980). Phenomena of hypnosis: 2. Posthypnotic amnesia. In G. D. Burrows & L. Dennerstein (Eds.), *Handbook of hypnosis and psychosomatic medicine* (pp. 85–103). Amsterdam: Elsevier/North-Holland.

Evans, F. J. (1981). Sleep and hypnosis: Accessibility of altered states of consciousness. *Advances in Physiological Sciences, 17*, 453–456.

Evans, F. J. (1986a). Hypnosis and behavioral compliance: Is the cup half empty or half full? [Commentary on N. P Spanos, "Hypnotic behavior: A social psychological interpretation of amnesia, analgesia and 'trance logic'"]. *Behavioral and Brain Sciences, 9*, 471–473.

Evans, F. J. (1986b). The importance and role of posthypnotic amnesia. In B. Zilbergeld, M. G. Edelstien, & D. L. Araoz (Eds.), *Hypnosis: Questions and answers* (pp. 173–180). New York: Norton.

Evans, F. J., Gustafson, L. A., O'Connell, D. N., Orne, M. T., & Shor, R. E. (1966). Response during sleep with intervening waking amnesia. *Science, 152*, 666–667.

Evans, F. J., & Kihlstrom, J. F. (1973). Posthypnotic amnesia as disrupted retrieval. *Journal of Abnormal Psychology, 82*, 317–323.

Evans, F. J., Kihlstrom, J. F., & Orne, E. C. (1973). Quantifying subjective reports during posthypnotic amnesia. *Proceedings of the 81st Annual Convention of the American Psychological Association, 8*, 1077–1078.

Evans, F. J., & Mitchell, W. A. (1977, October). *Interaction between neighbors during group hypnosis: The independence of social influence and hypnotizability*. Paper presented at the 29th Annual Meeting of the Society for Clinical and Experimental Hypnosis, Los Angeles.

Evans, F. J., & Thorn, W. A. F. (1966). Two types of posthypnotic amnesia: Recall amnesia and source amnesia. *International Journal of Clinical and Experimental Hypnosis, 14,* 162–179.

Geiselman, R. E., Fishman, D. L., Jaenicke, C., Larner, B. R., MacKinnon, D. P., Shoenberg, S., & Swartz, S. (1983). Mechanisms of hypnotic and nonhypnotic forgetting. *Journal of Experimental Psychology: Learning, Memory, and Cognition, 9,* 626–635.

Gheorghiu, V. (1967). Some peculiarities of posthypnotic source amnesia of information. In L. Chertok (Ed.), *Psychophysiological mechanisms of hypnosis* (pp. 112–122). New York: Springer.

Graham, K. R., & Patton, A. (1968). Retroactive inhibition, hypnosis, and hypnotic amnesia. *International Journal of Clinical and Experimental Hypnosis, 16,* 68–74.

Gregg, V. (1979). Posthypnotic amnesia and general memory theory. *Bulletin of the British Society of Experimental and Clinical Hypnosis, 2,* 11–14.

Hilgard, E. R. (1965). *Hypnotic susceptibility.* New York: Harcourt, Brace & World.

Hilgard, E. R. (1977). *Divided consciousness: Multiple controls in human thought and action.* New York: Wiley-Interscience.

Hilgard, E. R., & Cooper, L. M. (1965). Spontaneous and suggested posthypnotic amnesia. *International Journal of Clinical and Experimental Hypnosis, 13,* 261–273.

Hilgard, E. R., & Hommel, L. S. (1961). Selective amnesia for events within hypnosis in relation to repression. *Journal of Personality, 29,* 205–216.

Howard, M. L., & Coe, W. C. (1980). The effects of context and subjects' perceived control in breaching posthypnotic amnesiaa. *Journal of Personality and Social Psychology, 46,* 342–359.

Hull, C. L. (1933). *Hypnosis and suggestibility: An experimental approach.* New York: Appleton-Century-Crofts.

Kihlstrom, J. F. (1975). The effects of organization and motivation on recall during posthypnotic amnesia. *Dissertation Abstracts International, 36,* 2473B–2474B. (University Microfilms No. 75-240,82)

Kihlstrom, J. F. (1977). Models of posthypnotic amnesia. *Annals of the New York Academy of Sciences, 296,* 284–301.

Kihlstrom, J. F. (1978). Context and cognition in posthypnotic amnesia. *International Journal of Clinical and Experimental Hypnosis, 26,* 246–267.

Kihlstrom, J. F. (1980). Posthypnotic amnesia for recently learned material: Interactions with "episodic" and "semantic" memory. *Cognitive Psychology, 12,* 227–251.

Kihlstrom, J. F. (1983). Instructed forgetting: Hypnotic and nonhypnotic. *Journal of Experimental Psychology: General, 112*(1), 73–79.

Kihlstrom, J. R. (1985). Posthypnotic amnesia and the dissociation of memory. *Psychology of Learning and Motivation, 19,* 131–178.

Kihlstrom, J. F., Brenneman, H. A., Pistole, D. D., & Shor, R. E. (1985). Hypnosis as a retrieval cue in posthypnotic amnesia. *Journal of Abnormal Psychology, 94,* 264–271.

Kihlstrom, J. F., Easton, R. D., & Shor, R. E. (1983). Spontaneous recovery of memory during posthypnotic amnesia. *International Journal of Clinical and Experimental Hypnosis, 31,* 309–323.

Kihlstrom, J. F., & Evans, F. J. (1976). Recovery of memory after posthypnotic amnesia. *Journal of Abnormal Psychology, 85,* 564–569.

Kihlstrom, J. F., & Evans, F. J. (1977). Residual effect of suggestions for posthypnotic amnesia: A re-examination. *Journal of Abnormal Psychology, 86,* 327–333.

Kihlstrom, J. F., & Evans, F. J. (1978). Generic recall during posthypnotic amnesia. *Bulletin of the Psychonomic Society, 12,* 57–60.

190 *Induced and Spontaneous Models of Reversible Memory Disruption*

Kihlstrom, J. F., & Evans, F. J. (1979). Memory retrieval processes in posthypnotic amnesia. In J. F. Kihlstrom and F. J. Evans (Eds.), *Functional disorders of memory* (pp. 179–215). Hillsdale, NJ: Erlbaum.

Kihlstrom, J. F., Evans, F. J., Orne, E. C., & Orne, M. T. (1980). Attempting to breach posthypnotic amnesia. *Journal of Abnormal Psychology, 89,* 603–616.

Kihlstrom, J. F., & Register, P. A. (1984). Optimal scoring of amnesia on the Harvard Group Scale of Hypnotic Susceptibility, Form A. *International Journal of Clinical and Experimental Hypnosis, 32,* 51–57.

Kihlstrom, J. F., & Shor, R. E. (1978). Recall and recognition during posthypnotic amnesia. *International Journal of Clinical and Experimental Hypnosis, 26,* 330–348.

Kihlstrom, J. F., & Wilson, L. (1984). Temporal organization of recall during post-hypnotic amnesia. *Journal of Abnormal Psychology, 93,* 200–208.

Lavoie, G., & Sabourin, M. (1980). Hypnosis and schizophrenia: A review of experimental and clinical studies. In G. D. Burrows & L. Dennerstein (Eds.), *Handbook of hypnosis and psychosomatic medicine* (pp. 377–419). New York: Elsevier/North-Holland.

Lieberman, J., Brisson, A., & Lavoie, G. (1978). Suggested amnesia and order of recall as a function of hypnotic susceptibility and learning conditions in chronic schizophrenic patients. *International Journal of Clinical and Experimental Hypnosis, 26,* 268–280.

McConkey, K. M., & Sheehan, P. W. (1981). The impact of videotape playback of hypnotic events on posthypnotic amnesia. *Journal of Abnormal Psychology, 90,* 46–54.

Nace, E. P., Orne, M. T., & Hammer, A. G. (1974). Posthypnotic amnesia as an active psychic process: The reversibility of amnesia. *Archives of General Psychiatry, 31,* 257–260.

Neisser, U. (1967). *Cognitive psychology.* Englewood Cliffs, NJ: Prentice-Hall.

Nemiah, J. C. (1979). Dissociative amnesia: A clinical and theoretical reconsideration. In J. F. Kihlstrom & F. J. Evans (Eds.), *Functional disorders of memory* (pp. 303–323). Hillsdale, NJ: Erlbaum.

O'Connell, D. N. (1964). An experimental comparison of hypnotic depth measured by self-ratings and by an objective scale. *International Journal of Clinical and Experimental Hypnosis, 12,* 34–46.

O'Connell, D. N. (1966). Selective recall of hypnotic susceptibility items: Evidence for repression or enhancement? *International Journal of Clinical and Experimental Hypnosis, 14,* 150–161.

Orne, M. T. (1959). The nature of hypnosis: Artifact and essence. *Journal of Abnormal and Social Psychology, 58,* 277–299.

Orne, M. T. (1966). On the mechanisms of posthypnotic amnesia. *International Journal of Clinical and Experimental Hypnosis, 14,* 121–134.

Orne, M. T. (1979). On the simulating subject as a quasi-control group in hypnosis research: What, why and how. In E. Fromm & R. E. Shor (Eds.), *Hypnosis: Developments in research and new perspectives* (2nd ed., pp. 519–565). Chicago: Aldine.

Overton, D. A. (1968). Dissociated learning in drug states (state-dependent learning). In D. H. Efron, J. O. Cole, J. Levine, & R. Wittenborn (Eds.), *Psychopharmacology: A review of progress 1957–1967* (pp. 918–930). Washington, DC: U. S. Government Printing Office.

Pettinati, H. M. (1979). Selectivity in memory during posthypnotic amnesia. *Dissertation Abstracts International, 40,* 898B–899B. (University Microfilms No. 79-15, 840)

Pettinati, H. M., & Evans, F. J. (1978). Posthypnotic amnesia: Evaluation of selective recall of successful experiences. *International Journal of Clinical and Experimental Hypnosis, 26,* 317–329.

Pettinati, H. M., & Evans, F. J. (1980, October). *Qualitative analysis of the memory reports of amnesic and nonamnesic subjects.* Paper presented at the 32nd Annual Meeting of the Society for Clinical and Experimental Hypnosis, Chicago.

Pettinati, H. M., Evans, F. J., Orne, E. C., & Orne, M. T. (1981). Restricted use of success cues in retrieval during posthypnotic amnesia. *Journal of Abnormal Psychology, 90,* 345–353.

Radtke, H. L., & Spanos, N. P. (1981). Temporal sequencing during posthypnotic amnesia: A methodological critique. *Journal of Abnormal Psychology, 90,* 476–485.

Radtke, H. L., Spanos, N. P., Della Malva, C. L., & Stam, H. J. (1986). Temporal organization and hypnotic amnesia using a modification of the Harvard Group Scale of Hypnotic Susceptibility. *International Journal of Clinical and Experimental Hypnosis, 34,* 41–54.

Radtke-Bodorik, H. L., Planas, M., & Spanos, N. P. (1980). Suggested amnesia, verbal inhibition, and disorganized recall for a long word list. *Canadian Journal of Behavioral Science, 12,* 87–97.

Reed, G. (1979). Everyday anomalies of recall and recognition. In J. F. Kihlstrom & F. J. Evans (Eds.), *Functional disorders of memory* (pp. 1–29). Hillsdale, NJ: Erlbaum.

Roediger, H. L., & Crowder, R. G. (1976). A serial-position effect in the recall of United States presidents. *Bulletin of the Psychonomic Society, 8,* 277–278.

Rosenzweig, S. (1938). The experimental study of repression. In H. A. Murray (Ed.), *Explorations in personality* (pp. 472–490). New York: Oxford University Press.

Sarbin, T. R., & Coe, W. C. (1972). *Hypnosis: A social psychological analysis of influence communication.* New York: Holt, Rinehart & Winston.

Schuyler, B. A., & Coe, W. C. (1981). A physiological investigation of volitional and nonvolitional experience during posthypnotic amnesia. *Journal of Personality and Social Psychology, 40,* 1160–1169.

Schwartz, W. S. (1978). Time and context during hypnotic involvement. *International Journal of Clincal and Experimental Hypnosis, 26,* 307–316.

Schwartz, W. S. (1980). Hypnosis and episodic memory. *International Journal of Clinical and Experimental Hypnosis, 28,* 375–385.

Shor, R. E., & Orne, E. C. (1962). *The Harvard Group Scale of Hypnotic Susceptibility, Form A.* Palo Alto, CA: Consulting Psychologists Press.

Spanos, N. P. (1986). Hypnotic behavior: A social psychological interpretation of amnesia, analgesia and "trance logic." *Behavioral and Brain Sciences, 93,* 449–467.

Spanos, N. P., & Bodorik, H. L. (1977). Suggested amnesia and disorganized recall in hypnotic and task-motivated subjects. *Journal of Abnormal Psychology, 86,* 295–305.

Spanos, N. P., & D'Eon, J. L. (1980). Hypnotic amnesia, disorganized recall and inattention. *Journal of Abnormal Psychology, 89,* 744–750.

Spanos, N. P., Radtke, H. L., & Bertrand, L. D. (1985). Hypnotic amnesia as a strategic enactment: Breaching amnesia in highly susceptible subjects. *Journal of Personality and Social Psychology, 47,* 1155–1169.

Spanos, N. P., Radtke, H. L., Bertrand, L. D., Addie, L. D., & Drummond, J. (1982). Disorganized recall, hypnotic amnesia and subject faking: More disconfirmatory data. *Psychological Reports, 50,* 383–389.

Spanos, N. P., Radtke, H. L., & Dubreuil, D. L. (1982). Episodic and semantic memory in posthypnotic amnesia: A reevaluation. *Journal of Personality and Social Psychology, 43,* 565–573.

Spanos, N. P., Radtke-Bodorik, H. L., & Shabinsky, M. A. (1980). Amnesia, subjective organization and learning of a list of unrelated words in hypnotic and task-motivated subjects. *International Journal of Clinical and Experimental Hypnosis, 28,* 126–139.

Spanos, N. P., Radtke-Bodorik, H. L., & Stam, H. J. (1980). Disorganized recall during suggested amnesia: Fact not artifact. *Journal of Abnormal Psychology, 89,* 1–19.

Spanos, N. P., Stam, H. J., D'Eon, J. L., Pawlak, A. E., & Radtke-Bodorik, H. L. (1980). Effects of social-psychological variables on hypnotic amnesia. *Journal of Personality and Social Psychology, 39,* 737–750.

192      *Induced and Spontaneous Models of Reversible Memory Disruption*

Spanos, N. P., Tkachyk, M., Bertrand, L. D., & Weekes, J. R. (1984). The dissipation hypothesis of hypnotic amnesia: More disconfirming evidence. *Psychological Reports, 55,* 191–196.

St. Jean, R., & Coe, W. C. (1981). Recall and recognition memory during posthypnotic amnesia: A failure to confirm the disrupted-search hypothesis and the memory disorganization hypothesis. *Journal of Abnormal Psychology, 90,* 231–241.

Staats, J. M., & Evans, F. J. (1983, October). *Posthypnotic amnesia in four diagnostic groups of hospitalized psychiatric patients.* Paper presented at the 35th Annual Meeting of the Society for Clinical and Experimental Hypnosis, Boston.

Talland, G. A. (1965). *Deranged memory: A psychonomic study of the amnesic syndrome.* New York: Academic Press.

Thorn, W. A. F. (1960). *A study of the correlates of dissociation as measured by hypnotic amnesia.* Unpublished bachelor's (honours) thesis, University of Sydney, Australia.

Tulving, E. (1972). Episodic and semantic memory. In E. Tulving & W. Donaldson (Eds.), *Organization of memory* (pp. 381–403). New York: Academic Press.

Tulving, E., & Pearlstone, Z. (1966). Availability and accessibility of information in memory for words. *Journal of Verbal Learning and Verbal Behavior, 5,* 381–391.

Tulving, E., & Thompson, D. M. (1973). Encoding specificity and retrieval processes in episodic memory. *Psychological Review, 80,* 352–373.

Underwood, B. J. (1977). *Temporal codes for memories: Issues and problems.* Hillsdale, NJ: Erlbaum.

von Restorff, H. (1933). Über die Wirkung von Bereichsbildungen im Spurenfeld. *Psychologische Forschung, 18,* 299–342.

Wagstaff, G. F. (1977). An experimental study of compliance and post-hypnotic amnesia. *British Journal of Social and Clinical Psychology, 16,* 225–228.

Weitzenhoffer, A. M. (1953). *Hypnotism: An objective study in suggestibility.* New York: Wiley.

Weitzenhoffer, A. M., & Hilgard, E. R. (1959). *Stanford Hypnotic Susceptibility Scale, Forms A and B.* Palo Alto, CA: Consulting Psychologists Press.

Weitzenhoffer, A. M., & Hilgard, E. R. (1962). *Stanford Hypnotic Susceptibility Scale, Form C.* Palo Alto, CA: Consulting Psychologists Press.

Williamsen, J. A., Johnson, H. J., & Eriksen, C. W. (1965). Some characteristics of posthypnotic amnesia. *Journal of Abnormal Psychiatry, 70,* 123–131.

# 7

## Perception and Memory for Events during Adequate General Anesthesia for Surgical Operations

HENRY L. BENNETT
*University of California–Davis Medical Center*

Do patients remember what transpired during their surgery, either consciously or in the way their bodies recover after surgery? One man's auditory exposure during surgery might include the following conversation:

*One doctor*: Oh, yeah, he's a real loser (*referring to someone else*). He's not going to do very well.

*Other doctor*: Yeah. Is this bad (*asking nurse about a suture*)?

*Nurse*: Yeah, real bad (*to bad suture*). How is he (*referring to first person*) anyway?

*First doctor*: All screwed up. . . . This is just terrible (*referring to a fine point of surgical technique*). This is the worst bone graft ever; oh my God, this is just awful. . . . He's (*referring to the first person*) going to have a bad time in the future; I think he's going to do poorly. Very poorly.

*Second doctor*: No kidding. He's a goner. Maybe he'll leave town first.

One of the primary goals of anesthesia—amnesia—is achieved from the clinician's viewpoint if the patient does not have conscious recall of surgical events. The question still exists, however, as to whether the patient's self-report (and the anesthesiologist's observation) is accurate.[1] That is, can memories be recorded and can other changes in the nervous system take place (as learned responses to the environment) during the period when the patient

---

1. What is called "awareness during general anesthesia" in the anesthesiology literature is quite different. Within anesthesiology, a generic version of awareness is used—awareness of the environment. It is applied to cases of giving inadequate anesthesia: The patient is conscious but is otherwise unable or unwilling to communicate, or unsuccessful at communicating, this consciousness *of* the surgery. This outcome certainly exists in anesthesiology, and it is most unwelcome when it does. Every anesthesiologist would agree that "awareness" episodes can and do occur as results of inadequate anesthesia. Anesthesiologists currently lack an "awareness" monitor, and the most at-risk patients—trauma victims, the elderly, and Caesarian section patients—may have between 10% and 30% risk of being conscious *of* their surgeries. This can, in full-blown cases, be perhaps the most excruciatingly traumatic of all experiences, a truly torturous event (Anonymous, 1979). In adequate anesthesia these experiences are prevented; the patient does not report consciousness *of* anything. There is a reported incidence of less than 1% for conscious memories occurring following anesthesia, patients reliably demonstrate the amnesia required by adequate general anesthesia.

is anesthetized? And can methods like hypnosis be useful in helping us answer these questions? Before addressing these central questions, it is important to provide some background about the anesthetized state.

## GENERAL ANESTHESIA

Under general anesthesia, the patient appears unresponsive and comatose. The activities of the "old brain"—the hindbrain, the reticular activating systems, and the pontine structures—are the likely sites of adequate anesthesia using the potent inhalational agents (Clark & Rosner, 1973; Rosner & Clark, 1973; Winters, 1976). Remarkably, there is as yet no general theory of anesthetic action. Different substances with different loci of action are able to produce the same result. In defining adequacy of anesthesia, functional criteria are used: (1) The patient is unresponsive to painful stimulation; and (2) the patient is amnesic for the time period. These must coexist for general anesthesia to be successful. Despite immobility, however, there is during adequate general anesthesia a virtual storm of physiological activity going on within the patient.

### Neuroendocrine Variables and Learning

Increasing interest in neurotransmission and the physiochemical basis of memory has led to discussion of neuroendocrine responses (McGaugh, 1983; Pert, Ruff, Weber, & Herkenham, 1985). The stress responses to anesthesia and surgery are among the greatest acute physiological challenges. A neuroendocrine "window" is in effect, with high levels of circulating catecholamines, neuropeptides, and hypothalamic–pituitary–adrenal axis circuits ready to meet the crisis. Stress-related behaviors are known to influence the dose required to achieve surgical anesthesia. Anxious patients release more catecholamines into the bloodstream, resulting in more autonomic reactivity; therefore, higher levels of agents are needed to blunt cardiovascular and other observable responses ordinarily seen during stressful surgical events (Burnsten & Russ, 1965; Derbyshire *et al.*, 1983; Ramsay, 1982). For example, vasopressin (antidiuretic hormone, or ADH) has a stimulation effect in the central nervous system (CNS) and appears to act like catecholamine agonists (Doris, 1984; Strupp, Weingartner, Goodwin, & Gold, 1984). For the anesthetized patient, memory for intraoperative events may be modulated by a dynamic interplay between the centrally inhibiting agents used with anesthesia, such as the anticholinergics, and the patient's own central agonists, such as the catecholamines and neuropeptides. On the other hand, postanesthetic amnesia for declarative or episodic memories for surgery suggests that anesthetics and the amnestics supress efficient encoding by the hippocampal structures, and that this in turn suppresses intentional retrieval.

Learning new responses during deep anesthesia is possible, however. The connection to memory can be stated by a recently reported experiment. Profound depression of the CNS by high doses of barbiturates as confirmed by a flat electroencephalograph (EEG) allowed, nevertheless, for Pavlovian conditioning to an auditory signal in rats (Weinberger, Gold & Sternberg, 1984). The learning was behaviorally evident in a conditioned fear response which was elicited during the assessment of learning that took place on the 10th postanesthetic day. However, learning was demonstrated only in those animals who had been injected before training with epinephrine. The inclusion of neuroendocrine variables with learning during anesthesia may be a clue to the necessary and sufficient conditions for learning what is registered in the CNS through auditory pathways.

*Neurophysiology*

From the observation of the obtunded, tubed, catheterized, multiply IV-lined, split-open body of the patient during surgery, one may expect, *prima facie*, that the brain is idle, in neutral gear, unable, unwilling, unresponsive, and uncommunicative. One may expect that signals shot from the sense organs to the brain during this obtunded state simply do not register there, or that if they do, the signals have no consequence. Such an assumption may be further supported when the patient reports no memory for the surgical period.

EEG Recordings

EEG recordings have been enlightening to those believing that the CNS is inactive during anesthesia. While there is no recognized guide to the depth of anesthesia (at least to date) based upon an EEG, there is activity across the frequency domain. It is unclear, however, how the presence or absence of different frequency bands of electrophysiological activity relates to cognitive functioning.

A critical issue to claims that patients continue to "hear" during general anesthesia is whether the neuronal effects of general anesthesia obstruct the passage of auditory stimuli to areas subserving the processes of verbal comprehension. The effects of anesthetic agents on the EEG and the auditory evoked response (AER) of humans and animals have been well studied. Our understanding of the electrical events underlying the EEG and the AER is fragmentary and necessitates a cautious approach in correlating these neurophysiological indicators with the actual perception of auditory stimuli. Similarly, it should be noted that anesthetic agents are most often studied in isolation. In clinical practice, however, they are applied in conjunction with other drugs in a highly stressful setting, and such interactional effects are not well known.

## Sensory Evoked Responses

Evidence for the pharmacological and physiological locus of anesthetic action comes from electrophysiological work tracking sensory signals along pathways at different anesthetic concentrations. This work has produced the most direct link between the observable effects of anesthetic agents and the CNS activity supporting anesthesia. Averaged evoked response methodology has allowed relative precision in tracking sensory pathways and observing the activity of cells and cell clusters.

In terms of ongoing electrical activity in different parts of the brain during inhalational anesthesia, the reticular formation (RF) shows the most complete alteration, while the cochlear nucleus, geniculate nucleus, and auditory cortex are less affected. Cortical responses are attenuated, but waveform morphology persists; intracranial recordings demonstrate persistent neuronal firing patterns to auditory stimulation. The usual interpretation of diminished evoked response at the cortex involves both synaptic inhibition (leading to a loss of excitation reaching the cortex) and an anesthetic effect of cortical depression. However, depression of cortical neurons does not occur in isolated cortex during deep anesthesia (Mori, Winters, & Spooner, 1968; Winters, 1976).[2]

Late components of the AERs are changed under the influence of anesthetic agents. Late components of the AER are thought to reflect more intentional or decision-based activities. Earlier components represent pathways and early registrations of primary cortex. Rosner and Clark's (1973) model of anesthetic effects emphasizes drug differences in sequential regions of activity. Barbiturate effect is characterized as a rapid depression of the RF after which the nonspecific thalamic nuclei become "responsible" for control of the RF, in a cortico-thalamic feedback system. The same reversal of control occurs in ether anesthesia without the sudden depression of the RF and without producing hypersynchronization.

2. A methodological problem with evoked potentials is possible latency variability of the later components of the waveform. This makes interpretation of diminished late evoked potentials difficult. As Lader and Norris (1969) state, "The decrease in the amplitude of the evoked potential could reflect a decrease in the number of neuronal elements subserving 'associative' functions being activated by the stimulus. . . . Another possibility, stemming from the use of an averaging procedure, is that increased variability in the latencies of the individual waves being combined in the average produced the observed effect" (pp. 125–126).

Many researchers have investigated the involvement of the RF mecha-Rosner, 1973; Killam, 1962; Rosner & Clark, 1973; Winters, 1976; Winters, Mori, Spooner, & Kato, 1967). In general, these studies concur with Killam (1962): "The fact that the RF is the site common to the whole series of anesthetics forms the basis of the view that anesthetic properties of the compounds are dependent at least in part on depression of this region" (p. 194). Winters (1976) has proposed a multidirectional schema for the continuum of states of CNS excitability and depression in anesthesia. His schema follows the observation that low dosages of anesthetic agents produce increased excitability of the CNS. He proposes that high levels of RF unit activity in the early stages of anesthesia are necessary for cortical desynchronization: "As functional disorganization becomes more profound, the EEG pattern changes to the spiking phase and the bursting pattern of unit activity becomes more pronounced. At this time there is a profound loss of reticular modulation, the sensory input becomes markedly elevated, and the evoked responses in all brain areas are enlarged" (p. 42). This is descriptive of the early phases of Stage 2 anesthesia, an "excitement phase" through which the brain passes on toward deeper Stage 3 surgical anesthesia.

Responses at the cochlear nucleus are either augmented or not affected. This ties in well with the expected results of release from RF inhibition. Proceeding up the auditory pathway, the inferior colliculus shows marked depression of late potentials for most anesthetics. The early potentials are only moderately depressed. For the geniculate nucleus, there appear to be no decreases in signal strength or a modest decrease in amplitude, depending on the agent. This relay may represent a major intersection of routes, which may account for its response strength. Results from the auditory cortex are less clear. Overall amplitude of responses has been reported as slightly depressed to markedly depressed. An examination of the specific, early response components suggests that the amplitude and latency are both increased in lower inhalational doses, with amplitude falling off as the waveform morphology at later latencies deteriorates.

Recent work using AERs (Thornton *et al.*, 1983; Thornton, Heneghan, James, & Jones, 1984; Thornton, Heneghan, Navaratnarajah, Bateman, & Jones, 1985; Yeoman, Moreno, Rigor, & Dafny, 1980) indicates that the inhalational agents may have primary activity in the rostral hindbrain and brain stem, while the intravenous anesthetics affect cortical structures more profoundly. On the basis of the AER response, inhalational agents alter the latencies but not the morphology or amplitudes of the waves, while the potent intravenous agents affect the later cortical waves but not the early brainstem waves. Far from excluding the possibility, the results indicate that early sensory components of the auditory system are continuously active during general anesthesia.

## PERCEPTION AND MEMORY OF AUDITORY EVENTS DURING ANESTHESIA

Perception in the sense of phenomenal experience does not seem to occur during adequate anesthesia, but perception in the sense of the registration of sensory–neural events does. Memory, similarly, must be divided at least between (1) what are phenomenally represented as "episodic" memories for one's life experiences and (2) tendencies of the nervous system to change response patterns on the basis of reinforcing information. This latter form of memory is what has been neglected in most investigations of whether learning can occur during adequate anesthesia. For data about hearing during general anesthesia to be supported, a theoretical basis is advanced to support the claim that understanding language is highly automatic for pertinent information within structures activated early in the auditory system.

### Receiving Auditory Information

Sensory transmission of auditory information is either boosted or unchanged during what can exist as adequate clinical anesthesia. Deepening anesthesia does not produce a loss of sensory transmission for auditory information. But, the question remains, do these transmissions "sink in," or do they just "bounce off a wall" without any effect? The same question has been asked about other "unattended" sources of information.

### The Early-Selection Theory

For the past 30 years, research on selective attention has been concerned with how information from the environment is selected into consciousness. The inquiry was launched by Broadbent (1958, 1977), who proposed that strategies of searching the environment are analogous to a physical filter: Only those aspects that are selected into consciousness receive processing for meaning in the CNS. All else is discarded before there is any understanding as to what those signals signify. By this reasoning, a continuous effort of attention toward one source of information does not allow other sources of information to influence the nervous system if those sources require higher-level processing to understand their significance. Loud noises may catch our attention, but an adjacent conversation will not unless we happen to tune the filter to those physical characteristics of that conversation (pitch or direction of the voice). This view is called the "early-selection" theory of selective attention. What is critical to the theory is the position that unless there is selective attention paid to them, environmental signals cannot influence the nervous sytem based on the meaning of the signals (e.g., the meaning behind the sounds, "It's cancer; she's only got a few weeks left to live" is not understood unless active efforts of "paying attention" are made toward that signal). By this analysis, unselected auditory information is simply not processed by the nervous system for meaning and falls away like sound waves hitting a wall.

## The Late-Selection Theory

The major alternative to the early-selection theory is the "late-selection" theory of selective attention (Norman, 1968, 1976). Incoming signals are processed in parallel, and only then are they selected into focused attention for further processing or for action. The late-selection theory of attention allows for simultaneous sources of information to influence the nervous system, based on the full knowledge store. Only then is entrance into focused attention gained by the feedback influence of ongoing plans and the pertinence of the information. Consciousness *of* an event takes place after the knowledge base has already interacted with the incoming signals.

Work supports the capacity for multiple channels of auditory stimulus processing, sometimes regardless of awareness *of* the stimuli (Eich, 1984; Squire, 1982). It was learned that two verbal perceptual activities could be carried out in parallel simultaneously, yet there might be awareness *of* only one of them (Allport, Antonis, & Reynolds, 1972; Hirst, Spelke, Reaves, Caharack, & Neisser, 1980; Shaffer, 1975). In my own work, subjects who were consciously occupied in an auditory shadowing task were presented with an unattended message with direct statements to engage in a behavior (Bennett, 1980). Messages were maximally separated on the basis of physical characteristics of location and gender of the voice. Extensive debriefing of subjects revealed lack of awareness *of* the unattended message; however, covert videotaping documented a significant response to the unattended suggestion (". . . when you stop talking I want you to touch your nose"), compared with controls. Together, these experiments support the late-selection theory of selective attention. That is, language can be comprehended and responses initiated before conscious processes are activated. In other terms, conscious processes are not always necessary for highly skilled neurological and perceptual activities, which include language understanding (Schneider & Shiffrin, 1977; Shriffrin & Schneider, 1977, 1984). Therefore, it is possible to understand and respond to a linguistic message without awareness of that message.

For events taking place during adequate anesthesia and despite lack of conscious recall, there is compelling evidence that verbal perceptual processes continue during minimal (Adam, 1979), light (Bennett, Davis, & Giannini, 1985), and surgical (Goldmann, 1986; Millar & Watkinson, 1983; Stolzy, Couture, & Edmonds, 1986) levels of anesthesia. These perceptual processes have been demonstrated by persistence into the postoperative period of the effects of presentations of language messages during general anesthesia in the presence of a nearly uniform postanesthetic amnesia. Therefore, though obtunded, patients appear to be influenced by verbal messages they are asked to remember.

## Remembering Auditory Information from Surgery

The most potent claims for unconscious memory retention come from post-surgical recollections of some patients in hypnosis about events that occurred during surgery (Cheek, 1959, 1966, 1979; Levinson, 1965). Psychologists, in attempting to investigate such claims systematically, have come to the operating room with verbal recall and recognition tasks using word lists. Generally, their results have not added support for the retention of surgical events (Dubovsky & Trustman, 1976; Eich, Reeves, & Katz, 1985; Loftus, Schooler, Loftus, & Glauber, 1985). However, standard memory tasks may not be appropriate in such an emotion-laden or meaningful setting.

A surgical patient's nervous system facing general anesthesia must be presumed to be oriented toward surviving the acute event, alert to sources of information relevant to that survival. Information of current status and future prognosis is highly pertinent and in stark contrast to the content of standardized memory tests. Throughout the perioperative period—from before surgery until well into recovery from surgery—patients are concerned with their survival, and with assessments by the medical authorities of their condition and prognosis. Thus, less salient material (e.g., a word list) is not likely to be attended to, much less to be recalled later, while a patient's system may possibly be alert or overly sensitized to any remarks concerning his or her physical status. There is considerable evidence for this position.

## Pharmacological Studies of Memory and Amnesia

Many of the concomitant medications given during anesthesia have their own action that is likely to contribute differentially to what the patient might retain.

### Benzodiazepines

The clinical observation is that verbal retrieval is markedly depressed for material presented shortly after administration of the benzodiazepines or other "amnestics" (Dundee & Pandit, 1972a, 1972b; Pandit & Dundee, 1970; Pandit, Dundee, & Keilty, 1971; Pandit, Heistercamp, & Cohen, 1976; White, 1986). The psychopharmacological investigation of these drugs suggests, however, that there are not marked deficits in learning under the influence of the barbiturates or the benzodiazepines (Gray, 1982). Although clinically potent doses will usually result in complete conscious amnesia for events immediately following their administration in humans, it has been reported that these agents inhibit stimulus acquisition for items that are not very meaningful and/or are unrelated. When categorized lists or concrete as opposed to abstract word lists are learned, performance improves significantly (Lister, 1985). This suggests that the meaning of the items can affect their acquisition. In addition, experimental assessment of this amnesia has shown that cognitive skills will show savings from the learning trials in such tasks as backward-reading skills, mirror drawing, jigsaw learning, and reading a mirror image (Lister, 1985). To use the distinction between "knowing that" and "knowing how," declarative memory ("knowing that") can be selectively inhibited while procedural memory ("knowing how") is maintained.

Thus, the nervous system, though disrupted and selectively impaired by the "amnestics," does not cease acquiring material, nor are procedural tasks necessarily inhibited. Rather, the information that does enter the nervous system is less accessible to the systems of declarative memory for the episodes following administration. Given more retention for more organized and meaningful material, the issue of whether the benzodiazepines prevent later access to the content of meaningful stimulus presentations has not been adequately investigated in humans.

Anticholinergics

The central anticholinergic scopolamine has a more potent effect than the sedative/tranquilizers upon human cognitive abilities. Scopolamine blocks the reuptake of acetylcholine at the muscarinic receptors and thus limits the available neurotransmitters primarily in the frontal areas of the brain. Depending on their doses, atropine, glycopyrrolate, and scopolamine are effective in producing sedation and lack of vigilance.

Scopolamine, a belladonna alkaloid like atropine, has a reputation as a particularly potent amnestic. Pharmacological studies in humans have nevertheless found that "the apparent character of scopolamine-induced amnesia depended largely on the memory task used to define it" (Caine, Weingartner, Ludlow, Cudahy, & Wehry, 1981, p. 79). For example, subjects hearing 12 words controlled for imagery and frequency generated either semantic or acoustic associations after 0.8 mg of scopolamine (administered intramuscularly). In delayed-recall tests, both types of associations produced a 60–70% drop in memory, whereas cued recall for the same items showed only a 10% drop in memory performance. Therefore, retention was intact but effortful retrieval was impaired. "Evidently, the neurochemical processes disrupted by scopolamine are not involved in mediating the maintenance of information in memory" (p. 79). What scopolamine appears to do is to disrupt efficient encoding processes, leading not to an absence of retention but to a deficiency in effective retrieval. Intentional processes are disrupted by the amnestics, but the automatic processes of pattern recognition are not. Whether it is possible to prevent acquisition of particularly pertinent signals remains to be investigated.

## Muscle Relaxants

The widespread use of muscle relaxants in contemporary anesthesia has profoundly changed its conduct and allowed lesser concentrations of inhalational agents to be used during many surgeries. They act peripherally by blocking the transmission to the muscle at the end plate terminal. Since the synthesis of d-tubocurarine in 1942, both depolarizing and nondepolarizing muscle relaxants for skeletal paralysis have been introduced and are commonly used. It has been known for nearly 40 years that despite inducing a complete lack of movement from skeletal paralysis, muscle relaxants have no effect on cerebral function. Some surgeries that were performed solely with curare as the anesthetic resulted in patients' complaining of complete consciousness during surgery. Today, to be paralyzed and conscious of surgery is recognized as inadequate anesthesia and can produce a posttraumatic stress disorder requiring intensive psychotherapeutic intervention (Blacher, 1975, 1984).

### *Memory Retrieval: Case Reports*

A patient in one of our studies was having a laparoscopic tubal ligation under sufentanyl/nitrous oxide anesthesia. The following sequence of events was witnessed by three of us at the head of the operating table. The patient was intubated, and her eyes were taped closed. About halfway through the procedure, as the surgeons were examining her abdominal organs, the anesthesiologist asked them, "Is everything OK?" (referring to the patient's condition). The patient, until then lying still and with stable vital signs, quite intentionally nodded her head to indicate "Yes." We then calmly questioned her directly. She signaled with head movements that she was comfortable and was not having pain. She was reassured and remained still to the end of surgery. In the recovery room, and 2 weeks later in a postanesthetic interview, she had no recall (declarative memory) of the episode. Yet in the interview she responded vigorously to the intraoperative instruction that she signal having heard a message by tugging on her left ear in the interview (procedural memory).

   The history of anecdotal case reports in the anesthesiology literature shows that conscious memory is often not apparent until some significant time after surgery. Additionally, the report is invariably of a significant rather than a trivial incident. Not discussed here are cases of purely inadequate anesthesia where the patient remains fully conscious but is unable to do anything about it. Of interest to memory theory are cases selected when anesthesia is adequate and the patient reports no adverse effects or pain but simply remembers something. Levinson reports in his dissertation (1969) a case separate from his series in which a patient in hypnosis, following varicose vein stripping,

> stated that she could feel them working at the top of her left leg and was surprised that there was no pain. She heard her surgeon say to a lady doctor that she should do one leg and he would do the other. She described the surgeon standing on her left and the woman on her right. The surgeon was showing the other doctor how to do the operation. She could hear the anesthetist, Dr. Parkhouse, talking but could not recall exactly what he was saying. (p. 18)

Are such recollections accurate? Are they memory creations or recollections of actual events? The use of hypnosis is reviewed later. For now, the events reported by the patient in this case did occur.

## The "Fat Lady" Syndrome

The most common disparaging remark made in the operating room about the anesthetized patient is probably in reference to weight. The patient is over-weight and someone starts talking about it. There is also the "dirtball" phenomenon, which, if the thesis of auditory perception during general anesthesia is true, may be germane to these patients' later antisocial behavior. That is, particularly offensive and derogatory statements are made in regard to apparently unsavory patients and their immediate circumstances. Such statements would ordinarily incite some of these patients to attack the offenders. If there are memories of intraoperative events, especially pertinent ones, that can influence postoperative behaviors, insulting remarks toward these patients may generate antisocial postoperative behaviors.

But the existing literature shows only a tendency by overweight female patients to spontaneously recall disparaging remarks made about them. How might other reactions to demeaning or depersonalizing declarations during surgery take form?

In *Anesthesiology News* (Halfen, 1986), there is an anecdote of a woman remembering being called a "fat lady" while in surgery. The Eich *et al.* (1985) study describes a patient who recalled "fat lady" remarks. My own series included one patient with gross insults of the "fat lady" type and remarks about the patient's worthlessness. On the first postoperative day she suffered an unexplained myocardial infarction. Eight days after surgery, she broke off hypnotic regression to surgery in tears, without explanation or conscious reasons; she was the only patient among 55 to have been insulted so directly and the only patient to have an unexplained complication of surgery.

Another known case of the "fat lady" occurred recently with a usually respectful surgeon; the woman in this case also had an unanticipated postoperative myocardial infarction. A recent lawsuit was settled out of court in a case of "beached whale" remarks made by surgeons around an anesthetized woman. Interesting details of this case are that postoperatively the woman suffered numerous autonomic and vegetative disorders for several days until she stated to her nurse, "That bastard called me a beached whale." The nurse aided her recovery by checking with an operating nurse, who confirmed the insult. The fact that several days had elapsed when the patient recalled the insult is consistent with the experimental studies reviewed later. Insulting remarks by the surgeon and their postoperative effects on affect and vegetative processes are similarly described in Goldmann (1986).

Other Case Reports

Kumar, Pandit, and Jackson (1978) report a case of recall on the 10th postoperative day of intraoperative sounds and an awareness episode without a pain report. The patient had received a bolus of ketamine with a continuous infusion for successful open-heart surgery. Hilgenberg (1981) reports a case of awareness with fentanyl (90 $\mu$g/kg) and oxygen for open-heart surgery. The surgeon's words " . . . cutting down to the abdomen," which were used in instructing residents after sternotomy, were recalled. No pain reports were made. The report was made on the fourth postoperative day and was not distressful, nor were there autonomic or vegetative sequelae to surgery. Saucier, Walts, and Moreland (1983) describe an unusual case: A patient received a potent inhalational agent (halothane, 0.6–3.5%) for total hip arthroplasty revision, yet postoperatively reported continuous awareness of surgical conversations during several surgical periods when she received high concentrations of halothane. The precise content of the recall was confirmed. The patient reported feeling no pain during the case.

Levinson's (1969) dissertation contains several examples of patients who stated that they heard someone talking during surgery but were not able to report the content of what was said; yet the content of a temporarily similar conversation could be reported if it was personally relevant. This was also evident in a case of recall reported in the Eich *et al.* (1985) study.

Summary

In summary, the case report literature is informative about the issues of perception and memory for intraoperative events. On the one hand, nearly all adequate anesthetics produce an amnesia such that patients are satisfied that they cannot recall the events of surgery. On the other hand, auditory function is recognized as "the last to go" surrounding anesthesia for surgery. When unexpected recall occurs after apparently adequate anesthesia, it is for meaningful events. Responsiveness and high-level communication with patients can take place during some light anesthetics, yet there is amnesia following surgery. Given the theoretical framework based on the neurophysiological findings of intact early sensory components and the evidence favoring the late-selection theory of selective attention, verbal report data by patients may represent only the "tip of the iceberg." I now turn to the experimental investigations of learning and memory during states of general anesthesia.

## Memory Retrieval: Experimental Studies

Behavioral studies have assessed postoperative amnesia and found it to be quite impenetrable through normal memory assessments. Using stimuli such as letter–word pairs or repetitions of single words (Dubovsky & Trustman, 1976); a poem, a fire bell, and a list of words (Lewis, Jenkinson, & Wilson, 1973); and music (Brice, Hetherington, & Utting, 1970; Browne & Catton, 1973), both recall and recogition measures have supported the robustness of the amnesia that is familiar to those who have queried convalescent surgical patients. The findings from these studies have led to the conclusion that "discussion of clinical aspects of the patient's case need not be curtailed in the operating room and attempts at promoting healing through verbal suggestions during surgery will probably not be successful" (Dubovsky & Trustman, 1976, p. 701). That is, statements evaluative of the patient and his or her condition, can be made, according to the anesthesiology literature with impunity and without potential harm to the patient. More recently, another paper ends with a similar recommendation: "At present, however, the conclusion appears compelling that intraoperative events cannot be postoperatively remembered—either with or without awareness" (Eich *et al.*, 1985, p. 1147). Thus, surgical personnel are assured by these authorities that the patient can be safely considered psychologically inactive during anesthesia.

A review by Trustman, Dubovsky, and Titley (1977) serves as a watershed in the field, for it is the first methodologically rigorous review to make psychological sense of the claims relevant to intraoperative perception and memory. Reviews since 1977 (Bitner, 1983; Blacher, 1984) have echoed much the same interests in the questions that need addressing. The discussion that follows summarizes and integrates the results of several new studies that have been reported since the 1977 review (Barber, Donaldson, Ramras, & Allen, 1979; Bennett, Davis, & Giannini, 1984; Bennett *et al.*, 1985; Bonke, Schmitz, Verhage, & Zwaveling, 1986; Bonke & Verhage, 1984; Eich *et al.*,

1985; Loftus *et al.*, 1985; Mainord, Rath, & Barnett, 1983; Millar & Watkinson, 1983; Rath, 1982; Stolzy *et al.*, 1986).


Memory Assessed Verbally

Eich *et al* (1985) attempted intraoperatively to induce a spelling bias during postoperative tests. Their 48 patients participated in a 2 (dental surgery vs. major orthopedic surgery) × 2 (control vs. experimental group) design. Taped word lists without any personally relevant information were presented coincident with surgical incision. Sample stimuli and critical words were "a Grecian *urn*," "war and *peace*," "deep *sea*." The control group heard the word list prior to surgery. Recognition memory and spelling bias toward the presented word list was evident only in the control group. Criticisms that can be levied against this study include the following: The control group was not in any way amnesic, so their spelling bias may have been due to demand characteristics of the study; reliance upon intentional verbal retrieval processes made the likelihood of success remote; the lack of any personally relevant information in the taped presentation detracted from meaning; and presenting the word list only during the acute stimulation of surgical incision made generalization to the majority of surgical time without acute stimulation impossible.

Eich *et al.* (1985) report but do not discuss two cases of accurate intraoperative memory unrelated to their word lists. For example, a woman dental patient

> claimed that she had clearly heard the list of descriptive phrases, and had been pleasantly distracted by their presentation. Nevertheless, the patient could not recall any of the phrases, and her performance on the tests of homophone recognition and spelling did not exceed chance. More interestingly, the patient also claimed that shortly after the list had been presented and the headphones had been removed, she heard someone complain of difficulty in placing an intravenous tube in her arm and someone else complain about her weight. Two independent observers confirmed to us that these complaints had indeed been made. (p. 1146)

This accurate intraoperative recall demonstrates the point precisely. The memory test revealed complete amnesia, yet the "fat lady" comment was made only moments later. Despite this example of personal relevance and the early activation of knowledge structures, the authors claim at the closing of their article (as noted earlier) that "intraoperative events cannot be postoperatively remembered—either with or without awareness" (p. 1147). *Whose* amnesia is the question!

Millar and Watkinson (1983) conducted a sophisticated study using lists of unusual words and signal detection analysis. This study used a method of signaling from the patient called the "isolated forearm technique" (IFT) to assess responsiveness and only presented the words after all response had been lost. The IFT is a method of maintaining patient communication during muscular–skeletal paralysis by inflating a blood pressure cuff during administration of muscle relaxants and being careful not to totally paralyze the patient. With this method, finger signaling from the isolated arm is possible after the first passes of the relaxant through the system. Millar and Watkinson studied women having abdominal procedures under general anesthesia. Following the first incision, patients were presented either with radio static or with a personal statement of the importance of listening to the word list that followed. Anesthesia was maintained with between 0.25% and 1.00% halothane along with 66% nitrous oxide and 33% oxygen. There followed a list of 10 low-frequency words repeated four times, interspersed with requests that the patient signal by squeezing, straightening, and making a fist with the unparalyzed arm. Arm movements of patients compared with controls were equivocal. Recall by patients for any event during surgery was nil, and no patient reported memory for the word list or its content. Recognition guessing with 10 target words and 30 distractors was more accurate, and there were more correct rejections in the word-list groups than in guessing by controls. This yielded a statistically greater sensitivity measure, $d'$. Nonparametric analyses of the data were also significant. The authors conclude that a weak form of learning occurs during adequate surgical anesthesia.

Stolzy *et al.* (1986) used the same method. Thirty-one Veterans Administration Hospital patients with normal hearing agreed to participate. They heard a list of six uncommon words (experimental group; $n = 14$) or a list of six nonsense words (control group; $n = 17$) presented into their ears after a message indicated the importance of listening to the words. The list was repeated in different orders over a 15-minute tape. The isoflurane concentrations were between 0.8% and 2.0% during presentation of the word list. Patients were also breathing 50% nitrous oxide and 50% oxygen. They presented the word lists beginning 2 minutes after surgical incision. No patient recalled any surgical event, and recognition performance was based mostly on guessing. Correct recognition guesses, with 6 target words and 30 distractors were greater for the experimental than for the control group, $F(1, 20) = 10.16$, $p = .004$. Signal detection analysis was not applied.

Why was learning more easily demonstrated in the Stolzy *et al.* experiment? For one thing, the anesthesia was slightly different (Millar & Watkinson, 0.25–1.00% halothane with 66% nitrous oxide; Stolzy 0.8–2.0% isoflurane with 50% nitrous oxide). The higher nitrous oxide concentration could be a factor, but the data examining this point do not strongly support this proposition (Rosen, 1959). Second, the Millar and Watkinson patients were women approximately 40 years of age, while Stolzy *et al.*'s patients were Veterans Administration Hospital males between 28 and 78 years of age. The possibility of greater tolerance to the anesthetic agents in the latter group may exist. Rapport and motivation may also have been factors. Finally, testing time was later in the Stolzy *et al.* study (within 48 hours), compared to the Millar and Watkinson study (within 24 hours).

The Dubovsky and Trustman (1976) study was similar in design to the Stolzy *et al.* (1986) and Millar and Watkinson (1983) studies, relying upon a recognition test for a word list; however, they reported completely negative results, finding no basis for memory despite light anesthesia during list presentation. This led to the conclusion (cited earlier) that anesthesiologists should not worry about patients hearing them. The study enlisted 36 patients, most of whom were undergoing brief obstetrical procedures and were anesthetized to a stable level of anesthesia. When judged to be in a light plane of anesthesia, they had a message asking that they remember the following letter–word pairs. Then eight letter–word pairs were repeated for 15 minutes; for example, the voice on the tape said, "G is for game; S is for street," and so on. The stimulus word list was presented during Caesarian section, therapeutic abortion, or hysterectomy. During testing as soon after surgery as possible, patients were asked to choose the letters that had been presented from a randomized alphabet. Next, they chose from among four choices the word paired with each letter for each of the eight letter–word pairs. They also gave confidence ratings of their choices.

Possible criticisms of the Dubovsky and Trustman (1976) study are, first, that testing "as soon after surgery as possible" meant that residual anesthetics were in the patients' systems and, therefore, that their cognitive abilities were altered from normal. Second, the task was not well conceptualized. For example, it is well recognized that intentional and effortful mnemonic rehearsal is required for learning not very meaningful material in short-term memory processing. Automatic comprehension of pertinent discourse is an entirely different process. That is, the content might never have sufficiently engaged early knowledge systems. Therefore, even though Millar and Watkinson and Stolzy *et al.* used *unusual* words while Dubovsky and Trustman used *common* stimuli, there is no reason why common letter–word pairs should be easier to learn; in fact, they might be more difficult to retain, due to interference with established associative memory networks in automatic encoding processes during anesthesia (see also the discussion of the Loftus *et al.* study, below).

In a separate study reported in the same article, Dubovsky and Trustman also queried 12 dilatation and curettage (D&C) patients who had received during anesthesia a single word, "salami," presented every 5 seconds for 5 minutes; every 30 seconds for 5 minutes; then every 5 seconds again for 2 minutes. Within 24 hours, patients guessed from a sheet of 10 words as the taped voice repeated the words. Of the patients, 11 guessed incorrectly; the 12th patient said:

"Don't even show me the choices: the word was *salami.*" She remembered awakening during anesthesia, and her anesthesiologist reported that in the middle of the procedure, she had opened her eys *[sic]* and winked at him. Our only evidence for postoperative recall occurred in a patient who was not fully anesthetized! (p. 699)

The "salami" patient may or may not have remembered the word from the time she did open her eyes, as she had no memory of doing so (only the anesthesiologist recalled the event). If she had heard "salami" or remembered it from that instance, shouldn't she have said, "I remember opening my eyes, winking at you, and hearing the word 'salami'"? But she didn't. Like the woman my colleagues and I spoke to while she was under sufentanyl/nitrous oxide, she may have acted appropriately and not remembered it. On the other hand, why did she remember "salami"? It is circular reasoning to say that she was not anesthetized.

Thus, one likely explanation for the discrepancies among the three studies just described is the time of testing. As previously mentioned, in the Dubovsky and Trustman study, the memory testing commenced "as soon after surgery as possible." At this time, the patients almost certainly had residual anesthetic effects. On the other hand, testing 24 hours later by Millar and Watkinson resulted in a small effect. The Stolzy *et al.* patients were tested within 48 hours, and the investigators found a substantial effect—the largest of any verbal retrieval study. If memory improves with time, as these studies taken together seem to suggest, the extent that one can demonstrate a convincing memory effect for events occurring during anesthesia will depend in part on how long after anesthesia memory is tested. The experimental results for these studies imply a retrieval deficit, not a failure of perception.

Studies by Adam (1979) support this proposition. In a series of laboratory studies, Adam administered subanesthetic concentrations of different gaseous anesthetics to human volunteers. Through a learning–test–retest design, he estimated the savings of verbal and nonverbal material over time following recovery from the anesthetics. He discovered that amnesia was typically dense immediately following subanesthetic learning, but that recovery of material increased over time to the end of the 2-week test period. Thus, rather than a deficit of memory formation, Adam's results indicate a "permanent inaccessibility of traces" (p. 231). The memory existed but ordinary retrieval strategies were not able to access the information. We could say that the traces were dissociated from more intentional, declarative, and conscious processes.

The studies by Millar and Watkinson, Stolzy *et al.*, and Dubovsky and Trustman all used a verbal modality (i.e., word list) that has no relevance to surgical patients. With regard to the meaning of the stimulus material, the Loftus *et al.* (1985) case study is revealing. A noted expert on human memory and its distortions, Dr. Loftus had served as a consultant to a major hospital chain being sued by 169 female plaintiffs for admitted oral rape by an anesthesiologist during surgery. Many claims were filed on the basis of hypnotic recall obtained after the story broke in the newspapers. Skepticism turned to disbelief from some of the claims registered after hypnotic recall. There was a strong possibility of confabulation. Some years later, Dr. Loftus faced her own surgery. A true experimentalist, she arranged for a test of intraoperative hearing on herself. She and her colleagues called the trial a rigorous experimental test, but it fell short of this. The anesthesiologist read aloud 100 unrelated words during general anesthesia for an abdominal procedure. Anesthesia was maintained with 60% nitrous oxide and 1–3% isoflurane. One hour after anesthesia induction and 30 minutes after surgical incision, the list was read to Dr. Loftus at a rate of one word every 2 seconds. Chance-level performance resulted from testing at 28, 53, and 82 hours after exposure. The same list was used at each of three testings for guessing. Interestingly, a first-year resident who was present during the operation and exposed to the spoken list was given an unexpected memory test at the 82-hour test session. She also scored at chance levels. Though "aware" during surgery, the surgeons also found little pertinence to the words, and there was no early-structure activation by the word lists.

As with the Eich *et al.* (1985) patient who recalled talk of her fat but not the word groups presented immediately prior to this talk, early-structure activation will interact with the admittedly nebulous but clearly critical concern for *pertinence*. Early-structure activation may have more pertinence for evaluative and/or survival-type messages than for word lists. After the words were no longer read, conversation in the operating room resumed; perceptual mechanisms continued, though the experiment was over. Much more highly pertinent things than word lists are said in a person's surgery— an incredibly personal and vulnerable time, during which neurochemical activities are occurring at a feverish pace. If early perceptual structures can be said to operate during anesthesia, the operating room conversation has a better chance of being learned than a low-relevance word list.

The studies of postanesthetic verbal memory for intraoperative events can be summarized as follows: Stolzy *et al.* (1986) and Millar and Watkinson (1983) both found positive results. They did use *unusual* words in their lists, preceded by a message asking the patients to remember them, and they waited 24–48 hours to test for memory. In contrast, Eich *et al.* (1985), Dubovsky and Trustman (1976), and Loftus *et al.* (1985) found negative results. They used pairings or phrasings of *common* words, and they also did not introduce the lists with a request to the patients or call the patients by name. Too, the times of testing memory were relatively short following surgery—in the case of Dubovsky and Trustman, as soon after surgery as possible.

In a recent study, Goldmann (1986) gave a pretest of highly unique and obscure facts to patients. For example, the questions included "What is the blood pressure of an octopus?" Ten such obscure items were included in the 16-item test. Then, after a motivating consent interview and the pretest, he gave the correct answers to half the patients when they were anesthetized during surgery and then did postoperative retests 1–2 days postoperatively. There was a significant gain in scores for the experimental but not for the control group, $F = 6.20$, $p < .01$. No patient recalled or recognized having heard anything in surgery. However, one patient (a Russian immigrant), when asked how he had scored so much better on the posttest, stated, "There is more in my head now than there was before."

## Memory Assessed Nonverbally

Even though verbal recall and recognition of surgical conversations are difficult if not impossible, the fact that a few patients will recall conversations, especially if highly motivated (Yeakel, 1974), signifies the potential for information to be assimilated into the CNS. Can this information affect the status of the body and psychological well-being, even though the information never enters consciousness? This is the intent of research that recognizes the dense declarative/episodic/conscious/verbal postoperative amnesia, yet seeks to ask whether high-level stimulus registration may continue during anesthesia with postoperative results. In this approach, there is a relinquishing of the burden on verbal retrieval as the sole criterion of stimulus acquisition.

One easily utilized and well-established way of activating response tendencies by verbal means is through the use of suggestions. Suggestions act as procedural instructions that, when combined with a delay in time until their activation or retrieval, qualify as memories. In addition, given their effortlessness of experience, suggestions may act by engaging early preattentive levels of the knowledge base. Word lists require effortful rehearsal. Thus, on the basis of evoked potential data, the early structures may be sensitive to verbal suggestions, while later intentional processes, such as verbal rehearsal, are most certainly obliterated by anesthetics.

Parallels exist in sleep research. A behavioral response to a verbal message administered to sleeping subjects was successfully carried out over adjacent and temporally remote sleep periods up to the 6-week period of the experiments. A suggestion followed by a cue word was spoken to highly suggestible subjects who were confirmed to be in Stage 1 (REM) sleep. The cue word elicited the suggested behavior, as confirmed by film records of subjects' sleep behavior (Evans, 1979; Evans, Gustafson, O'Connell, Shor, & Orne, 1966, 1969). The sleep state went undisturbed during the learning and testing trials—always Stage 1 REM sleep. Further replications have been successful and support the original conclusions (Aarons, 1976; Perry, Evans, O'Connell, Orne, & Orne, 1978). Subjects were amnesic for the suggestions, though sleep periods tested days and even weeks later confirmed that the verbal cue was still effective in eliciting the suggested behavior. Memory inquiries included the use of hypnosis. In none of them was hypnosis or any other inquiry able to produce the original suggestions that were still behaviorally active. This indicates, according to the late-selection theory of selective attention, that the knowledge base is at least partially located neurologically and temporally before consciousness *of* the event. Consciousness arises after knowledge has already intervened. Thus, the knowledge base can be activated *early* rather than *late* in the processing sequence. By this analysis, the late-selection theory applies with the sleep suggestion studies: Effects of verbal suggestions were acted upon behaviorally (neurologically) by early rather than by late perceptual processes. Completely new information was not learned in these studies; rather, existing knowledge was activated. Memory in terms of conscious recollection may indeed be amnesic when neurological processes act autonomously in early rather than late structures in the nervous system. There is *no* identity presumed, however, between natural circadian sleep and general anesthesia. Rather, a behavioral response was demonstrated in these studies to verbal suggestions in the presence of a dense amnesia during the time when the effects of the suggestions were still active within the nervous system. This functional result is equivalent to what has been claimed for perception during general anesthesia: postanesthetic effects in the presence of amnesia.

Hutchings (1961) claimed highly therapeutic benefits from presenting positive suggestions addressed personally to 200 anesthetized surgical patients. Hutchings's clinical series used the same tactic (direct physiological suggestions) as the Wolfe and Millet (1960) series of 1,500 patients had; but it still lacked a control group, though the absolute levels of postoperative pain medications in milligrams of meperidine (Demerol) were impressively low. Postoperative responses to minor surgical procedures were reportedly more successfully improved by intraoperative suggestion than were the outcomes to major surgery.

Barber and colleagues (1979) tested hypnotic suggestions for nonverbal responses during exposure to 20–40% nitrous oxide as compared to 100% oxygen. The patients breathing nitrous oxide responded better to a posthypnotic suggestion later, as they left the experiment, than the oxygen-breathing controls. However, this concentration of nitrous oxide was lower than that commonly used in surgery (50–67%).

Mainord *et al.* (1983) had the operating surgeon make the following statements to half of 24 patients undergoing back surgery: "Mr./Ms. ———, the operation has gone well and we will soon be finishing. You will be flat on your back for the next couple of days. When you are waiting it would be a good idea if you would relax the muscles in the pelvic area as this will enable you to urinate and it will not be necessary to use a catheter" (p. 4). The surgeon said this in the latter part of neurosurgical procedures on the spine during a fairly deep level of anesthesia (Stage 3, Level 2). Both early time to micturation (urination) and the need for a postoperative urinary catheter were significantly improved in the instruction condition; 8 of 12 controls required postoperative urinary catheterization, whereas none of the 12 suggestion patients did. A replication and extension done by Rath (1982) found similar results and added a preoperative variable. The design was a 2 × 2 randomly assigned analysis-of-variance model. A total of 44 general surgery patients were first divided into two groups: preoperative relaxation training or preoperative social history (irrelevant to surgery). The second variable was intraoperative presentation of either specific suggestions and instructions on recovering from surgery or irrelevant suggestions and instructions. In both cases, Rath spoke each patient's name clearly into his or her ear and personally delivered the message in the operating room during closure, approximately 15 minutes before potent agents, nitrous oxide, and skeletal paralysis were reversed. The patients were probably in a light plane of adequate anesthesia. The intraoperative suggestions that were delivered were simple and direct statements about the importance of muscle relaxation in the operative site; ability to urinate easily; expectations of a comfortable recovery; and the fact that the patient would soon be back in his or her room, awake and pleased at how well everything had gone. There was a main effect for the group receiving intraoperative direct suggestions to show fewer analgesic requirements, lower pain ratings, and earlier discharge from the hospital. There was no statistically significant interaction with preoperative relaxation training. The preoperative group receiving instructions showed only a trend in that direction. However, the preoperative relaxation group did not receive specific suggestions or instructions—only nonspecific relaxation training without instructions on how to apply this training to recovery from surgery. In this case, intraoperative suggestions for specific physiological and involuntary responses had a greater effect than preoperative information on postoperative involuntary physiological processes. Whether the same direct suggestions and instructions given preoperatively would have been as effective remains unanswered. The conclusion that can be drawn once again suggests that the use of nonverbal indicators that are directly suggested during anesthesia may show strong postoperative effects, despite complete conscious amnesia. One further aspect of Rath's study concerns his method of memory assessment for the intraoperative messages. The intriguing results of this method are discussed in a later section.

A study by Bonke and Verhage (1984) closely paralleled our studies (Bennett *et al.*, 1984, 1985) in presenting continuous reassurances and suggestions for improved outcome to anesthetized patients. However, use of prerecorded therapeutic tapes was not effective in changing postoperative outcome in the three studies (two by our group, one by Bonke & Verhage), except for the outcome in one of Bonke and Verhage's groups. The other conditions in the Bonke and Verhage study—music, operating room sounds, and prerecorded positive suggestions—made no difference in recovery. No evidence of postoperative improvement could be found from 45 minutes or 120 minutes of taped suggestions and music in our two studies.

It should be emphasized that the prerecorded tapes were highly artificial. The messages in our studies were hypnotic-like suggestions interspersed with classical and contemporary music and metaphorical stories for recovery. There was a great deal of content repetition over the 45-minute (Study 1) and 120-minute (Study 2) tapes; indeed the content was interesting and culturally relevant only to us. One patient undergoing hypnotic recall, after several items of vague recall, spontaneously exclaimed, "There's something else . . . like someone reading a script . . . telling me to relax. . . . I didn't like it . . . it was in the way." Similarly, in the Bonke and Verhage series of 91 patients, the "therapeutic message" tape consisted of two statements about the patient's good condition and excellent recovery, then continuous white noise, and then repetition of the same two fragments; in all, there were six repetitions per hour of the phrases. The more or less equivocal results on involuntary physiological recovery may have resulted in these three studies from the messages' lack of pertinence, believability, and excessive redundancy—a "broken record" syndrome. In a reanalysis of their data, Bonke *et al.* (1986) found that there had been a positive effect on the convalescent period in older patients exposed to the therapeutic suggestions.

Our two studies (Bennett *et al.*, 1984, 1985), though failing to demonstrate an effect of prerecorded suggestions on recovery, also utilized a personalized request that the patients indicate having heard the message by engaging in a cued behavior during the postoperative interview. Suggestion patients did so signficantly more often than controls. Though taped suggestions did not aid recovery, personalized instructions were effective. These studies are described in more detail below.


## ROLE OF HYPNOSIS IN STUDIES OF ANESTHESIA AND SURGICAL MEMORIES

Hypnotic inductions have been used in age-regressed reproductions of intraoperative events. Strong claims of the utility of hypnosis to uncover "unconscious surgical memories" have been advanced (Cheek, 1959, 1966, 1979) without adequate experimental investigation. The clinical reports in the late 1950s and early 1960s chronicled cases of catharsis by hypnotic age regressions to surgical anesthesia. The patients' complaints, like those of the early hypnotic cases of the 18th and 19th century, were primarily autonomic and vegetative physical disorders of the body. The case reports involved the smooth musculature and the autonomic, vegetative, and hemostatic systems. The techniques used for uncovering the traumatic events were similar to current therapeutic treatments, including hypnotherapeutic treatments, for posttraumatic stress disorder: a trusting-facilitating environment, the use of verbal methods, and working through of the traumatic memories. The results claimed by Cheek and others were of complete symptom remission when the unconscious memory from surgery was revealed.

At the outset, memory distortion must be acknowledged as possibly the primary effect of hypnotic age regression (O'Connell, Shor, & Orne, 1970; Orne, 1979). Given this, if unambiguously positive evidence comes forth for validated memories of events that occurred intraoperatively and that the patient has previously denied knowing the existence of, hypnotic recall can be claimed successful. The writings of Cheek must serve as an advisory role for controlled investigation. Perhaps his clinical experience provides a brilliant method that nevertheless has been utterly lacking in independent confirmation?

A well-known study by Levinson (1965) staged a mock "surgical crisis" when by EEG criteria patients were in deep (Stage 3) ether anesthesia. None of the 10 dental patients recalled the event, though in hypnosis 4 patients were reported to give verbatim or near-verbatim recall of the crisis. The Levinson study is cited widely as an example of the lessons of perception during general anesthesia, but unfortunately the methodology included no control group, nor was Levinson blind when he induced the hypnotic regression to the operation.

The verbatim hypnotic recall of the specific and unusual intraoperative "crisis," however, is reproduced in a transcript in Levinson's dissertation (1969). The data have high face validity. The near-verbatim recall in 4 of the 10 patients is subject only to the criticism of possible cueing after surgery but before hypnotic retrieval, as the words of the hypnotist indicate care and deliberation with knowledge of possible cueing. Clearly the topic, despite ethical and methodological flaws, deserves more than the complete lack of attention it has received for 20 years.

We (Bennett *et al.*, 1984, 1985) followed the recommendations of Trustman *et al.* (1977), who had emphasized the need for a double-blind placebo control design. Hypnotic recall followed double-blind criteria and was matched against the actual intraoperative events as transcribed from recordings taken at the patients' ears or from the recordings that had been presented into the patients' ears.

Our first two studies of 23 and 32 patients used hypnotic regression, according to the Cheek (1959, 1960) method as taught by him. The hypnotically obtained data constituted a major focus of the studies. Hypnotically obtained data in general are not particularly helpful scientifically; the substance of hypnotic recall is in a free-recall context and as such is difficult to evaluate objectively, despite the face validity of the evidence. Much more persuasive are data that utilize more objective measures. Experimental urging to patients under anesthesia to remember in ways not relying upon intentional verbal retrieval have been reviewed above. These types of requests to patients were made in Studies 1 and 2 reviewed below.

## Studies 1 and 2

### Patients and Location

A total of 55 patients were recruited and adequate data collected on each over the two studies. Ages of the participants ranged from 18 to 60, with a mean age of 34.8 years ($SD = 13.7$). Three hospitals participated: a public teaching hospital (University of California–Davis Medical Center in Sacramento, CA), a private teaching hospital (Stanford Hospital in Stanford, CA), and a private hospital (O'Connor Hospital in San Jose, CA).

### Design

The design was a 2 (hernia vs. gall bladder surgeries) $\times$ 2 (suggestions vs. operating room sounds) double-blind design presented to patients under anesthesia. The presurgical consent interview explained that throughout surgery, patients would receive over headphones at a normal listening volume one of two conditions: either a prerecorded tape or the actual operating room sounds and voices. A convalescent interview would determine their memory and would involve hypnosis as a possible memory aid. In addition, hypnotic ability was assessed by the Stanford Hypnotic Clinical Scale (SHCS; Hilgard & Hilgard, 1979).

### Procedure

Surgical procedures were limited to inguinal hernia repair and cholecystectomy (gall bladder removal). This was meant to provide a variable of depth of anesthesia. (Cholecystectomy required entering the peritoneal cavity, a more stimulating surgical procedure than hernia repair, which involves tissue superficial to the peritoneum.) During the last months of the second study, eight orthopedic patients were added due to the lack of target surgeries.

Standard anesthetic practices were followed with all patients. A question following surgery, "Did the patient at any time achieve awareness during surgery?" asked the anesthesiologist for a qualitative opinion of the adequacy of anesthesia. In all cases, the anesthesiologists gave a negative response to the question. All types and quantities of anesthesia were recorded from the anesthesia record, including preoperative medications. Induction of anesthesia was by thiopental, followed by muscle relaxants, nitrous oxide, and enflurane or halothane.

After the induction of anesthesia, headphones were placed over the patient's ears. In the control condition (operating room sounds condition, or ORSC), stereo microphones in the outer shell of the earphones recorded these events while the earphones maintained them at the ears at the ambient volume. In the suggestion condition (SC), a prerecorded tape was played at a normal listening volume. Beginning with the initial incision, the tape played continuously, suggesting rapid healing and comfort interspersed with music. So that patients might recognize it, the voice on the tape belonged to the presurgical consent interviewer. In the first study, the tape played for the initial 45 minutes of the surgery. In the second study, the 2-hour tape was stopped 5 minutes before the reversal of anesthesia was begun. If surgery exceeded 2 hours, the tape was started again from the beginning.

A special suggestion was included in the prerecorded tape. In Study 1, this suggestion stressed the importance of lifting the index finger of the left hand during the convalescent interview when the interviewers requested the patient to close his or her eyes and imagine having feelings of hunger. In Study 1, the message occurred twice, at 5 and at 40 minutes after the initial surgical incision. In Study 2, the message was made more personal by recording the suggestion for each patient after the consent interview. The suggestion in Study 2 was simpler and asked, along with suggestions for a comfortable recovery:

> [Patient's name], when we come to talk with you it is very important that you pull on your ear so that I can know you have heard this. It is very important that you pull on your ear when we come to speak with you so that doctors and nurses can know that you can hear in surgery. Your ear might itch a little and you will need to pull on it or you might just know to pull on your ear. That way we will know you have heard this. (Bennett *et al.*, 1985, p. 175)

This message was played only once, 5 minutes before the reversal of anesthesia was begun.

These suggestions allowed for a nonverbal response to intraoperative verbal statements. If patients responded to the suggestion by spontaneous behavior during the blind postoperative interview, support would be provided for the potentially suggestive effect of intraoperative conversation. On the other hand, if patients did not respond, the amnesia might be due to an inability of the nervous system to comprehend and/or store verbal input under the influence of anesthetic agents.

All medical personnel remained blind to the condition in effect for each patient and were not involved with the study. The assistant operating the tape recorder in the operating room had no other contact with the patient or with other members of the research team until after the postoperative interview. Even then, blind conditions were enforced until completion of the study. Interviewers similarly were blind to all patients' experimental conditions until after each study had been completed.

The postanesthetic interview was conducted at least 2 days postoperatively and up to 2 weeks after surgery. The two-person team always included the investigator who had obtained the patient's consent and whose voice was on the suggestion tape, though neither interviewer knew whether any patient had received the SC or the ORSC. The interview was standardized and contained five parts:

   1. Assessment of present status and all memories for before, during, and after surgery.
   2. Assessment of hypnotic ability with the SHCS (Hilgard & Hilgard, 1979).
   3. In the waking state, a discussion of the experience with the scale and permission to investigate intraoperative memories through additional hypnosis.
   4. A hypnotic regression to the operation, with strong suggestions that memories for events from surgery would become conscious. Because there were claims for its usefulness for such a task, an ideomotor signaling system was incorporated into the standard interview (Cheek & LeCron, 1968) in the hope that it would facilitate recovery of intraoperative memories.
   5. A discussion and debriefing.

Being blind to the events during a patient's surgery, the interviewers did not bias the suggestion or control groups differently. Observation of the suggested nonverbal response took place after the regression in Study 1 and throughout the interview in Study 2. Observation of these responses was reliably observed by the interview team ($r = .92$).

Results

In Study 1, 23 patients were interviewed (the SHCS was administered to only 19 of them). In Study 2, there were 32 patients (SHCS scores were obtained from 29). No patient in either study could remember anything from the period following induction of anesthesia to awakening at the end of anesthesia in the recovery room or on the ward.

In Study 1, 10 of 13 SC patients (77%) demonstrated the nonverbal response during the blind convalescent interview; 3 of 9 ORSC patients also responded to the cue by lifting their fingers (33%). Unfortunately, the response was confounded by the interview technique, which utilized ideomotor finger signaling. Thus, the false positives were later realized to be a consequence of the interview technique, and the entire group of nonverbal response results was set aside as confounded.

In Study 2, the response suggested to each patient during the last 5 minutes of anesthesia was to touch or pull his or her ear during the interview. Here the results were methodologically valid. Of the SC patients, 9 of 11 (82%) showed at least one ear touch during the interview, compared to 9 of the 21 ORSC patients (43%). An exact $2 \times 2$ frequency table of the number of patients in each group who touched their ear produced a Fisher's exact $p$ of 1.04 (1-tail). This represented a point biserial correlation between specificity of response and group of .57. The difference of 6.0 ear touches per interview for SC patients to less than 1 ear touch per patient for ORSC patients was significant on a Mann–Whitney $U$ test ($U = 49$, $n_1 n_2 = 231$, $p < .02$). Patient postoperative behavior was significantly affected by verbal statements made during general anesthesia in the presence of a complete conscious amnesia. No SC patient recalled the ear-touching suggestion during any portion of the interviews, in spite of strong suggestions for memories to become conscious at interview.

When hypnotically regressed back to the operation, none of the SC patients in either study recalled the suggestion for nonverbal behavior (finger lift in Study 1, ear touch in Study 2). The lack of memory, even in hypnosis, confirmed the dense postanesthetic amnesia, but we interpreted it as a retrieval failure rather than a failure of formation because the ear-touching suggestion in Study 2 was successful even though attempts to retrieve the memory were not.

Despite the amnesia for the nonverbal suggestion in the SC, hypnotic regression to the operation for patients in both conditions was successful in eliciting instances of recall of meaningful events during anesthesia. However, there was often difficulty in verifying the recall material generated by a patient, even with the aid of transcripts of the sounds reaching the patient's ears during anesthesia. How were free-recall statements to be assessed if they consisted, of "a knife" (scored as no recall), or "A doctor says to pass the gauze. . . . 'Drop that gauze' . . . 'wrong kind of gauze' . . . he wanted roll-out, not round pieces [of gauze]" (scored as accurate recall). The hypnotic recall that was judged accurate was also meaningful to the patient, compared to a random sampling of the content of the tape-recorded conversation. Some 100 pages of transcribed conversation over the surgeries in the operating room sounds conditions revealed instances of meaning to the patient: "This is the worst bone graft ever. . . . Oh, Lord, this is awful," or "Well, this is just [patient's first name]; she's our 'blue plate special' for today." The memory assessments from surgeries where pessimistic or derogatory conversation occurred were qualitatively different from the others.

The "worst bone graft ever" patient, a 31-year-old female, had the longest postoperative hospital stay and more pain medication requirements (72 doses) than any other. In hypnosis, she stated something was disturbing, "something to do with my leg. It's not going to work right. The doctor said it wasn't going to work the way it should." But can this be unambiguous evidence for memory?

The "blue plate special" patient, in her late 50s, had just prior to that remark been referred to as obese, unattractive, and not worthy of the surgical team's spending much time sewing her up after her cholecystectomy. (She has been mentioned earlier in connection with the "fat lady" syndrome.) She had the second longest convalescence because of a postoperative myocardial infarction on the first postoperative day—the only heart attack in the series of 55. She stated in the postoperative interview that she had chosen her surgeon because he was "the nicest of them all" around the hospital office where she had worked. It was he who made the disparaging remarks, and yet there was no recall of the episode. Hypnosis was terminated when, upon approaching the surgical period during regression, the patient began to weep; she later stated that her sadness (which she attributed to her son's housing situation) had just risen up in her. The two longest recoveries from surgery were by these patients whose surgeons had made intraoperative pessimistic or derogatory statements.

Given the nonverbal response results, instances of recall that were unique and that matched unique operative events spanning all operations within a study were scored as successful recalls. The recall productions that were judged accurate were not clearly related to patients' hypnotizability.

SHCS scores could not be statistically related to medical variables, except for a finding associating higher hypnotizability scores with shorter postoperative stays following hernia repair ($n = 20$, $r = .81$). In the assessment of memory, scores on the SHCS were related to the accurate hypnotic recall of intraoperative events if the recalled event was unique among all surgeries or was specifically present in the experimental suggestion tape. Recall was related to hypnotic ability, defined in terms of scores on the SHCS and its individual items, in the following ways:

1. SHCS scores correlated .24 with the accuracy of hypnotic recall of surgery.
2. SHCS scores correlated .09 with the presence of the suggested nonverbal behavior.

3. SHCS scores correlated .13 with the number of semantic units[3] produced during hypnotic recall of surgery.

4. The number of semantic units in the SHCS "dream" item correlated .26 with the number of semantic units in the hypnotic recall of surgery ($p = .07$).

5. The number of semantic units in the SHCS "dream" item correlated .24 with the accuracy of hypnotic surgical memory.

6. The number of hours after surgery that hypnotic recall was attempted correlated .17 with accuracy of the recall.

7. The number of semantic units produced during hypnotic recall correlated .36 ($p = .009$) with the accuracy of the recall.

As a trend, patients who had more hypnotic ability as assessed by the SHCS were more successful in recalling intraoperative events, though SHCS scores were not related to elicitation of the nonverbal response. An exception was a 22-year-old Hispanic male who had an SHCS score of 1 and did not respond to the ear-touching suggestion during interview. However, his mother had taught him trance techniques and, from within his own self-generated trance, after many minutes of deepening and machinations, he recalled the composer and musical selection played just prior to the ear-touching suggestion. He was also at the same level of anesthesia for both events and, though clearly not suggestible, recalled "a male voice speaking to me telling me to relax" and "soothing music—by Chuck Mangione, the same that I hum to myself." This man had a high anesthetic requirement at 3% enflurane during these events.

A better predictor of recall accuracy was production of semantic units on the dream itself of the SHCS. Patients who had more to say about a suggested dream also had more to say when it was suggested that they would produce events from their surgery. Accuracy was related to the number of these productions; the more data (semantic units) the patient produced in hypnosis, the more likely the data were to be judged accurate for some of the productions.

## Study 3

The studies just described revealed that ordinary memory inquiries, including hypnotic recall efforts, were not as reliable as a nonverbal signal in indicating

3. The term "number of semantic units" refers to a content-analytic count of the unique items produced in hypnosis for recall of surgical events. The count does not necessarily reflect accuracy, merely production of units of meaning. Thus, "I hear bells clanging and someone talking" equals two units (bells clanging and someone talking are independent events), whereas "I see a green and white spotted calf standing in an open space" equals one unit (the calf).

that an auditory message was acquired during surgical anesthesia. It was now important to extend the presentation time of the suggestion for the nonverbal behavior further into the operative period. Presentation of experimental information was confined in previously successful studies (including our own) to one discrete point during the anesthetic: either during stable surgical anesthesia (Millar & Watkinson, 1983; Stolzy *et al.*, 1986), or just before emergence (Bennett *et al.*, 1985). Study 3 was designed to test differences in auditory acquisition as a function of the time the patient was under anesthesia and the anesthetic agents administered. A standardized meaningful message was presented to patients during different phases of clinical anesthesia, followed by postoperative interviews that assessed verbal and nonverbal memories of the experimental message.

Methods

A total of 48 patients aged 19–63 years, scheduled for elective surgery and in generally good health, were chosen. Each consented to be a participant, and institutional approval from the Human Subjects Review Committee was obtained. Patients were told that surgical personnel often assume that the patient will not comprehend their conversations. The patient was told to listen for a special message during anesthesia. To increase the meaning of the neutral study message, patients were also told that a personal message for their good recovery would precede the study message. The interviewer made a tape recording for each patient, which included (1) the patient's preferred name, (2) personalized statements of well-being regarding the specific operation, (3) suggestions for recovery, and (4) a statement on the importance of engaging in a specific behavior during a postoperative interview. The behavior was randomly assigned among patients from among four choices: touching the right or left ear, or lifting the left or right index finger.

Patients requiring general anesthesia for gastrointestinal, gynecological, orthopedic, or plastic surgeries were studied. No attempt was made to control the anesthetic technique. All patients received nitrous oxide (40–67%) and isoflurane (0.25–1.50) ($n = 29$), halothane (0.5–2.0%) ($n = 11$), or enflurane (1–3%) ($n = 8$). Anesthetic intravenous agents included diazepam, fentanyl, and morphine sulfate. The anesthesiologist confirmed that patients were adequately anesthetized and clinically stable. Heart rate and blood pressure did not observably change with presentation of the message. All anesthetic agents and their doses were recorded in relation to the time of message delivery. Presentation of the experimental message was via tape recorder through stereo earphones fitted by a separate experimenter and monitored to insure adequate presentation over a separate set of earphones. Postoperative interviews were conducted 1–20 days following anesthesia. The two interviewers recorded all instances of the four nonverbal target behaviors throughout the 30-minute interview, at the end of which the entire taped message was played to the patient, breaking the blind condition for the experimenters. The presence or absence in the interview of the specific behavior mentioned in the experimental message was taken as evidence for or against learning during general anesthesia.

Preoperative and intraoperative variables were recorded in regard to patients, anesthesia doses, and presentation of the message. Amounts of medications, induction agents, and anesthetics; the time that the message was played to the patient after induction and before emergence; anesthetics present at that time; preoperative and intraoperative hemodynamics; and postoperative interview responses (including nonverbal responses) were recorded. A mathematical model (logistic regression) was developed from these data to determine which variables correlated with the presence of the suggested behavior in the postoperative interview.

Results

Time of message presentation varied from 15 to 293 minutes after induction (10 to 219 minutes before emergence). The mean time to message presentation was 93 minutes after intubation ($SD = 64.3$ min.) and 59 minutes before emergence ($SD = 58.2$ min.).

Interview questioning revealed that no patient verbally recalled the experimental message or any intraoperative event. Interview observation of patients' nonverbal behavior revealed responses to the intraoperative message in 33 cases and a lack of a specific response in 15 cases. The statistical model found two variables associated with the postoperative nonverbal behaviors (1) presentation of the message for that behavior ($p < .02$), and (2) a nonsignificant trend for intraoperative intravenous diazepam to suppress the response ($p = .13$) if it were given before the message. A noteworthy finding was a *lack of correlation* between nonverbal response and time of presentation, levels of inhalational agents, or hemodynamic variables. From this series, the data suggest that time of presentation does not modulate stimulus acquisition during anesthesia. Time of the postoperative interview to assess the effects of the message was also not related in this series to elicitation of a response. This was also the case in Studies 1 and 2 but the time of the interview may have had an effect in the semantic memory experiments by other investigators, where patients tended to be interviewed very soon postoperatively. In our three studies we tended to interview patients later—from 24 or even 48 hours after surgery to several weeks postoperatively.

The success of a nonverbal behavior as an indicator of intraoperative perception throughout the surgical period when adequate clinical anesthetics are used, and in the uniform presence of a dense postoperative amnesia, has recently been replicated in patients having open-heart surgery in England and receiving a narcotic-balanced anesthetic (Goldmann, 1986). Thirty patients were given highly motivating consent interviews the evening before surgery. After coming off cardiopulmonary bypass and being warmed to 38° C, they were presented with personalized messages of the importance of touching their chins during the postoperative interview (this study was a fairly direct replication of Studies 1 and 2 above). Suggestion patients ($n = 21$) touched their chins more ($M = 4.3$ chin touches, $SD = 5.9$) than control patients ($n = 9$) ($M = 2.4$, $SD = 2.4$), $F = 5.91$, $p < .01$. Hypnotic recall was also successful, but hypnotizability scores were not obtained. This replication adds further support to the reliability of nonverbal assessments of learning during anesthesia.

The Rath (1982) study used a unique, and, for present purposes, highly pertinent memory task to assess retention after surgery for the intraoperative messages (discussed earlier; these were "live" relevant or irrelevant instructions and suggestions for postoperative recovery delivered 15 minutes before the reversal of anesthesia). As is typical of these studies, no patient had recall for the intraoperative message. Memory was assessed between 4 and 24 hours after the end of surgery. Rath had patients listen to every sentence from both relevant and irrelevant messages, though any one patient had been exposed to only one set of these. He told them, "During surgery I talked to you," and went on to explain the importance of remembering the statements he had made. Aware of the need for blind memory assessment, he had patients listen with their eyes closed to a prerecorded tape. Rath told the patients further that, because they did not consciously remember anything, perhaps another part of their mind could signal which phrasings they had heard by lifting a finger—one finger for "Yes" and another for "No"—after each phrase on the tape. The patients' motor response accurately discriminated between presented and nonpresented phrases, and the results were highly statistically significant. This result is particularly interesting in light of claims by Cheek for the utility of motor signaling to questions as a way of uncovering surgical memories. Similarly, we used the ideomotor finger response in Studies 1 and 2 as a means of testing Cheek's claims. That verbatim hypnotic recall was at least partially obtained through such means underlies the validity of the existence of memory systems that are highly resistant to verbal systems but accessible through nonverbal means.


## OVERALL DISCUSSION

What, then, is the nature of postanesthetic amnesia, and can it be breached? The method in part determines the answer. If by a "breach" one means verbal recall, episodic memory, or declarative memory, then there is no or very little "memory" for what transpires under adequate general anesthesia. However, lack of conscious recall, which is the clinical endpoint, does not appear to be a criterion for lack of auditory registration during anesthesia; this underscores the need for careful evaluation of learning, with appropriately sensitive assessment instruments. Verbal retrieval *of* what is learned (i.e., declarative memory) can be absent, while behavioral measures (i.e., procedural memory) can reflect that learning occurred (Squire, 1982). Thus far, theories of anesthesia have not made the distinction in memory processes between conscious recall of information and physical and/or behavior changes as a result of assimilating information presented under anesthesia.

A theoretical model, that of neodissociation theory (Hilgard, 1977), may offer a psychological basis for explaining the curious anomalies of the problems of perception during general anesthesia. In the day-to-day behavior of operating room personnel, there exists the anesthetized patient amidst conversations of considerable importance to that patient. This creates a real-world model where neodissociation theory may be tested. That is, if these conversations are automatically monitored, as the evidence suggests, then it is the nature of the amnesia rather than stimulus acquisition under anesthesia that is the proper subject of investigation in the postanesthetic surgical patient. Given the profound conscious amnesia of the convalescent surgical patient, the consequences of such registrations would be expected to be dissociated from conscious processes.

The evidence we have examined fits such a model quite well. Behavioral nonverbal indices have successfully been activated in response to intraoperative suggestions when verbal retrieval strategies have uniformly failed to indicate any evidence of memory for intraoperative events. The two studies using word lists (Millar & Watkinson, 1983; Stolzy *et al.*, 1986) were successful, then, because they introduced the message by asking that the patient remember it; they used unusual words as stimuli, thus activating semantic memory uniquely; and they tested verbal memory late rather than early after anesthesia. Similarly, Goldmann's (1986) elegant study provided answers to previously cued but obscure questions and activated semantic memory with unique information. The Barber *et al.* (1979) study of potentiating posthypnotic suggestions during nitrous oxide exposure; the Mainord *et al.* (1983) study of specifying pelvic muscle relaxation and easy urination; Rath's (1982) study of specifying a smooth recovery from surgery; Goldmann's (1986) study of chin touching; and our three studies have all used suggestions for nonverbal behaviors as a model of assessing perception. Because they did not rely upon intentional, verbal memory, these studies could demonstrate considerably more retention.

Dixon's (1971) proposed physiological model for subliminal perception may also be relevant to anesthesia. Particularly pertinent is that Dixon no longer uses the word "subliminal," but has revised the conceptual framework and has labeled it "preconscious processing" (Dixon 1981). Dixon states that the critical mechanism for retention without consciousness involves classical afferent transmission, which activates cortical processes for determining *the content of* consciousness, but does not activate reticular systems that mediate awareness. Thus, in a review of unconscious processes, Shevrin and Dickman (1980) postulate—on the basis of selective-attention theory and subliminal-perception work—the existence of cognitive activities that are independent of consciousness of these activities and their contents. Dichotic-listening work, in particular, requires central preattentive processes that come before the consciousness *of* the material being tracked to account for the experimental data. The physiological speculations are intriguing because they involve the same structures that are active and inactive in anesthesia: intact sensory receptors, afferent fibers, and cortical association areas, and abnormal activity in reticular systems. The same is true for the several studies reviewed on behavioral response to suggestions during REM sleep.

The experimental data from research on selective attention, investigations of subliminal perception, sleep studies, basic neurophysiology, classical sensory mapping in anesthetized animals, and the anesthesiology literature converge upon the conclusion that early knowledge structures may respond to pertinent linguistic information under anesthesia while later intentional processes are amnesic. Given the probable loci of the potent inhalational agents' anesthetic action in reticular structures, the evidence points toward the validity of the proposition that the nervous system picks up auditory information and can therefore be changed by the content of conversation in the operating room.

Access to these memory structures is, according to the present theory, better through more automatic or early processes than through later, more deliberative ones. In addition, these influences are not technically subliminal, but are dissociated from consciousness *of* them or their influence. While hypnosis can be a tool for becoming conscious of such influence, such practices are fraught with methodological difficulties that make scientific conclusions impossible in the absence of controlled research designs. When such designs are tested, hypnosis is no more or less magical than in any other context. Valid recall of otherwise unconscious information did occur in our first two studies, but in some cases the material was too vague to confirm accuracy (e.g., "knife"); in other cases, it was accurate but mixed together with unconfirmable material, so as to render the judgment of accuracy impossible without independent confirmation. Thus, hypnosis by itself adds little to the data besides revealing to the patient images, sensations, and recollections of the perioperative period. Though usually not distressing, these reminiscences are powerful stimuli and should be approached with caution.

In summary, the processes of selective attention show rather conclusively that the nervous system can respond *automatically* to a pertinent linguistic message. Second, research in memory and amnesia shows that intentional verbal retrieval measures based on conscious memory searches do not necessarily predict the presence or absence of prior learning. In fact, it is clear that verbal retrieval from conscious searches is exquisitely sensitive to anesthetics, but that memory can still be present. Third, hypnosis provides a possible means of gaining access to otherwise dissociated memory structures of events during general anesthesia. However, the demand characteristics and falsifiability of the subsequent data must be clearly spelled out; free-recall data of actual operating room events are difficult to assess objectively. Fourth, the hypnosis and suggestion literatures unequivocally show that visceral, autonomic, and vegetative processes are sensitive to verbal suggestion. By this connection with physiology, memory can be dynamic and active in, for example, smooth musculature. This final area takes the issue from the mundane to the serious, because patients exposed to physiologically active verbal statements during surgical conversations are potentially at risk.

## ACKNOWLEDGMENTS

I would like to thank Candia Smith for her contribution; John Eisele, MD, and Wally Winters, PhD, MD, for their support; and Carrie Grady and Muza Kenning for their editorial assistance. Hamilton Davis, MD, former Chairman of Anesthesiology at the University of California–Davis Medical Center, provided expertise and support that gave birth to this work. His presence is missed but his contributions remain.

## REFERENCES

Aarons, L. (1976). Sleep-assisted instruction. *Psychological Bulletin, 83*, 1–40.

Adam, N. (1979). Disruption of memory functions associated with general anesthetics. In J. F. Kihlstrom & F. J. Evans (Eds.), *Functional disorders of memory* (pp. 219–238). Hillsdale, NJ: Erlbaum.

Allport, D. A., Antonis, B., & Reynold, P. (1972). On the division of attention: A disproof of the single-channel hypothesis. *Quarterly Journal of Experimental Psychology, 24*, 225–235.

Anonymous. (1979). On being aware [Editorial]. *British Journal of Anaesthesia, 51*, 711–712.

Arduini, A., & Arduini, M. G. (1954). Effect of drugs and metabolic alterations on brain stem arousal mechanisms. *Journal of Pharmacology and Experimental Therapeutics, 110*, 76–85.

Barber, J., Donaldson, D., Ramras, S., & Allen, G. D. (1979). The relationship between nitrous oxide conscious sedation and the hypnotic state. *Journal of the American Dental Association, 99*, 624–626.

Bennett, H. L. (1980). *Selective attention: The expression of suggested actions in an unattended message.* Unpublished doctoral dissertation, University of California–Davis.

Bennett, H. L., Davis, H. S., & Giannini, J. A. (1984). Nonverbal response to intraoperative conversation. *Anesthesia and Analgesia, 63*, 185. (Abstract)

Bennett, H. L., Davis, H. S., & Giannini, J. A. (1985). Nonverbal response to intraoperative conversation. *British Journal of Anaesthesia, 57*, 174–179.

Bitner, R. L. (1983). Awareness during anesthesia. In F. K. Orkin & L. H. Cooperman (Eds.), *Complications in anesthesiology* (pp. 349–354). Philadelphia: J. B. Lippincott.

Blacher, R. S. (1975). On awakening paralyzed during surgery: A syndrome of traumatic neurosis. *Journal of the American Medical Association, 234*(1), 67–68.

Blacher, R. S. (1984). Awareness during surgery [Editorial]. *Anesthesiology, 61*(1), 1–2.

Bonke, B., Schmitz, P. I. M., Verhage, F., & Zwaveling, A. (1986). Clinical study of so-called unconscious perception during general anaesthesia. *British Journal of Anaesthesia, 58*, 957–964.

Bonke, B., & Verhage, F. (1984). *A clinical study of so-called unconscious perception during general anesthesia.* Unpublished manuscript.

Brice, D. D., Hetherington, R. R., & Utting, J. E. (1970). A simple study of awareness and dreaming during anesthesia. *British Journal of Anaesthesia, 42*(6), 535–542.

Broadbent, D. E. (1958). *Perception and communication.* Oxford: Pergamon Press.

Broadbent, D. E. (1977). The hidden preattentive processes. *American Psychologist, 32*(2), 109–118.

Browne, R. A., & Catton, D. V. (1973). A study of awareness during anesthesia. *Anesthesia and Analgesia, 52*, 128–152.

Burnsten, B., & Russ, J. J. (1965). Preoperative psychological state and corticosteroid levels of surgical patients. *Psychosomatic Medicine, 27*, 309–316.

Caine, E. D., Weingartner, H., Ludlow, C. L., Cudahy, E. A., & Wehry, S. (1981). Qualitative analysis of scopolamine-induced amnesia. *Psychopharmacology, 74*, 74–80.

Cheek, D. B. (1959). Unconscious perception of meaningful sounds during surgical anesthesia as revealed under hypnosis. *American Journal of Clinical Hypnosis, 1*(3), 101–103.

Cheek, D. B. (1966). The meaning of continued hearing sense under general chemo-anesthesia: A progress report and report of a case. *American Journal of Clinical Hypnosis, 8*(4), 275–280.

Cheek, D. B. (1979, November). *Awareness of meaningful sounds under general anesthesia: Consideration and a review of the literature 1959 to 1979.* Paper presented at the 22nd Annual Scientific Meeting of the American Society of Clinical Hypnosis, San Francisco.

Cheek, D. B., & LeCron, L. M. (1968). *Clinical hypnotherapy.* New York: Grune & Stratton.

Clark, D. L., & Rosner, B. S. (1973). Neurophysiologic effects of general anesthetics: I. The electroencephalogram and sensory evoked responses in man. *Anesthesiology, 38*(6), 564–582.

Derbyshire, D. R., Chmielewski, A., Fell, D., Vater, M., Achola, K., & Smith, G. (1983). Plasma catecholamine responses to tracheal intubation. *British Journal of Anaesthesia, 55*, 855–860.

Dixon, N. (1971). *Subliminal perception.* New York: McGraw-Hill.

Dixon, N. (1981). *Preconscious processing.* New York: Wiley.

Doris, P. A. (1984). Vasopressin and the central integrative processes. *Neuroendocrinology, 38*, 75–85.

Dubovsky, S. L., & Trustman, R. (1976). Absence of recall after general anesthesia: Implications for theory and practice. *Anesthesia and Analgesia, 55*(5), 696–701.

Dundee, J. W., & Pandit, S. K. (1972a). Anterograde amnesic effects of pethidine, hyoscine and diazepam in adults. *British Journal of Pharmacology, 44*, 140–144.

Dundee, J. W., & Pandit, S. K. (1972b). Studies on drug-induced amnesia with intravenous agents in man. *British Journal of Clinical Practice, 26*(4), 164–166.

Eich, E. (1984). Memory for unattended events: Remembering with and without awareness. *Memory and Cognition, 12*(2), 105–111.

Eich, E., Reeves, J. L., & Katz, R. L. (1985). Anesthesia, amnesia, and the memory/awareness distinction. *Anesthesia and Analgesia, 64,* 1143–1148.

Evans, F. J. (1979). Hypnosis and sleep: Techniques for exploring cognitive activity during sleep. In E. Fromm & R. E. Shor (Eds.), *Hypnosis: Developments in research and new perspectives* (2nd ed., pp. 139–183). New York: Aldine.

Evans, F. J., Gustafson, L. A., O'Connell, D. N., Orne, M. T., & Shor, R. E. (1966). Response during sleep with intervening waking amnesia. *Science, 152,* 666–667.

Evans, F. J., Gustafson, L. A., O'Connell, D. N., Orne, M. T., & Shor, R. E. (1969). Sleep-induced behavioral response: Relationship to susceptibility to hypnosis and laboratory sleep patterns. *Journal of Nervous and Mental Disease, 148*(5), 467–476.

Goldmann, L. (1986). *Awareness under general anaesthesia.* Unpublished doctoral dissertation, Cambridge University.

Gray, J. A. (1982). *The neuropsychology of anxiety: An enquiry into the functions of the septo-hippocampal system.* New York: Oxford University Press.

Halfen, D. (1986, March 12). What do "anesthetized" patients hear? *Anesthesiology News,* p. 12.

Hilgard, E. R. (1977). *Divided consciousness: Multiple controls in human thought and action.* New York: Wiley.

Hilgard, J. R., & Hilgard, E. R. (1979). Assessing hypnotic responsiveness in a clinical setting: A multi-item clinical scale and its advantage over single-item scales. *International Journal of Clinical and Experimental Hypnosis, 27,* 137–149.

Hilgenberg, J. C. (1981). Intraoperative awareness during high-dose fentanyl–oxygen anesthesia. *Anesthesiology, 54,* 341–343.

Hirst, W., Spelke, E. S., Reaves, C. C., Caharack, G., & Neisser, U. (1980). Dividing attention without alteration or automaticity. *Journal of Experimental Psychology: General, 109*(1), 98–117.

Hutchings, D. D. (1961). The value of suggestion given under anesthesia: A report and evaluation of 200 consecutive cases. *American Journal of Clinical Hypnosis, 4,* 26–29.

Hutchinson, R. (1960). Awareness during surgery–a study of its incidence. *British Journal of Anaesthesia, 33,* 463–469.

Killam, E. K. (1962). Drug action on the brain-stem reticular formation. *Pharmacological Reviews, 14,* 175–223.

Kumar, S. M., Pandit, S. K., & Jackson, P. F. (1978). Recall following ketamine anesthesia for open-heart surgery: Report of a case. *Anesthesia and Analgesia, 57*(2), 267–269.

Lader, M., & Norris, H. (1969). The effects of nitrous oxide on the human auditory evoked response. *Psychopharmacology* (Berlin), *16,* 115–127.

Levinson, B. W. (1965). States of awareness during general anaesthesia. *British Journal of Anaesthesia, 37,* 544–546.

Levinson, B. W. (1969). *An examination of states of awareness during general anaesthesia.* Unpublished doctoral dissertation, University of Witwatersrand, South Africa.

Lewis, S. A., Jenkinson, J., & Wilson, J. (1973). An EEG investigation of awareness during anaesthesia. *British Journal of Psychology, 64*(3), 413–415.

Lister, R. G. (1985). The amnesic action of benzodiazepines in man. *Neuroscience and Biobehavioral Reviews, 9,* 87–94.

Loftus, E. F., Schooler, J. W., Loftus, G. R., & Glauber, D. T. (1985). Memory for events occurring under anesthesia. *Acta Psychologica, 59,* 123–128.

Mainord, W. A., Rath, B., & Barnett, F. (1983). *Anesthesia and suggestion.* Paper presented at the 91st Annual Convention of the American Psychological Association, Los Angeles.

McGaugh, J. L. (1983). Hormonal influences on memory. *Annual Review of Psychology, 34,* 297–323.

Millar, K., & Watkinson, N. (1983). Recognition of words presented during general anesthesia. *Ergonomics, 26*(6), 585–594.

Mori, K., Winters, W. D., & Spooner, C. E. (1968). Comparison of reticular and cochlear multiple unit activity with auditory ER during various stages induced by anesthetic agents: II. *Electroencephalography and Clincial Neurophysiology, 24,* 242–248.

Norman, D. A. (1968). Toward a theory of memory and attention. *Psychological Review, 75*(6), 522–536.

Norman, D. A. (1976). *Memory and attention* (2nd ed.). New York: Wiley.

O'Connell, D. N., Shor, R. E., & Orne, M. T. (1970). Hypnotic age regression: An empirical and methodological analysis. *Journal of Abnormal Psychology Monographs, 76*(3, Pt. 2).

Orne, M. T. (1979). The use and misuse of hypnosis in court. *International Journal of Clinical and Experimental Hypnosis, 27*(4), 311–341.

Pandit, S. K., & Dundee, J. W. (1970). Pre-operative amnesia. *Anaesthesia, 25*(4), 493–499.

Pandit, S. K., Dundee, J. W., & Keilty, S. R. (1971). Amnesia studies with intravenous premedication. *Anaesthesia, 26*(4), 421–428.

Pandit, S. K., Heistercamp, D. V., & Cohen, P. J. (1976). Further studies of the anti-recall effect of lorazepam. *Anesthesiology, 45*(5), 495–500.

Perry, C. W., Evans, F. J., O'Connell, D. N., Orne, E. C., & Orne, M. T. (1978). Behavioral response to verbal stimuli administered and tested during REM sleep: A further investigation. *Waking and Sleeping, 2,* 35–42.

Pert, C., Ruff, M., Weber, R. J., & Herkenham, M. (1985). Neuropeptides and their receptors: A psychosomatic network. *Journal of Immunology, 135*(2), 820–826.

Rath, B. (1982). *The use of suggestions during general anesthesia.* Unpublished doctoral dissertation, University of Louisville.

Ramsay, M. A. E. (1972). A survey of pre-operative fear. *Anaesthesia, 27*(4), 396–402.

Rosen, J. (1959). Hearing tests during anaesthesia with nitrous oxide and relaxants. *Acta Anaesthesiologica Scandinavica, 3,* 1–8.

Rosner, B. S., & Clark, D. L. (1973). Neurophysiologic effects of general anesthetics: II. Sequential regional actions in the brain. *Anesthesiology, 39*(1), 59–81.

Saucier, N., Walts, L. F., & Moreland, J. R. (1983). Patient awareness during nitrous oxide, oxygen, and halothane anesthesia. *Anesthesia and Analgesia, 62,* 239–240.

Schneider, W., & Shiffrin, R. M. (1977). Controlled and automatic human information processing: I. Detection, search, and attention. *Psychological Review, 84*(1), 1–66.

Shaffer, L. H. (1975). Multiple attention in continuous verbal tasks. In P. M. A. Rabbitt & S. Dornic (Eds.), *Attention and performance V* (pp. 157–167). New York: Academic Press.

Shevrin, H., & Dickman, S. (1980). The psychological unconscious: A necessary assumption for all psychological theory? *American Psychologist, 35*(5), 421–434.

Shiffrin, R. M., & Schneider, W. (1977). Controlled and automatic human information processing: II. Perceptual learning, automatic attending, and a general theory. *Psychological Review, 84*(2), 127–190.

Shiffrin, R. M., & Schneider, W. (1984). Automatic and controlled processing revisited. *Psychological Review, 91*(2), 269–276.

Squire, L. R. (1982). The neuropsychology of human memory. *Annual Review of Neuroscience, 5,* 241–273.

Stolzy, S., Couture, L. J., & Edmonds, H. L., Jr. (1986). Evidence of partial recall during general anesthesia. *Anesthesia and Analgesia, 65,* S154. (Abstract)

Strupp, B., Weingartner, H., Goodwin, F. K., & Gold, P. W. (1984). Neurohypophyseal hormones and cognition. *Pharmacology and Therapeutics, 23*, 179–191.

Thornton, C., Catley, D. M., Jordan, C., Lehane, J. R., Royston, D., & Jones, J. G. (1983). Enflurane anaesthesia causes graded changes in the brainstem and early cortical auditory evoked response in man. *British Journal of Anaesthesia, 55*, 479–486.

Thornton, C., Heneghan, C. P. H., James, M. F. M., & Jones, J. G. (1984). Effects of halothane or enflurane with controlled ventilation on auditory evoked potentials. *British Journal of Anaesthesia, 56*, 315–323.

Thornton, C., Heneghan, C. P. H., Navarantnarajah, M., Bateman, P. E., & Jones, J. G. (1985). Effect of etomidate on the auditory evoked response in man. *British Journal of Anaesthesia, 57*, 554–561.

Trustman, R., Dubovsky, S., & Titley, R. (1977). Auditory perception during general anesthesia—myth or fact? *International Journal of Clincial and Experimental Hypnosis, 25*(2), 88–105.

Weinberger, N. M., Gold, P. E., & Sternberg, D. B. (1984). Epinephrine enables Pavlovian fear conditioning under anesthesia. *Science, 223*, 605–607.

White, P. F. (1986). Pharmacologic and clinical aspects of preoperative medication. *Anesthesia and Analgesia, 65*(9), 963–974.

Winters, W. D. (1976). Effects of drugs on the electrical activity of the brain: Anesthetics. *Annual Review of Pharmacology*, 413–426.

Winters, W. D., Mori, K., Spooner, C. E., & Kado, R. T. (1967). Correlation of reticular and cochlear multiple unit activity with auditory evoked responses during wakefulness and sleep: I. *Electroencephalography and Clinical Neurophysiology, 23*, 539–545.

Wolfe, L. S., & Millet, J. B. (1960). Control of post-operative pain by suggestion under general anesthesia. *American Journal of Clinical Hypnosis, 3*, 109–112.

Yeakel, A. E. (1974, November). Recall of events while under general anesthesia. *Pennsylvania Medicine*, pp. 47–49.

Yeoman, R. R., Moreno, L., Rigor, B. M., & Dafny, N. (1980). Enflurane effects on acoustic and photic evoked responses. *Neuropharmacology, 19*, 481–489.

# 8

## Hysteria and Memory

MARC H. HOLLENDER
*Vanderbilt University School of Medicine*

"Hysteria," in the title of this chapter, refers to two distinctly different phenomena. One is a symptom picture, the so-called Dissociative Disorders of the Diagnostic and Statistical Manual of Mental Disorders, third edition (DSM-III); the other is a character picture, the so-called Histrionic Personality Disorder of DSM-III. Just as hysteria refers to two distinctly different phenomena, so too does the involvement of memory.

### DISSOCIATIVE DISORDERS

"Dissociation" has been defined as an unconscious defense mechanism involving the segregation of any group of mental or behavioral processes from the rest of the person's psychic activity (Kaplan, Freedman, & Sadock, 1980). A Dissociative Disorder is defined in DSM-III as "a sudden, temporary alteration in the normally integrative functions of consciousness, identity, or motor behavior" (American Psychiatric Association, 1980, p. 253). The amnesia of a Dissociative Disorder involves an active process, a repression of disturbing memories. Once repressed, access to these memories is temporarily cut off.

In the first three Dissociative Disorders of DSM-III–Psychogenic Amnesia, Psychogenic Fugue, and Multiple Personality—a memory disturbance is a central feature. These three disorders are defined and described first. Two other types of disorders, disorders in which there is amnesia for recent aberrant behavior, are also defined and described. They are the culture-bound syndromes (which are not included in DSM-III, but are discussed here along with the DSM-III diagnoses) and a disorder called Alcohol Idiosyncratic Intoxication in DSM-III (formerly Pathological Intoxication).

232

*Psychogenic Amnesia*

Description

Psychogenic Amnesia is a sudden inability to recall important personal information; this inability is too extensive to be explained by ordinary forgetfulness and is one for which no organic mental disorder is found. It is probably the most common of the DSM-III Dissociative Disorders. An emotionally disturbing event often precedes an episode.

In Psychogenic Amnesia, four types of disturbance in recall can be delineated:

> In *localized* (or circumscribed) amnesia . . . there is a failure to recall all events occurring during a circumscribed period of time, usually the first few hours following a profoundly disturbing event. . . . [*S*]*elective* amnesia [is] a failure to recall some, but not all, of the events occurring during a circumscribed period of time. [Other types of disturbance in recall] are *generalized* amnesia, in which failure of recall encompass the individual's entire life, and *continuous* amnesia, in which the individual cannot recall events subsequent to a specific time up to and including the present. (American Psychiatric Association, 1980, p. 253)

In Psychogenic Amnesia, in which a memory defect is pivotal, there is no fundamental impairment in the memory processes of registration and retention, as can be demonstrated when the amnesia is overcome. The impairment is in recall or in access to stored or repressed memories. This impairment protects against the emergence into consciousness of the painful memories, emotions, or ideas associated with profound loss or fear, disabling rage, or humiliating shame.

Case Report

The following case report illustrates the type of memory disturbance encountered in Psychogenic Amnesia. A 32-year-old salesman, Mr. A, was transferred to a psychiatric unit after spending 6 days on a medical unit where an extensive workup failed to reveal significant organic pathology. He had been admitted to the hospital after being found slumped over the steering wheel of his car; the car was parked but with the motor running. At that time he did not know who he was, how he came to be where he was found, or where he was going.

When admitted to the psychiatric unit, Mr. A was calm and coherent but unable to remember anything about his life after 1959 (the year at this time was 1974). The present episode, involving the memory disturbance, followed his wife's announcement on Christmas Eve that she planned to divorce him. After an unsuccessful attempt on Christmas Day to persuade her to remain with him, he left home and later was found 20 miles away as described above.

As an infant, Mr. A had been abandoned by his mother. He did not know for sure who his father was. Until he graduated from high school and went to work, he was shuttled among members of his mother's family. At the age of 20 he married a high school classmate. They had two sons, aged 10 and 8.

During two Amytal Sodium (amobarbital sodium) interviews, 2 days apart, Mr. A was able to recall the events leading up to his hospitalization. From then on, and without the further use of Amytal Sodium, he gradually was able to remember more and more of what had transpired since he left home. By his 12th day on the psychiatric unit, his memory was intact.

In this instance, the amnesic state followed an emotionally upsetting event and served to block it out of awareness. Early life experiences made Mr. A especially vulnerable to reacting with great intensity to rejection. He was unable to remember anything after 1959, the year he was 17 and the year he regarded as the happiest one in his life. With the use of Amytal Sodium and in a supportive environment, it was possible to gain access to memories that had been blocked out. Mr. A, with the help of his therapist, was gradually able to face and deal with the painful circumstances that preceded the onset of his dissociated state.

The types of amnesia in this case were as follows: When the patient was first hospitalized, it was generalized. Later, when only events after 1959 could not be remembered, it was continuous.

### Psychogenic Fugue

Psychogenic Fugue should perhaps be regarded as a special subtype of Psychogenic Amnesia. The main feature is sudden, unexpected travel away from home or one's customary place of work, with an inability to recall one's previous identity or one's past. In some instances there may be the assumption of a completely new identity. According to DSM-III, "The individual may give himself or herself a new name, take up a new residence, and engage in complex social activities that are well-integrated and do not suggest the presence of a mental disorder. . . . In all cases of fugue . . . the individual's travel and behavior must appear more purposeful than the confused wandering that may be seen in Psychogenic Amnesia" (American Psychiatric Association, 1980, p. 255).

In Psychogenic Fugue, complete amnesia is the rule, but there may be vague memories of wandering. Fenton (1982) commented,

The most common clinical picture is of the patient finding himself at some distant place, astonished and puzzled at his own inability to explain how he got there. There is usually amnesia for personal identity as well. The person may wander long distances. . . . [I]n general he is able to look after himself, avoids common dangers, and eats adequately as long as his money lasts. . . . The few patients who have actually been observed during the fugue state behave normally except that they may fail to recognize friends and relations.

## Multiple Personality

### Description

In Multiple Personality there are two or more distinct personalities within a person, each of which is dominant at a particular time. According to DSM-III, "Each personality is a fully integrated and complex unit with unique memories, behavior patterns, and social relationships that determine the nature of the individual's acts when that personality is dominant" (American Psychiatric Association, 1980, p. 257). As in the other Dissociative Disorders, an organic mental disorder must be ruled out.

### Case Report

The following case report (from Mathew, Jack, & West, 1985) is an example of the clinical picture encountered in patients with Multiple Personality. Ms. B, 31 years old and married, was admitted to a psychiatric unit because of frequent, abrupt, and total personality changes noted during a 2-week period. Ms. B had been in treatment for alcoholism, anxiety, and depression for the previous 2 years. The appearance of multiple personalities, which occurred shortly after childhood memories of severe verbal, physical, and sexual abuse by her father and his friends, were reactivated in treatment.

When admitted to the hospital, Ms. B had three personalities. She was unaware of the "other two personalities" but complained of "missing time." In her original personality she was anxious and depressed and expressed concern about the effect her disability had on her family. She was well behaved and conversed easily. Her second personality was that of a 7-year-old girl, agitated, fearful, and plagued by visions of her sexually abusive father. While in this personality, her voice and handwriting were childish. A third personality, seen only infrequently, was of a harsh, aggressive, foul-mouthed woman. This person was angry and hostile most of the time.

The transitions from one personality to another were abrupt and unpredictable. After 8 weeks of inpatient treatment using supportive and uncovering psychotherapy, the three personalities began to fuse. At the time of discharge, Ms. B was relatively stable and had come to terms with her unpleasant childhood memories (Mathew *et al.*, 1985).

The diagnosis of Multiple Personality may be suggested by memory gaps and time distortions. In Ms. B's case, she complained of "missing time." The diagnosis can be made on the basis of "multiple amnestic episodes together with the presence of alternating separate and distinct identities" (Putnam, Loewenstein, Silberman, & Post, 1984). Ms. B fulfilled the requirements for the diagnosis.

In terms of memory in the person with multiple personalities, recall is appropriate for the personality that is holding sway at a given time. This personality may or may not know about the other personalities. In Ms. B's case, she was not aware of the other two personalities originally, and consequently there were amnesic periods or gaps that she described as "missing time."

## Summary for Dissociative Disorders Centrally Involving Memory Disturbance

In summarizing information about amnesia, Gifford, Murawski, Kline, and Sachar (1977) stated:

> 1) Periods of amnesia can occur spontaneously, last from a few hours to many months, and may include events limited to the amnesic interval or covering an entire lifetime; 2) in most cases memories of these events are simply dissociated from conscious perception and not irrevocably destroyed; 3) memories return spontaneously or can be recovered by hypnotic techniques with varying degrees of completeness; 4) the individual was observed during the amnesic interval "behaving normally" and carrying out the complex, purposive actions of traveling, finding lodgings, obtaining information, and so on; and 5) various types of personality change accompanied these amnesic disturbances, from an acute sense of loss of identity to the assumption of one or more distinct new identities or the emergence of complex "multiple personalities." (p. 102)

## Culture-Bound Syndromes

### Description

The culture-bound syndromes, which include latah, amok, wihtigo, and piblokto (Arctic hysteria), are also dissociative disorders, although not included in DSM-III. Characteristically, they appear in the members of the group within a culture subjected to much pressure and confronted by tasks they cannot master. Under these circumstances, they have recourse to a culturally tolerated or sanctioned safety valve, an outlet provided in almost all societies. Although each of the culture-bound syndromes has distinctive features, there are several shared features. Many of these syndromes contain elements of aggressiveness, bizarre behavior, and loss of control (Hollender, 1976). West (1967) included "hysterical fit" under "frenzied or violent states of dissociated behavior," regarding it as the European or American counterpart of states such as amok or latah. Most culture-bound syndromes are of sudden onset, brief duration, and abrupt termination, with amnesia for much if not all of the attack.

## Case Report of Negi Negi

The following description was given for an episode of negi negi, a culture-bound syndrome, encountered in the Bena Bena tribe living in the highlands of New Guinea (Langness, 1965). A young man became agitated, ran toward people, and made threatening gestures with a wooden club. It took four men to subdue him. His eyes were glazed and his skin cold to the touch. He breathed in deep, panting gasps and gave no indication that he could hear or understand what was said to him. (There is amnesia for episodes such as this one.)

Negi negi occurs exclusively in males, usually between the ages of 22 and 32 years, has its onset at night, lasts 3–24 hours, and often is associated with the recent death of a person who was a member of the same subclan. The Bena Bena, in whom the fear of ghosts is ubiquitous, important, and very genuine, believe that the person affected is the victim of a malevolent ghost. Accordingly, no stigma is attached to the episode, there is no public censure, and the outburst is soon forgotten.

The Bena Bena social system places considerable pressure on young men. In the case cited above, the man was resentful because his desires were being thwarted by his clansmen and his wives. Yet there was no way in which he could vent his anger and resentment directly, because aggression toward clansmen was expressly and strongly forbidden. The only outlet provided and implicitly sanctioned was an attack of negi negi. Such an outburst discharges aggression and sends a message. It expresses unconsciously what cannot be stated in words: "Do not expect so much of me. The outburst in which I discharge feelings, including anger, is not of my doing; it is the ghost that is responsible."

## Alcohol Idiosyncratic Intoxication

### Description

Alcohol Idiosyncratic Intoxication, formerly called Pathological Intoxication, has been defined and described in the following manner in DSM-III:

> The essential feature is a marked behavioral change—usually to aggressiveness—that is due to the recent ingestion of an amount of alcohol insufficient to induce intoxication in most people. There is usually subsequent amnesia for the

period of intoxication. The behavior is atypical of the person when not drinking—for example, a shy, retiring, mild-mannered person may, after one weak drink, become belligerent and assaultive. During the episode the individual seems out of contact with others. (American Psychiatric Association, 1980, p. 132)

There is good reason, however, to contend that Alcohol Idiosyncratic Intoxication is actually a Dissociative Disorder (Hollender, 1979). If the small amount of alcohol were left out of the description in DSM-III, the description would certainly be compatible with a diagnosis of Dissociative Disorder. Like culture-bound syndromes and so-called "hysterical fits," and unlike Psychogenic Amnesia and Psychogenic Fugue, it is a Dissociative Disorder in which aggressive and destructive behavior is likely to be prominent.

## Case Report

The following case report (from Kosbab & Kuhnley, 1978), written to alert clinicians to Pathological Intoxication (as it was then called), would seem to illustrate the contention that Alcohol Idiosyncratic Intoxication is actually dissociative in nature. A 22-year-old college student, Mr. D, became markedly agitated while attending a party. When he returned to his home he physically pushed family members around, verbally abused them, destroyed household furnishings, and then ran into the street clothed only in his underwear. He proceeded to preach from atop a parked car. Four hospital attendants were unable to control him because he showed "unusual strength." It was noted that he had "wild, gleaming eyes" and that his complexion was "much darker than usual." His conduct was characterized as totally inconsistent with his usual behavior. When Mr. D was finally subdued, he was in a daze, confused, bewildered, and noncommunicative. After a "deep sleep," he was alert, appropriate, and cooperative and almost completely amnesic for the events of the previous night.

In taking Mr. D's history, it was learned that much tension and discouragement had preceded the episode of disturbed behavior. He was concerned that he might be flunking out of college, beset by internal and external pressures to make it through school, and having difficulties in financing his education; he was especially concerned about losing eligibility for the GI Bill because of shortcomings in his scholastic performance. At the same time, he felt under great pressure from his woman friend, to whom he was devoted and whom he wished to marry. There were also other pressures within his home and immediate family. To top things off, he had had to attend military reserve duties that particular weekend, and by the time he arrived at the party, he was feeling "upset" and tense.

On psychological testing, it was noted that Mr. D primarily dealt with primitive aggression by denial and avoidance. No evidence for an organic brain syndrome was found. Because the episode beginning with aggressive behavior and ending with deep sleep and amnesia for the outburst occurred after Mr. D had drunk a single bottle of malt liquor, Kosbab and Kuhnley (1978) made the diagnosis of Pathological Intoxication. They did so in spite of the fact that Mr. D acknowledged that he previously drank an occasional beer or two a month without untoward effects.

There is ample reason to conclude that in this case and in similar cases the diagnosis should be one of Dissociative Disorder and that the small amount of alcohol imbibed is incidental rather than causal. May and Ebaugh (1953) stated, "Critical study of the various descriptions of pathological intoxication tends to create the suspicion that a naive and credulous belief in the magic powers of alcohol and the diagnostic value of amnesia has resulted in a blending of the symptoms and characteristics of different reaction types to create an entity that bears more relation to legendary composite figures such as the minotaur and centaur than to clinical reality." (p. 200) Amnesia could, of course, be consistent with a diagnosis of either Dissociative Disorder or Alcohol Idiosyncratic Intoxication.

## HISTRIONIC (HYSTERICAL) PERSONALITY

The following criteria have been set down in DSM-III for the diagnosis of Histrionic Personality Disorder:

> A. Behavior that is overly dramatic, reactive, and intensely expressed, as indicated by at least three of the following:
> (1) self-dramatization, e.g., exaggerated expression of emotions
> (2) incessant drawing of attention to oneself
> (3) craving for activity and excitement
> (4) over-reaction to minor events
> (5) irrational, angry outbursts or tantrums
> B. Characteristic disturbances in interpersonal relationships as indicated by at least two of the following:
> (1) perceived by others as emotionally shallow and lacking genuineness even if superficially warm and charming
> (2) egocentric, self-indulgent, and inconsiderate of others
> (3) vain and demanding
> (4) dependent, helpless, constantly seeking reassurance
> (5) prone to manipulative suicidal threats, gestures, or attempts (American Psychiatric Association, 1980, p. 315)

Chodoff (1982) contends that at a phenomenal level there is a rough consensus among clinicians about the characteristics delimiting the hysterical (or histrionic) personality. Some debate, I would suggest, might occur, however, about whether the pattern described is a disorder or a life style. Be that as it may, the two cardinal features of the clinical picture are histrionic and seductive behavior.

Histrionic (or Hysterical) Personality Disorder is a diagnosis applied almost exclusively to women. Those women so labeled are usually attractive and personable as well as histrionic and seductive. They have a predilection for vivid colors and much makeup. Bodily movements are sexually suggestive. Some women, like poor actresses, overplay their roles, while others, like star performers, are more convincing. Their mood tends to be shallow and their affect labile and volatile. A bubbly effervescence may suddenly and unexpectedly be followed by a fall into the depths of despair. Their world contains little gray; almost everything is black or white (Hollender, 1971).

In describing the characteristics seen in the hysterical personality, Chodoff (1982) stated that they manifest a high degree of overt emotionality. He added,

> In their interactions with men, hysterics tend to be attention-seeking and sexually seductive, although it has frequently been noted that this behavior has a superficial quality and is not in fact intensely erotic. Above all, and consistent with the DSM-III name change, hysterics are histrionic. They are always on stage and in performance, sometimes to such an extent that they have difficulty distinguishing fantasy from reality.

Cultural forces that favor the development of childlike women foster the hysterical personality life style, but cultural forces in themselves are not sufficient. An attractive physical appearance (face and figure according to popular standards) and a particular emotional or personality makeup (vivacious and personable) are also required. If in addition psychological problems favor the development of this pattern, the process may be much intensified.

Some women may behave in a childlike manner because such behavior is expected, or even required, of them; others may behave in this manner because their emotional development was arrested and they are incapable of behaving otherwise. There is a fundamental difference between the woman who elects to play an assigned role and one who has no other choice. If the external situation changes, as it did for Scarlett O'Hara in *Gone with the Wind* (Wells, 1976), an individual who is playing the role of the hysterical personality may quickly discard it and replace it with behavior better adapted to current needs. The truly childlike person may lack such adaptive ability, and, as a consequence, the demands of a new external situation are likely to cause an emotional disturbance expressed as depression or in psychosomatic symptoms. Concentration and memory, then, are likely to be impaired as long as the state of decompensation persists.

Cognitive style is pivotal in terms of understanding memory in a person with the life style of the hysterical personality. According to Shapiro (1965), the following characteristics of the cognitive style are striking: (1) an incapacity for persistent or intense intellectual concentration, (2) the distractibility or impressionability that follows from it, and (3) the nonfactual world in which hysterical personalities live.

Shapiro (1965) also pointed out that hysterical cognition in general is global, relatively diffuse, and lacking in sharpness, particularly in sharp detail. In a word, it is impressionistic. Persons with hysterical personalities tend to respond quickly and are highly susceptible to what is immediately impressive, striking, or merely obvious. Instead of expending intellectual effort, the person who has a hysterical personality uses hunches or "inspirations." Hunches, which might appropriately serve as steps in thinking or reaching a conclusion, become the final, conscious cognitive product.

Psychological test results are generally consonant with clinical findings (Pope & Scott, 1967). The person with a hysterical personality produces quick, thoughtless responses on the Wechsler Adult Intelligence Scale. Also, scores on the Performance scale may be higher than those on the Verbal scale, reflecting relative overemphasis on action and underemphasis on thinking. With projective techniques, impulsiveness may appear in a kind of intellectual laziness—a tendency to develop responses spontaneously and impressionistically and with an attitude of carelessness to perceptual accuracy.

Related to memory in the hysterical personality is the issue of affective truth. By "affective truth," it is meant that the "facts" as stated depend in some measure on what feels right at a given moment. Thus, one set of "facts" may be presented one day and a somewhat different set the next day. Often the person who operates at the level of affective truth is accused of lying. This is not likely to be intentional; there is no wish to deceive. The person merely has a different approach—an approach that is subjective rather than objective, impressionistic rather than precise.

Based on the following description, it seems likely that for the 19th-century actress Adah Isaac Menken, truth was a subjective phenomenon (Falk, 1934): "We must not assume from the various examples of Menken's fancy that she was an inveterate liar. Nearer the truth, and kinder to her memory, is it to assume that when she found dull realism too monotonous for her poetical imagination, she was disposed to apply a little embroidery. It was just poetic license" (pp. 141–142).

For the reasons just stated—affective truth and poetical imagination—it may appear that the person with a hysterical personality suffers from a memory defect, but memory is not actually tested. It has also often been noted that the person with a hysterical personality is relatively lacking in intellectual curiosity and as a consequence possesses a paucity of factual knowledge. The paucity of factual knowledge applies not only to the well-known naiveté of these individuals in regard to sexual information, but also to areas that are not highly charged emotionally. On psychological tests, deficiency in general factual information is a relatively reliable diagnostic indicator; persons with hysterical personalities gather impressions, not facts (Shapiro, 1965). In drawing a word picture, persons with hysterical personalities will describe their affective experiences and responses in considerable detail, but say little in factual terms about what transpired. What happened is of much less interest to them than how they felt about what happened (Lorenz, 1955).

As the result of the focus of the person with a hysterical personality, the registration of events as memories is highly selective and sharply limited. It is not that the apparatus for gathering and storing information is defective; it is that inattention or indifference results in a spotty or incomplete registration and limited retention of factual information. There may even be a cavalier attitude about and a disdain for bothering to remember what occurred, especially in regard to details or minutiae. Thus, a particular cognitive style may account for what is often labeled as "poor memory."

## SUMMARY

Although amnesia is involved in all of the Dissociative Disorders, it serves a somewhat different function in Psychogenic Amnesia, Psychogenic Fugue, and Multiple Personality as one group of these disorders than it serves in culture-bound syndromes, hysterical "fits," and so-called Alcohol Idiosyncratic Intoxication as the other group. In the former, its role is to protect the person and to keep him or her from facing a painful or distressing situation. In the latter, its role is to shield the person from blame or guilt for an aggressive outburst that has erupted in response to unbearable stress. In the first type of disorder, amnesia is a primary reaction, and no physical violence is involved. In the second type of disorder, amnesia is a secondary reaction, and physical violence is a major component of the primary response.

In Histrionic Personality Disorder, the involvement of memory is on an entirely different basis from that in a Dissociative Disorder. Attitude, not amnesia, is crucial, and motivation and cognitive style are major determinants. Persons with the life style of histrionic (hysterical) personality may make relatively little effort to register or retain information, and as a consequence they may recall the general thesis but garble the facts. They are likely to treat this failure to recall facts in a cavalier manner; it is not regarded as important enough to merit a special effort. In most instances the mental apparatus involved in memory is intact but shows the effects of disuse.

## REFERENCES

American Psychiatric Association. (1980). *Diagnostic and statistical manual of n orders* (3rd ed.). Washington, DC: Author.

Chodoff, P. (1982). The hysterical personality disorder: A psychotherapeutic ap A. Roy (Ed.), *Hysteria* (pp. 277–285). New York: Wiley.

Falk, B. (1934). *The naked lady*. London: Hutchinson.

Fenton, G. W. (1982). Hysterical alterations of consciousness. In A. Roy (Ed. (pp. 229–246). New York: Wiley.

Gifford, S., Murawski, S, Kline, N. S., & Sachar, E. J. (1977). An unusual adverse self-medication with prednisone: An irrational crime during a fugue-state. *Ir Journal of Psychiatry in Medicine, 7*, 97–122.

Hollender, M. H. (1971). The hysterical personality. *Contemporary Psychiatry, l*

Hollender, M. H. (1976). Hysteria: The culture-bound syndromes. *Papua New Gi cal Journal, 19*, 24–29.

Hollender, M. H. (1979). Pathological intoxication—is there such an entity? *Clinical Psychiatry, 40*, 424–426.

Kaplan, H. I., Freedman, A. M., & Sadock, B. J. (Eds.). (1980). *Comprehensive psychiatry* (3rd ed.). Baltimore: Williams & Wilkins.

Kosbab, F. P., & Kuhnley, E. J. (1978). Pathological intoxication. *Psychiatric* 35–38.

Langness, L. L. (1965). Hysterical psychosis in the New Guinea Highlands: A example. *Psychiatry, 28*, 258–277.

Lorenz, M. (1955). Expressive behavior and language patterns. *Psychiatry, 18,*

Mathew, R. J., Jack, R. A., & West, W. S. (1985). Regional cerebral blood flov with multiple personality. *American Journal of Psychiatry, 142*, 504–50!

May, P. R. A., & Ebaugh, F. G. (1953). Pathological intoxication, alcoholic hal other reactions to alcohol. *Quarterly Journal of Studies on Alcohol, 14,*

Pope, B., & Scott, W. H. (1967). *Psychological diagnosis in clinical practic* Oxford University Press.

Putnam, F. W., Loewenstein, R. J., Silberman, E. J., & Post, R. M. (1984). M ality disorder in a hospital setting. *Journal of Clinical Psychiatry, 45*, 1

Shapiro, D. (1965). *Neurotic styles*. New York: Basic Books.

Wells, C. E. (1976). The hysterical personality and the feminine character: A sti O'Hara. *Comprehensive Psychiatry, 17*, 353–359.

West, L. J. (1967). Dissociative reaction. In A. M. Freedman & H. I. F *Comprehensive textbook of psychiatry* (p. 885). Baltimore: Williams &

# CLINICAL STUDIES OF MEMORY ENHANCEMENT WITH HYPNOSIS AND RELATED STATES

# 9

## The Clinical Use of Hypnosis in Aiding Recall

FRED H. FRANKEL
*Beth Israel Hospital and Harvard Medical School*

## THE ROLE OF REMEMBERING IN PSYCHOTHERAPY

Since the dawn of dynamic psychiatry, a dramatic revelation, an emotional catharsis, or the uncovering of painful secrets has been a major goal of the therapy. It is difficult if not impossible to pay tribute to all who might have shaped the concepts of dynamic psychotherapy, but several influences, both direct and indirect, are obvious. To begin with, the religious confession of hidden evil had for centuries testified persuasively to the value of sharing deep secrets. Then, as the early discovery of the unconscious unfolded, the Marquis de Puységur in his expanded work with Mesmer's animal magnetism demonstrated the accessibility of important secrets during somnambulistic states. The very first patient in whom the Marquis induced magnetic sleep, Victor Race, informed him of a conflict he had had with his sister, about which he would never have dared speak when in a normal state (Puységur, 1784/1785). A century later, Benedikt wrote of the relevance of painful secrets in the genesis of hysterical symptoms (Benedikt, 1894), and Charcot pointed to the existence of unconscious isolated ideas as the nuclei of certain neuroses (Charcot, 1890). Although others, too, had contributed to the development of this theme, it burgeoned when Freud, Janet, and Jung, all following their own respective conceptual pathways, pursued the importance of gaining access to unconscious hidden or repressed material, generally laden with emotion. Thus, revisiting an individual's personal history, whether touching on experiences in reality or on wishful fantasies and painful conflicts, became the keystone of the psychotherapeutic method. The life blood of the procedure sprang from the continuity, the connectedness, or the determinism that causally linked the personal history to the current problems.

Ellenberger (1970) highlights the difficulties encountered in trying to define the precise history of ideas in this regard. Few developments take hold unless the intellectual world is prepared for their arrival. The ideas of creative thinkers are generally shaped by those of their predecessors. Examples of patients achieving cures after bringing unconscious hidden ideas or unconscious conflicts back to consciousness and working them through are abundant in the psychoanalytic literature of Freud and his followers, as well as in the writings of Janet and a number of others (see Ellenberger, 1970). Prior to this, although it does not appear from Mesmer's writings that he himself promoted recall of the past, he did establish the importance of rapport between magnetizer and patient (Ellenberger, 1970); in view of the dramatic emotional accompaniments of his "crises," it is possible that he contributed more to laying the groundwork for the practice of dynamic psychotherapy than is generally acknowledged. Regardless of the speculation surrounding Mesmer's influence on the practice of modern therapy, his associate the Marquis de Puységur, in his discovery of secrets in the trance, surely helped to pave the way for the expectation of hypermnesia in hypnosis.

## Hypnosis as a Means of Accessing Hidden Experiences

The notion that patients after hypnotic induction are able to recall considerably more of their past than when in the waking state has been universally viewed as a major advantage provided by hypnosis. While evidence for this belief is still being examined, this idea is firmly rooted in traditional psychiatric theory.

The new dynamic psychiatry that ushered in the 20th century was confronted by the knowledge that although Freud and Breuer had initially depended on the use of hypnosis to gain access to the past (Breuer & Freud, 1895/1955), Freud had then abandoned its use to pursue the development of his theories and the use of free association as a substitute technique. Janet, on the other hand, had reported that he had not only gained access to the memories of past traumas in hypnosis, but had used the opportunity to offer strong contrary suggestions designed to dismantle and reshape the memories, thus making them more acceptable (Janet, 1889). Janet claimed that he had reversed the memory of past psychic injuries for one of his patients by adding suggestions in hypnosis to persuade her that she had in fact *not* interrupted her first menstrual period by plunging into cold water; that she had *not* witnessed a fatal bloody accident at the age of 16; and that the child with whom she was compelled to share a bed at the age of 6 was indeed healthy and did *not* have impetigo over the entire left side of her face. The results of this unusual technique of trying to reverse memories in hypnosis receive further attention later, in connection with the reliability of recall in hypnosis. The reshaping of memories, with little finesse, is now not generally accepted as being helpful to the therapy.

The psychological damage to the troops in World War I provided the impetus for renewed interest in hypnosis. Clinical reports reaffirmed the use of hypnosis in facilitating recall. Shell-shocked soldiers were helped in hypnosis to remember and relive their traumatic experiences, with a beneficial effect on their symptoms (Wingfield, 1920).

Reorientation of the patient to an earlier period or a younger age level was felt to enhance hypermnesia. The therapeutic use of increased hypnotic recall grew, as underscored by the growing number of published clinical reports (Erickson, 1943; Erickson & Kubie, 1941; Lindner, 1944; Smith, 1936–1937; Taylor, 1923). In the mid-20th century hypnosis was fairly frequently used to recover forgotten experiences and their associated emotions, which, it was believed, acted as potent sources of conflict. Wolberg (1948), in his detailed description of the technique, reported on his clinical experience of its effectiveness in recovering information.

Psychoanalysts who departed from the customary Freudian mistrust of hypnosis came to recognize the usefulness of hypnotic rapport in augmenting the transference. The procedure, by catalyzing the activation of intense emotional reactions, was thought to revive the earliest affects and the determinants of the neurosis. Today, so firm is the belief in the genuine uncovering effects of hypnosis that therapists often feel the need to protect their patients upon awakening from being overwhelmed by the memories they have just retrieved. Patients are urged during hypnosis to remember when they awaken only those aspects of the past experiences that they can tolerate.

Techniques have been developed to hasten the activation of early memories. Among these, Watkins proposed the "affect bridge" (Watkins, 1971), with which he attempted to lead the patient directly from currently experienced affect to similar feelings in the past; and Barnett (1981) attempted to facilitate associations to past events by having the patient respond to questions posed in a strictly prescribed fashion.

## Questions about the Accuracy of Hypnotic Recall in the Clinical Setting

While the discussion above reflects events at the center of the interest in hypnosis, professionals and the public alike, more peripherally and in greater numbers, have at times been half-hearted in their trust in hypnosis as a gateway to the past. Almost paradoxically, elements of scorn have intermingled with the wish for the magic that hypnosis is assumed to hold. Even the courts, frequently rational to a fault, have in many instances been persuaded in recent years that hypnosis can uncover the incontrovertible truth (see Orne, Whitehouse, Dinges, & Orne, Chapter 2, this volume). Traditional psychoanalysts and therapists, while uneasy at the prospect of engaging in the use of hypnosis themselves, have on occasion requested colleagues experienced in its use to interview their patients in an effort to get around an impasse in the therapy. While greater numbers of clinicians have in recent years turned to the adjunctive use of hypnosis in both symptom removal and the uncovering process, some have tended to approach the subject with greater objectivity and an appreciation of the art and the science involved—a reflection of the *Zeitgeist* that permits and encourages the use of psychological treatment methods, while simultaneously requiring that those who use such methods demonstrate their validity. The questions are inevitable: How accurate is recall in the clinical context without or with hypnosis? Does hypnosis affect the ease with which past events can be recalled? Is the hypnotic induction procedure essential to the process, and, if so, what does it contribute?

While the improved methodologies of the experimental psychologists have enabled them to challenge a number of deeply rooted beliefs about hypnosis, none of their findings directly addresses the value of hypnosis as an aid to recall in psychotherapy. Laboratory analogue studies, while answering what they set out to investigate, have not helped in clarifying the processes under discussion here. So, for example, while it is clear that nonsense syllables are not remembered more easily in hypnosis and that recognition of previously learned material is not enhanced (Council on Scientific Affairs, American Medical Association, 1985), the recall of meaningful, potentially emotion-laden, personal memories remains a clinical exercise that is not easily duplicated in a laboratory setting.

## Accuracy of Nonhypnotic Recall in the Clinical Setting

A subject that must be addressed before discussing concerns about the factual accuracy of hypnotic recall is the factual accuracy of any material recalled in analysis or therapy *without* the aid of hypnosis. Some investigative studies on factors influencing recall are particularly illustrative. Wulf (1922/1938), commenting on how his subjects sharpened or leveled certain aspects of the original visual perceptions when these were reproduced, concluded that not everything that is perceived will be retained, and that the physiological "engram" cannot be thought of as an unalterable impression that can only fade and blur. With time, he claimed, deviations from the original occur.

Similarly, Bartlett (1932) regarded remembering as an active process of reconstruction, not a mechanical revival of static engrams. Hartmann, Kris, and Loewenstein (1946) addressed the level of maturation and psychic development at the time an event is experienced as a factor in determining what is retained by the individual. Subsequent experiences may influence and alter the original memory and bring it to conscious awareness in a changed form. What is remembered is more often a constellation of events than any single, unchanged, and completely intact memory trace.

In summarizing their review of conceptions of memory, Reiff and Scheerer (1959) emphasized that learning and memory are not considered completely synonymous. In addition, learning is a selective process dependent upon individual and environmental factors; the act of recall is one of contemporary reconstruction of the past event, and is to a large extent dependent on the state of a person at the time of the recall. Any learning or recall thus occurs in a context that exerts an influence on the process.

In a penetrating assessment of the truth or fiction uncovered by the psychoanalytic method, Spence (1982) pointed out that much is taken for granted that should not be. The data on which important elements of psychoanalytic theory rest are not self-evident. He argued that the choice of a particular linguistic construction, whether by the analyst or the analysand, fixes the form of the event or memory that is being sought. Spence set out to show that the verbal construction that the analyst helps to create in the analysis (or therapy) not only shapes both analyst's and analysand's views of the past, but also *becomes* the past, although it is a creation of the present. He drew attention to the extent to which Freud made therapists aware of the persuasive power of a coherent narrative, and in particular of the way in which an aptly chosen interpretation or reconstruction can fill the gap between two apparently unrelated events and, in the process, make sense out of nonsense. He concluded that therapists have been significantly influenced by Freud in how they listen to patients. As a consquence, the process that they follow fails to distinguish what is historically accurate from the narrative that is presented. Because the system encourages the belief that the patient has privileged access to the past, what the patient tells and what the therapist hears are assumed to be a piece of history, an account of the way things were. Despite this confusion between narrative and historical truth, Freud believed that every interpretation always contains a piece of historical truth, and that this kernel makes the interpretation effective. This reasoning does not take into account the effect of comments by the therapist, intended to aid the memory of the patient, which (whether done wittingly or unwittingly) can supply details to make the story somehow coherent. The ultimate result is that what really happened does not always correspond to what was remembered.

By the end of his career, Freud seemed to be more satisfied with the principle that what was in fact being produced was a new construction rather than a reconstruction:

> The path that starts from the analyst's construction ought to end in the patient's recollection; but it does not always lead so far. Quite often we do not succeed in bringing the patient to recollect what has been repressed. Instead of that, if the analysis is carried out correctly, we produce in him an assured conviction of the truth of the construction, which achieves the same therapeutic result as a recaptured memory. (Freud, 1937/1964, pp. 265–266)

If recall in customary analysis or therapy is only questionably accurate, why does it appear to be therapeutically effective? The answer can only be speculative. The therapeutic force may derive from the interpersonal or other aspects of the procedure, and really may not be entirely dependent on what is recalled. Furthermore, "an interpretation may bring about positive effect not because it corresponds to a specific piece of the past but because it appears to relate the known to the unknown, to provide explanation in place of uncertainty" (Spence, 1982, p. 290). Certain kinds of statements produce changes in behavior by virtue of being stated, regardless of their veridicality.

### What Advantages to Aiding Recall Might There Be in Adding Hypnosis to the Therapy?

I have already touched on the uncertainty in the assumption that a patient will arrive at the truth by free-associating, and I have described how this nonetheless leads to his or her belief in the accuracy of what is recalled. If the accuracy of wakeful recall is questionable, there is probably little to support any greater truth in statements that are produced in hypnosis. Experimental studies strongly suggest that leading questions in hypnosis can lead to confabulation, and do (Council on Scientific Affairs, American Medical Association, 1985). Personal motivation of the patient can similarly lead to confabulation. Thus, there is no evidence that the use of hypnosis must lead to the truth. Furthermore, there have been no reliable studies (only case reports) that directly relate to remembering accurately affectual personal experiences.

We should, thus, guard even more against the effects of the following example of statements that typify how recall is initiated in hypnosis:

> You can recall any fact or memory, no matter how long ago, no matter how unpleasant. Nothing is ever forgotten. You can remember and you will. You are going back in time to an important event. You are going back to the date and the time. You can feel your breathing getting faster as you re-experience that very special moment.

Because we know that patients who are hypnotizable are very likely to respond to suggestion, phraseology such as that given above can surely lead to very creative memories, influenced by the fantasies of both the therapist and the patient—"memories" that are probably wide of the truth. Janet's restructuring of the past, previously referred to (Janet, 1889), is a telling demonstration of the extent to which memories in hypnosis can be shaped.

### A CONCEPTUAL MODEL

In light of the fact that the accuracy of hypnotic recall may play little or no role in therapeutic success, it may be helpful to outline what factors justify continued clinical use of hypnosis as an aid to recall.

Transference, which is regarded as a major means of re-enacting affects and experiences of the past, is hastened and deepened in hypnosis. This derives not only from the intense trust and the archaic or primitive elements that permeate the relationship, but also from the very nature of the dissociated state, cut off from the critical and monitoring functions of the ego. This disconnection also permits a freer flow of affect and of fantasy. Primary process has an unusual opportunity to emerge, and affect is often unexpectedly strong.

With resistance and defenses somewhat lessened, and the affect as an important bridge to the past, emotionally charged material appears to emerge much more readily. Because of increased suggestibility and responsiveness, many of the memories produced may equally well be fused or distorted. However, the affects associated with the true or false memory are then negotiated for the first time or renegotiated in a situation that provides a greater degree of mastery and control for the subject, now secure in the comfort of the supportive hypnotic relationship. If the false memories are reflective of deep-seated wishes and fears, the negotiation or working through under reassuring circumstances is clearly relevant and helpful. Furthermore, the narrowed focus of interest and attention throughout the procedure enhances communication.

Because hypnotic procedures are applied clinically with scant attention to the formal assessment of hypnotizability, we may also ponder the role of "hypnosis" when the system is used with patients who are only moderately or minimally responsive to induction procedures. Clinical opinion supports the view that patients who experience dramatic events in hypnosis are usually those who are at least fairly hypnotizable and who are capable of altered states of awareness and dissociation. Furthermore, for those who are not, and who yet participate in the procedure, some effects of a positive kind seem to accrue. The experience is different from that of most clinical encounters, even in the absence of a dissociative trance. As alluded to above, the interaction is supportive and soothing, rarely confrontative, and generally optimistic and encouraging. Few adult interactions outside of family and deep personal mutual commitments offer as much caretaking and concern. It would seem, then, that the benefits of introducing hypnosis to aid the uncovering process may theoretically be considered in three tiers:

1. The first tier derives from the nonspecific therapeutic momentum generated by any clinical encounter. Merely interacting with another individual who is perceived as a therapist or a healer, and who behaves as such, contributes to improvement (Frank, 1961).

2. The second tier is the more specific benefit from the hypnotic context itself, in which the patient closes his or her eyes, abdicates initiative, and waits to be directed for his or her own good by the therapist. Optimistic phrases imply that the patient has skills that can be harnessed to recover memories

that will be useful. The setting is contrived and out of the ordinary; even when stripped of magic and mysticism, it conveys messages about the distinct relationship between patient and therapist, and about the effectiveness of the latter in helping to marshall the skills of the former. Even if the trance does not occur, transference is affected, the defenses are mollified, and the therapeutic momentum is boosted.

3. The third tier reflects the specific therapeutic factors that flow from the occurrence of the trance itself. These, as outlined earlier, affect transference even more; because of the dissociative process, they impinge on memory, mood, and perception in ways that help to reconstruct the past or to create it even more dramatically than does analysis or therapy in the absence of trance.

## CLINICAL CASES

Very practical reasons for the continued clinical use of hypnosis as an aid to recall can be seen in the following brief clinical illustrations. Clearly, some distinctive quality attaches to the clinical process when hypnosis is introduced, even when the trance per se is minimal. The first case illustrates the point that while obtaining more details of a traumatic memory was the patient's purpose in requesting hypnosis, whether or not the added details she acquired during hypnosis in fact actually happened was immaterial to her feeling better. The second case reports the forceful influence of hypnosis on transference. The remaining three cases demonstrate unusual effects on recall, not only when uncovering was the intended purpose, but even when it was not.

### Case 1

A 25-year-old musician, raped 2 years earlier, was referred by her current therapist to determine whether hypnosis would help her resolve her problems. Although engaged in psychotherapy for much of the period since the rape, she continued to experience occasional flashbacks, disturbing dreams, and a high level of anxiety. She dwelled for lengthy periods of time on questions regarding her role in the rape, particularly whether she could have escaped or done anything else to prevent it. She was especially concerned that her passivity and compliant style had been seen by her assailant as encouragement. She requested hypnosis in the hope that it would enable her to recall the event in greater detail and establish for her what the facts had indeed been.

The rape had taken place in a remote building on a college campus, where she worked alone. After returning to her floor from a visit to the restroom downstairs, she had come upon her assailant, masked and armed, crouching at the door to her office. He had spotted her as she entered the corridor, moved rapidly toward her, and, getting behind her, placed his right hand over her mouth as he placed the gun in his left hand against her neck. She had felt paralyzed and rooted to the spot as he walked her into the office, demanding the keys to the safe and the money. He had forced her to search through her desk and her pocketbook, all the while standing close up against her, threatening and verbally abusing her in a hoarse whisper; she then realized that he had an erection. With the gun at her neck she had felt forced to undress at his command, and had been subjected to sexual assault. She had felt frozen throughout the event and shattered by it. With the act completed, he had left with the money, leaving her to telephone her husband to come to pick her up and begin the arduous course of trying to put her life together again with a visit to the nearest emergency ward several miles away.

Despite what she described as useful therapy for almost 2 years, she continued to wonder whether she had indeed had time to flee from the hallway when she first spotted him at the door of her office, and whether her subservience had not led him to shift his intentions from robbery alone to include rape as well.

Her own tendency to passivity had been a problem for her since adolescence—a problem initiated by her struggle to come to terms with her verbally abusive father. She had sought therapy during her late teens and had developed a fair understanding of her ambivalent feelings toward him. Having been his favorite until she reached puberty, she now recognized that the shift in his attitude was related in some way to her physical maturity. She knew from her discussions in therapy since the rape that she had seen similarities between her father's style and the demands of the rapist.

In other respects, her personal history revealed sympathy for her mother, whom she saw as browbeaten, and a long-standing ambivalence regarding authority figures. She was a college graduate with keen intellectual interests, and had married at age 21; her husband was a geologist 6 years her senior.

The patient was intent on revisiting the traumatic episode in hypnosis, in order to determine whether she could recall it or describe it under those circumstances in a manner that would help her resolve her major questions: namely, had she in some way caused the event to happen, and could she have escaped it? Despite her commitment to the procedure, she recognized that she was likely to interpret hypnosis as another version of a rape, with herself passive and under the control of someone else. To obviate this, the second and third sessions were devoted to discussing hypnosis and modeling it. When in the fourth session an induction procedure was introduced, she was invited to keep her eyes open or to open them whenever she chose, as she became accustomed to the events that were to lead to relaxation and recall. In the subsequent six sessions, constant and firm but gentle emphasis was placed on the fact that she was entitled to feel relaxed, and that although in hypnosis she was nonetheless at liberty to recall only as much as she chose to. Furthermore, she was invited to share only that which she felt comfortable sharing. She acknowledged that she was deeply embarrassed at the thought of describing the details of the assault, and was encouraged to report only those details that she felt she could.

In the fifth visit, with the aid of hypnosis, she recounted the events of the rape with considerable affect. She described how she had loathed doing what he demanded of her, and she argued back and forth about how much she could or could not have resisted the muzzle of the gun at her neck. She pleaded for patience and assistance in the therapy while coming to terms with the event. In subsequent hypnotic sessions much of the same ground was covered; she repeated some of the same details, but was able to do so with less distress. She required constant reassurance and reminders of the fact that whatever had taken place during the rape had occurred under duress.

In discussions before the hypnosis in each session, and then during hypnosis, time was spent dealing with her resentment at having to accept the rape as part of her experience. She discussed at length how her previous two therapists had encouraged her to accept the rape as a part of herself and her history, and to attempt to integrate it. Her desire was to keep it outside of herself; it might perhaps be attached to her body or limbs, but because of its evil nature she preferred it to remain outside of (or on the exterior of) her body rather than be part of her. In discussion she tried to think of it as a corn or a callus, extraneous, somewhat bothersome, but not capable of influencing or shaping the whole of her self-image and her future.

By the 12th session she described feeling considerably easier about the problem, although not yet totally at peace about it. The turning point had come after the sixth session, when she experienced a dream in which she had found herself reporting that she had aborted the rape. This encouraged her optimistic belief that she would be able to accept as much of the rape as she had to, and yet be able to survive.

She described the most valuable part of the procedure as being her ability to view the hypnotic event as a protected situation. Behind this protective screen, once she had gone through the induction procedure, she felt she could examine the history of the details closely, gain familiarity with them, and then emerge from the protective environment of the trance with as much of the rape as she chose to carry out with her. She appreciated the permission not to have to say everything that came into her mind, and the acknowledgment that in some way she could own the feelings she felt before having to describe them. This all provided a means for her to exert some mastery over the memories and over the event, which had seemed until then to be totally beyond her control.

*Case 2*

A competent, unmarried internist in her mid-30s was referred by her therapist, a senior woman analyst who had been working with her for 3 years, for
assistance through hypnosis in gaining control over her retching and vomit-
ing—behavior associated with symptoms resembling anorexia nervosa. This
pattern was sometimes associated with overeating, but her diet was usually
very limited and she weighed only 105 pounds. She was the second of four
siblings born to a Midwestern farm couple somewhat rigid in their outlook.
While her father was warm and demonstrative, her mother was severely
restricted, depressed, and resigned. Self-sacrifice, self-criticism and poor self-
esteem were much in evidence in both the patient and her mother. The eating
disorder had started when the patient was in her late teens.

We used the hypnosis as a means of uncovering and enhancing the
positive memories of childhood; of facilitating the behavioral techniques
aimed at having her visualize herself at the weight she hoped to achieve; and
of having her feel relaxed and reassured before and after her meals that her
body could comfortably absorb the food. Most of her pleasant memories
involved her father's warmth and concern for her. Her interaction with him
had been one of her few sources of emotional comfort as she was growing up.
She responded especially well to the admonition that her stomach could take
care of itself and that she should devote her energies to other things. Her
progress with regard to eating and general confidence was apparent early in
the therapy, and continued. She also continued to see her regular therapist
twice a week, and visited me at first weekly and then less frequently. Her
therapist and I talked occasionally, and I took care not to have the content of
our sessions usurp what belonged to her regular therapy.

The issue of transference had been raised by her therapist on several
occasions, at which times the patient was adamant in her refusal to acknowledge that either her therapist or I played any significant role in her mental
life. She turned down any of the more elementary suggestions that she was
disturbed by the therapist's having to be out of town occasionally.

The course of therapy in both systems reached a plateau at about 8
months after I first saw the patient. She had had some relief and gained a
little weight, but there was more to accomplish. It was then that the outside
world lent a hand. A student with the same name as mine was assigned to her
department on rotation. She felt an instantaneous interest in him and sought
information from him about our relationship. She was immediately im-
pressed by his style of interacting with patients which she found unusually
compassionate and concerned. She mentioned this to me in passing, but
dwelled on it much more expansively with her other therapist. She found
herself preoccupied with his manner and his work on the service and was
compelled to call him one night at 11 P. M. Embarrassed, she mumbled a

garbled apology for having disturbed his privacy and the next day proceeded to unburden herself to her therapist. She was perplexed and overwhelmed by the nature and intensity of her feelings for this man, 10 years her junior, whom she had met but recently, and who, she admitted, had in no way actively encouraged her interest. It was a most unusual and dramatic turn of events in her rather austere life which thus far had been largely devoted to her professional work. She was discomforted and puzzled by it all until over the course of a few weeks she was able to acknowledge the relevance of the event to the transference in the therapy and in hypnosis.

Some months after this event, she found herself in considerably greater control of her eating habits; she had gained 10 pounds; and by mutual agreement she ended the therapy with hypnosis but continued in treatment with her therapist.

## Case 3

The British Broadcasting Corporation (BBC) recently made a television documentary on hypnosis (Barnes, 1982). The director wished to film a teaching seminar on hypnosis, and requested an opportunity to film an induction procedure with someone who had never been hypnotized before. I agreed to do this, because he was concerned about the response of the viewers to the fact that all the British clinicians he had filmed thus far were demonstrating with patients whom they already knew and had hypnotized previously. He wanted something different, and provided the subject, who was a young English woman on a visit to her sister in Canada. She flew to Boston with the specific purpose of participating in the seminar. I spent 15 minutes with her ahead of time to confirm that she was an intelligent, interested, and well-put-together young woman, not about to decompensate under bright lights in the presence of trainees and the BBC camera crew. We agreed to work together, and the result is on film.

After inducing hypnosis, I had the subject levitate her arm, which she could not return to the arm rest until given permission to do so, and then proposed to intensify the trance. I asked her to cast her mind back over her past to recall any very happy and relaxing experiences she had had; the reliving of the experiences in her mind's eye would help her to get even more relaxed and comfortable.

When she nodded her head to signify that she had found a happy memory, I asked her whether she wanted to share it with us. She again nodded assent, and with her eyes closed she began to recount the day, when she was 9 years old, that her younger sister was born. Watching her closely at this time, I could see the glistening tears begin to roll down her cheeks through the happy smile. (Viewers of the documentary can see this for themselves.) I said, "You are so happy it appears to have made you cry," with which she agreed. The tears continued to roll; I offered her the chance to back away from the issues and come out of trance, and she readily agreed. I attempted to lead her, when out of trance, to a recognition of some of her ambivalence, but she would have no part of it. She emphasized how very happy that day was, and also how frightening it had been at age 9 to wake in the morning to find her mother gone to the hospital to give birth to a younger sister. She admitted that she sometimes had thought of that day before now, but found this experience thinking of it somewhat different.

## Case 4

A woman in her mid-50s was referred for hypnosis to help in the alleviation of Raynaud phenomenon. Both her hands and feet would become cold and blue in the winter; in fact, even the anticipation of going out in the cold could precipitate a bout of vasospasm. Her response to hypnosis was impressive, and she learned to practice on her own, in anticipation of going out in the cold weather. She could encourage a dilatation of the vessels in her hands and feet, and create enough warmth to sustain her when she was outside, well protected by her boots and mittens. Because this result is also readily achievable through biofeedback, I thought it would be interesting to measure her hypnotizability on a rating scale.

I selected the Stanford Hypnotic Clinical Scale (Morgan & Hilgard, 1978–1979), a five-item measure that takes 15–20 minutes to administer. It is a series of instructions read aloud in a very systematized and prosaic fashion. The first item on this scale is a sensory–motor one, in which a suggestion is given to the subject that his or her outstretched arms are moving closer together. The second item involves having the subject have a dream in hypnosis, and then reporting on the vividness of the imagery. In the third item, the subject is asked to return to a day in the third, fourth, or fifth grades associated with a happy memory. The subject in this case first chose the fourth grade, then changed it to the third. She described being in class with a favorite teacher, and then flushed as the tears began to flow. When asked to explain her experience and behavior, she was at first at a loss; then she added that it had been the last day of the year, and because she had been a favorite of this teacher, the parting had been extremely sad for her.

We concluded the other two items, a suggestion for amnesia and a posthypnotic suggestion. She had scored 4 our of a possible 5, clearly in the high range. We then discussed the event. She was astonished that the memory should have affected her to this extent. The event had taken place almost half a century earlier, and she had never to her knowledge given it a second thought. We had by then had about eight sessions, during most of which we had focused on the imagery to do with overcoming the Raynaud symptoms, and had paid very little attention to her personal history.

## Case 5

A 35-year-old married woman, the mother of two, was referred for the symptomatic treatment of a flight phobia that had bothered her for 15 years—so much so that she had not flown in all this time, despite numerous opportunities and more than ample financial means to do so.

She had been born in Europe, but had come to the United States at the age of 18 to attend college. At 20 she had boarded a plane to return to the States after a visit home that was seriously marred by her father's ill health. The flight had encountered bad weather and had been especially fearsome for her. An attempt soon after had resulted in a similarly anxiety-provoking experience, and that was the last time she had flown. Vacation and business trips were acceptable to her only if she could drive or go by train. As stated above, she had not flown in 15 years.

She was an only child. After completing college, she had married a fellow student, settled in this country, and brought her parents over to share her home. Her father, an engineer, was effective and bright; they had a good relationship. Her mother was immature, dependent, and intrusive. The patient had two boys, aged 10 and 8, and a very comfortable marriage. She pursued her own professional career as an artist.

Four years prior to seeing me, the patient had entered therapy in an attempt to resolve differences in the relationship between herself and her mother. About a year after the commencement of the therapy, she had discovered a lump in her breast, undergone a mastectomy, and spent the major part of the remaining 3 years in therapy discussing her reactions to the surgery and her concerns about the prognosis. She had paid little attention to the flight phobia during the therapy. When she heard from others about the success of hypnosis in the treatment of phobias, she raised the possibility with her former therapist, who was very supportive of the idea.

The patient related warmly and well, and was enthusiastic about the treatment. I undertook to help her with imaginal desensitization in hypnosis, and obtained her permission to videotape all the treatment sessions for teaching purposes. Her response to hypnosis was very satisfactory, and treatment proceeded. By the eighth session she was able to imagine herself undertaking a flight without becoming anxious as she pictured herself boarding the plane, strapping herself into her seat, taxiing down the runway, and taking off. We had decided that she would go from this eighth session (armed with her new confidence and an ability to practice self-hypnosis should she become anxious) directly to the airport to board a flight. She got to her seat on the plane, fastened her seat belt, and immediately entered a self-hypnosis exercise, which entailed sitting with her eyes closed as if in deep thought. The passenger seated next to her wondered out loud what she was doing. When she told him, he immediately reassured her that there was nothing to worry about. He was a pilot, he said, and he told her how his airline sent them on a course every 6 months to refresh their skills in emergency landings. "Absolutely nothing to be concerned about," he assured her.

The consequences of this exchange were disastrous to the therapy. She could no longer concentrate on all she'd been taught, had a frightful trip, and came home by train. Her next session with me focused on her anger at me for allowing her to go on the trip before she was ready. "What is more," she added, "I have been unable to concentrate on the exercise of self-hypnosis since then. My mind just won't relax!" I tried to assist her here first by discussing her disappointment in me. Then, after inducing hypnosis, I attempted to re-establish her skill with self-hypnosis by suggesting that she simply let pleasant thoughts or memories come from the back of her mind to provide her with restful and peaceful scenes. Because she was an artist, I added that images of color or textures and patterns might be helpful, too.

After a few minutes the patient signaled that she had conjured up a pleasant memory, and indicated her willingness to share it with me. She recalled with much warmth a nanny she had had during her childhood, a warm, comforting person who had cared for her tenderly. She could recall her smell and the texture of her clothes. She was deeply involved in the memory. I suggested she dwell on it and in the future use it as a bridge or entry into the trance state in self-hypnosis exercises. There was then a long pause and a light moan; clearly something was wrong. I pursued it, and she said, "I've just remembered—I can't believe it—for the first time I've remembered that she was the first person I ever knew who had a mastectomy. I've never discussed this before."

The therapeutic strategy underwent an unanticipated change; I tried to help her to hold on to whatever positive memories she had about the nanny and then suggested that she come out of trance. In the discussion that followed she animatedly declared that she was astonished that in all the years of her therapy discussing her own mastectomy, she had *never* referred to the woman in this way, never made the connection, and never associated her feelings about her own surgery with the fact that this much-loved woman who had been a mother surrogate had gone through the same procedure when the patient was 12. She had never recalled that her first exposure to the subject had been in association with this woman, who had remained in the service of the family until the parents left to come to the United States. One might try to explain this discovery in several ways, but it is noteworthy that the patient herself was astonished that only in hypnosis had she been able to make the connection.

## DISCUSSION

The rape victim described in Case 1 provided the best description of the value of hypnosis in her case. She expressed her relief at discovering the extent to which she herself could control the uncovering process. She described a sense of protection in hypnosis, as if she were behind a screen where she could revisit past memories at her own pace, and emerge from the shelter of hypnosis with as much memory as she chose. She also found that she had an opportunity to come to terms with the experiences and their accompanying affects before having to share them with me. Gradually, she permitted herself to experience increasing degrees of discomfort, confident that she could retreat behind the "hypnotic screen" should she prefer to do so. This ultimately allowed her to see the rape as aborted, as not her responsibility, and as an external attachment assigned to the role of a corn or a callus.

It is difficult to deny the importance to this patient of the altered perception in hypnosis, in allowing her to feel protected and in control to this extent. However, in evaluating the role of hypnosis in this case, one must also weigh the use of therapeutic techniques that have little to do with hypnosis per se, but are part of many forms of therapy based on compassionate understanding. She was introduced in stages to the new procedure; she was supported and encouraged in remembering only that which she felt prepared for; and she was given permission to share only the information that she chose to share. All of these criteria will contribute to a trusting relationship and in many instances to an effective treatment process, regardless of the particular form of therapy used. Nonetheless, it is difficult to conceive of a setting as helpful as the hypnotic induction in providing a context for this nonconfrontative style.

The case history of the anorexic physician (Case 2) captures the dramatic way in which positive features of the transference are precipitated and forced to unfold in the presence of the hypnotic relationship. While remaining aloof in her therapy, she was unable to ignore her strong preoccupation with the care and concern shown to patients by a medical student on her floor, particularly as this was closely related to the work being done in hypnosis. It is difficult to ignore the strong likelihood of displacement. Consciously, she had been able to deny the transference issues in both systems of therapy, until confronted by her extraordinary behavior.

The unexpected floods of affect in the third and fourth cases (the subject filmed by the BBC and the woman with Raynaud phenomenon) amply demonstrate the ready availability of strong emotions during hypnosis. Memories in both situations that seemed initially to be primarily happy were precipitously permeated by sadness. The ambivalence that must have attended both of those events—the birth of a younger sibling and the sadness of the separation entailed in promotion to the next grade—was nowhere in conscious evidence when the subjects chose quite voluntarily to return to those memories. In the presence of the dissociated state, other factors emerged, to the great surprise of both individuals. The Raynaud patient was astonished at the force of the experience, to which she had given no attention whatsoever in close to half a century.

The fifth case (the woman with the flight phobia and the sudden memory of her childhood nurse) provides a truly dramatic illustration of the fact that the use of hypnosis *can* facilitate recall of an accurate memory. It is, of course, noteworthy that it was not intended that the procedure should facilitate memory, and that the accuracy of the memory per se would be unrelated to its clinical value. Of special interest was the patient's astonishment at the rediscovery that her nurse had indeed undergone a mastectomy when she (the patient) was 12 years old. She had succeeded in totally repressing that fact for years, even when given the opportunity to recall it during the years of therapy following her own surgery. Only in hypnosis—and then unbidden in a sense, because the therapy was not aiming to uncover any such aspect of her history—did the memory emerge.

We are forcefully reminded here that theories and the data from experimental studies, relevant as they are to the growth of the field, might best be regarded as beacons, not barriers. Part of their purpose is to illuminate, not to dictate, the paths that we follow clinically. Because of rather than despite the data accumulated thus far, hypnosis will probably continue to lay claim to its use as an aid to recall in therapy, because not infrequently it seems to do just that.

## REFERENCES

Barnes, M. (Director). (1982). *Hypnosis on trial* [Television program]. London: British Broadcasting Corporation.

Barnett, E. A. (1981). *Analytical hypnotherapy: Principles and practice.* Kingston, Ontario: Junica.

Bartlett, F. C. (1932). *Remembering.* Cambridge, England: Cambridge University Press.

Benedikt, M. (1894). Das seelenbinnenleben des gesunden und kranken menschen [Second life]. *Wiener Klinik, 20,* 127–138.

Breuer, J., & Freud, S. (1955). Studies on hysteria. In J. Strachey (Ed. and Trans.), *The standard edition of the complete psychological works of Sigmund Freud* (Vol. 2, pp. 1–305). London: Hogarth Press. (Original work published 1895)

Charcot, J. M. (1890). Lecons sur les maladies du système nerveux. In *Oeuvres complètes* (Vol. 3, pp. 335–337). Paris: Progrès Médical.

Council on Scientific Affairs, American Medical Association. (1985). Scientific status of refreshing recollection by the use of hypnosis. *Journal of the American Medical Association, 253,* 1918–1923.

Ellenberger, H. (1970). *The discovery of the unconscious.* New York: Basic Books.

Erickson, M. H. (1943). Hypnotic investigation of psychosomatic phenomena: A controlled experimental use of hypnotic regression in the therapy of an acquired food intolerance. *Psychosomatic Medicine, 5,* 67–70.

Erickson, M. H., & Kubie, L. S. (1941). The successful treatment of a case of acute hysterical depression by a return under hypnosis to a critical phase of childhood. *Psychoanalytic Quarterly 10,* 592–609.

Frank, J. D. (1961). *Persuasion and healing: A comparative study of psychotherapy.* Baltimore: Johns Hopkins University Press.

Freud, S. (1964). Constructions in analysis. In J. Strachey (Ed. and Trans.), *The standard edition of the complete psychological works of Sigmund Freud* (Vol. 23, pp. 255–269). London: Hogarth Press. (Original work published 1937)

Hartmann, H., Kris, E., & Loewenstein, R. M. (1946). Comments on the formation of psychic structure. *Psychoanalytic Study of the Child, 2,* 11–38.

Janet, P. (1889). *L'automatisme psychologique.* Paris: Alcan.

Lindner, R. M. (1944). *Rebel without a cause: The hypnoanalysis of a criminal psychopath.* New York: Grune & Stratton.

Morgan, A. H., & Hilgard, J. R. (1978–1979). The Stanford Hypnotic Clinical Scale for Adults. *American Journal of Clinical Hypnosis, 21,* 134–147.

Puységur, A. M. J. Chastenet, Marquis de. (1784–1785). *Mémoires pour servir à l'histoire et à l'établissement du magnetisme animal* (2 vols.) Paris: Cellot.

Reiff, R., & Scheerer, M. (1959). *Memory and hypnotic age regression: Developmental aspects of cognitive function explored through hypnosis.* New York: International Universities Press.

Smith, G. M. (1936–1937). A phobia originating before the age of three cured with the aid of hypnotic recall. *Character and personality, 5,* 331–337.

Spence, D. P. (1982). *Narrative truth and historical truth: Meaning and interpretation in psychoanalysis.* New York: Norton.

Taylor, W. S. (1923). Behavior under hypnoanalysis, and the mechanism of the neurosis. *Journal of Abnormal and Social Psychology, 18,* 107–124.

Watkins, J. G. (1971). The affect bridge: A hypnoanalytic technique. *International Journal of Clinical and Experimental Hypnosis, 19,* 21–27.

Wingfield, H. E. (1920). *An introduction to the study of hypnotism.* London: Balliere, Tindall.

Wolberg, L. R. (1948). *Medical hypnosis: Vol. 2. The practice of hypnotherapy.* New York: Grune & Stratton.

Wulf, F. (1938). Tendencies in figural variation. In W. D. Ellis (Ed.), *A source work of gestalt psychology.* New York: Humanities Press. (Original work published 1922)

# 10

## Recovery of Memory and Repressed Fantasy in Combat-Induced Post-Traumatic Stress Disorder of Vietnam Veterans

LAWRENCE C. KOLB
*Veterans Administration Medical Center and Albany Medical College*

"Narcosynthesis," the intravenous administration of a hypnotic drug to elicit repressed memories and emotional abreaction, was so named during World War II by Grinker and Spiegel (1945). The use of intravenous medication to treat psychiatric disorders was introduced much earlier, however, by Black-wenn (1931). Grinker and Spiegel, and many other psychiatrists in the allied forces, applied the technique in order to obtain a quick reduction of the seriously disorganizing symptoms of the acute stress disorders induced by combat. The technique was found to be particularly effective in reduction of amnesic and confusional states, mutism, and various conversion-like paralytic conditions. Grinker and Spiegel were of the opinion that this technique was more effective than hypnosis, which apparently was first used for such conditions during World War I (Simmel, 1921).

With both techniques, narcosynthesis and hypnosis, there is uncertainty as to whether the recovery of memories, the emotional abreaction, or the combination of both is responsible for the therapeutic outcomes. Too, the issue of the veridical nature of the disclosed memories exists in both cases. Gerson and Victoroff (1948) reported attempts as early as 1931 to obtain criminal confessions from subjects when under the influence of drugs. They questioned the validity of the data so procured, and pointed out that such confessed material is limited by a subject's own fantasies and delusions. Only a few years later, their position was verified by an experiment conducted by Redlich, Ravits, and Dession (1951), who found that subjects who were requested to maintain lies under drug-induced altered states of consciousness varied in their ability to do so, depending upon their pre-existing personality organization, their psychological defensive structure, and their underlying unconscious state.

My recent work (Blanchard, Kolb, Pallmeyer, & Gerrardi, 1983; Kolb, 1984b; Kolb & Mutalipassi, 1983) in treatment of the symptom complex now designated in the American Psychiatric Association's *Diagnostic and Statistical Manual of Mental Disorders*, third edition (DSM-III) as Post-Traumatic Stress Disorder (PTSD), Chronic or Delayed, provides some data that support the position taken by Gerson and Victoroff (1948) and by Redlich *et al.* (1951) as to the potential distortion of observed behavior and of verbal reports obtained through suggestion or verbal stimulation in altered states of consciousness induced by parenteral administration of a barbiturate. My observations also raise the question as to potential differences in the quality of the material obtainable through altering consciousness by means of hypnosis versus that obtainable through the induction of light barbiturate narcosis. The patients in this series, including the two whose cases I report in this chapter, were combat veterans with histories of serious repeated dissociative states (flashbacks) and startle reactions, followed by acting out in a threatening or violent manner. These symptoms had been unrelieved by previous treatments. In the course of treatment, these veterans, after reporting a sense of self-estrangement, revealed a hitherto "hidden" amnesia.

## DESCRIPTION OF THE TECHNIQUES USED

### Method of Narcosynthesis Induction

The standard protocol for drug administration in this type of treatment (Blanchard *et al.*, 1983) was used. A slow intravenous injection of a barbiturate (Amytal Sodium or Pentothal) was given to the point where the individual's brain function was impaired, as measured by a failure in the capacity to count backward and by the development of slurred speech. However, rather than verbal suggestion as the abreactive stimulus, each subject was exposed to a sound track of 30 seconds of music followed first by 30 seconds of silence and then by 30 seconds of Vietnam combat sounds played at moderate intensity. The subject's behavior was videotaped. After recovery from the trance state (usually the following day), the patient was brought to view his behavioral response (Kolb, 1984a).

Thus, the standard technique of narcosynthesis induction was altered, in that abreaction was induced by means of a short but meaningful audiosignal consisting of a track of combat noises of modern warfare (helicopter, rifle, mortar fire, and machine gun fire). It was further modified by audiovisual recording of the evoked abreactive behavior to allow me, after the patient had recovered full consciousness, to be able to confront the patient with his elicited but repressed affective state and associated behavior.

## Abreaction and the Role of the Therapist

I conceive of abreaction and the therapeutic working through thereafter (Kolb, 1984a) as going beyond the simple discharge of massively repressed emotion to subsequent patient–therapist interaction through confrontation, clarification, and interpretation. All confrontations with the videotapes were arranged so that I was present to offer empathic support and understanding, as well as to seek further clarification and afford interpretation (Kolb, 1983). The patients were prepared for abreaction beforehand through my description of the process and the potential suggestion of a yet unknown response. They further committed themselves to respond through signing releases for both the induction procedure and the videotaping.

As I see it, the psychiatrist as therapist fills the role not only of a medical technician, but also of a surrogate superego, established as such through the patient's willingness to participate with him or her as the observer of denied emotion and behavior. It is this role of surrogate superego that carries the therapeutic relationship beyond one of technical derepression of retained emotion. To be sure, the patient reports an immediate sense of relief of tension after abreaction. Much, however, has to do with the therapist's willing, noncritical acceptance of the patient's evoked affect and behavior. Both the internally and externally feared criticism of the emotional response are experienced with another, who, through noncritical acceptance and support, alleviates the shame, guilt, or disgust that may be aroused in the patient's later thinking of the catastrophic event. Audiovisual confrontation of the abreaction with therapeutic support establishes a psychotherapeutic frame for further "working through" and integration of the hitherto repressed complex and overwhelming emotional crises, and the subsequent personality responses thereto. The use of pharmaceuticals to alter the state of consciousness also offers a permissive and accepting milieu for the abreaction, as the drugs used are recognized as altering brain functioning and reducing conscious control and restraint.

In all, 18 combat veterans were so treated, and 14 immediately responded with time regression to an emotionally traumatic war experience. The initial behavioral responses noted may be classified as fighting, cringing, or fleeing, followed by gross affective display of fear, rage, indignation, sadness, or guilt, and by verbal re-enactment of their actions and later thoughts as to the traumatic experience. During the session, I stimulated verbal elaboration through clarifying questions as I listened to the catharsis.

CLINICAL CASES

## Case 1

The fact that other than actual combat experience may be re-enacted during such narcosynthetic abreaction is demonstrated fully in Case 1.

### Background

A 35-year-old combat veteran of Vietnam was referred for consultation to determine whether he suffered from PTSD. He told me that he had a nervous condition, seemed to be shaking most of the time, was unable to concentrate, and felt worse when he was unoccupied. He reported that he had repetitive attacks of shortness of breath and dizziness, as well as insomnia and nightmares recreating the overrun of his unit by the enemy in Vietnam. He had served as a jet engine mechanic in a Marine support unit. He remained overly sensitive to noises recalling small-arms fire, and flinched when he heard such. He recounted his near loss of life when on guard in a perimeter infiltrated by the enemy; he had struggled with a man whom he eventually killed by slashing his throat. His best friend had been killed at this time. Since his discharge from the military, he withdrew from social contacts, was easily provoked to rage, and had lost his first wife in divorce due to his moodiness and outbursts of temper.

### Treatment

Narcosynthetic treatment was initiated with the intravenous administration of Amytal Sodium. His speech became slurred when approximately 350 mg of the drug had been administered. Then, as described earlier, he was exposed to 30 seconds of musical sound stimulation. There was no behavioral response. Following the brief period of silence, the combat soundtrack was introduced. The patient immediately attempted to flee. He commenced crying out and talking about his buddy's head being blown off, his fright and hatred of the enemy, his sense of responsibility for the action, and his inability to protect his friend. As he awakened quickly, I administered a further 250 mg of Amytal Sodium. He became unarousable. On recovery of arousability, he cried out many times that he not be tortured, that he not be cut, and that he be let go. These pleadings and cries persisted over a 6½-hour period, in spite of many attempts to terminate the abreaction by telling him the actual time and place. The patient finally regained orientation and immediate conscious contact with me and others. He slept soundly thereafter throughout the night.

The following morning, the patient was questioned as to what was going on during the later portion of the abreaction, as it related to no known incidents reported earlier as taking place. He then recounted his fears of being captured by the Viet Cong at a time when he and three buddies had been ambushed shortly after they left a Vietnam village to return to camp. Previously, he had seen the badly mutilated bodies of some Americans who had been captured, tortured, and killed. The patient recalled his fantasies of capture and terror of torture while in hiding, as well as his sense of guilt and responsibility for his buddies, whom he felt he had led into the trip. He stated that he had never in real life been captured or tortured.

Following this cathartic treatment, the patient continued in individual therapy while he attended school and until he moved to another part of the country.

## Comment

This case makes it clear that repressed but terror-filled fantasies may form a sizable portion of the material released through abreactive derepression in certain individuals. The abreaction obtained provided for me a clearer perception of the affects motivating this patient. This man was both terror- and shame-ridden—affective states not recognized during the initial diagnostic interviews.

## *Case 2*

The second case reported here demonstrates the deleterious effect of continued amnesia upon self-perception and representation (self-image) and the power of repression to reassert itself in order to obscure the suffering of powerful affect.

## Background and Preliminary Treatment

The patient, a 34-year-old multicombat veteran, was referred for consultation. He complained of increasing periods of depression, bouts of crying, and thoughts of death and suicide; in addition, he complained of many repeated attacks of stomach trouble and diarrhea, a sense of shaking, pressures in the head, and startle reactions to loud noises reminiscent of gunfire. On questioning, he admitted that his sleep was broken frequently by repetitious nightmares of combat and imagined wounding and dismemberment. At times he awakened screaming for a medic following dreams of his own wounding. During the daytime he had intrusive thoughts of the death of his closest friend after a mine explosion and a mistaken attack by American artillery on his platoon. Finally, he reported increasing anxiety on his job in the past 5 years, as well as conflicts with his wife.

The patient's developmental history disclosed that he was a healthy boy, the second son of two, who had been an average student and had completed high school. His parents were alive and well; he described them as sound, good people, the mother being the disciplinarian. On his return from Vietnam the patient had married and now lived with his wife and two daughters. He was regularly employed with the local fire department. On mental status examination, he appeared as a neatly dressed, lean man, clear and coherent in his responses but tremulous and tearful in describing his combat experiences. Other than the symptoms mentioned in his present illness, no other psychopathology was noted.

The patient was entered in a stress group meeting and weekly individual psychotherapy. Then exposed to auditory stress (combat noise), he responded excessively on all systems examined by psychophysiological monitoring, which is typical of patients with PTSD. For this reason, together with his general symptomatology, he was started on an antidepressant; this resulted in improvement in sleep and a reduction of his gastrointestinal problems. Later, his irritability and other somatic symptoms (including nightmares) were modified following a course of propranolol. After the initiation of the individual psychotherapy, improvement was noted in both his vocational and his marital problems.

Despite his improvement, the patient finally revealed that he felt estranged from himself—that there was something forgotten from his Vietnam experiences. After his friend had been killed on a mission in which they had tossed a coin to decide who would go out, and he had reacted emotionally on hearing of the friend's death, he stated that the other men in his company had begun acting strangely toward him. He could not recall why they thought that he was odd. He had come to think of himself as disliked and disliked himself. He wanted to avoid others and behaved shyly. This was reflected in several of his interpersonal relationships when he detached himself from others. He indicated his wish to recover, stating he would not become "himself" until this was accomplished. The patient was advised that this might be done by continuing in individual psychotherapy. If this proved unsuccessful, the amnesia might be reduced in a hypnotic trance, or, failing that, narcosynthesis. He chose the first course (individual psychotherapy), which continued over a year without resolution of the amnesia. I attempted later to use hypnosis but this failed; also, the patient scored 0 on the Stanford Hypnotic Clinical Scale (SHCS).

Narcosynthesis

The patient was twice scheduled for a Pentothal interview but failed to appear for the treatment, apologizing for his forgetting the appointment time. On the third scheduling, he appeared. Following the induction of light barbiturate narcosis, the patient again recounted tossing the coin with his buddy to choose who would go on the mission. With great sobs and many tears, he described the shocking way in which he had been told of the killing of his friend by another man who returned from the mission in a helicopter. He had not been able to believe the news. He then was brought to describe how for several days thereafter he had rushed out to each returning helicopter sobbing and screaming his buddy's name. He wept a great deal and felt overwhelmed with rage at another man who he was told had not carried out his mission and had exposed his buddy. The patient went on to describe his evacuation to an aid station, his return, and his exposure to teasing by his former buddies for his behavior. He continued crying and sobbing in the trance state, repeatedly calling the name of his buddy; this behavior persisted over an hour and was terminated by giving him an intramuscular injection of Valium.

After the patient recovered consciousness, he was shown the videotape of his early responses. Unfortunately, the later responses of crying and sobbing were not recorded. He was told of these responses and was provided with an interpretation of his behavior as due to overwhelming grief, guilt and despair, leading to an interruption of his capacity for retaining reality. The patient then went on to report the continuation of his unusual behaviors in Vietnam, after which he had fallen and fractured his fibula, and had been evacuated again. At the aid station, his pain and the fracture had been denied by his attendants for a time, until a perceptive physician examined him. Treated over a period of time, he had once again returned to combat duty; he was given a protected assignment, but the sense of estrangement from self and others continued, reinforced by the avoidance he sensed in his former buddies.

Due to the inability to record the full abreaction, the patient's audiovisual confrontation with his abreactive behavior was incomplete. Without direct confrontation with a videotaped record, the patient expressed his continuing doubts of what had happened. He was unable initially to accept the report or the interpretation. After a number of weeks of continuing psychotherapeutic work, he developed "gun-barrel" vision, which was resolved only after interpretation of his possible unwillingness to see the truth. Over subsequent weeks of working through, he came to accept cognitively his breakdown of emotional control on the battlefield. In the next year he appeared to integrate the repressed material as he became much more socially active at home, at work, and in a service organization.

## Comment

This clinical experience demonstrates the powerful and continuing force of psychological repression in retaining highly distressing emotions of acute grief and shame, and thus impairing memory—in this case, resulting in an enduring amnesia that further distorted the patient's sense of self. In spite of the patient's expressed desires to recover his lost memory and repair his self-image, he "unconsciously" forgot his appointments for the arranged narco-synthesis. After the event, he found himself unwilling to accept my verbal report and later developed a partial amblyopia. The latter disappeared as he worked through and integrated the experience cognitively in continuing psychotherapy. The absence of direct confrontation via videotape allowed the continuation of repression and denial over an extended period of time following narcosynthetic intervention.

## DISCUSSION

On the basis of the World War II experience mentioned earlier (Grinker & Spiegel, 1945), I initially elected to use the narcosynthetic technique rather than hypnosis. As I was working with a population of men with the chronic and delayed expressions of PTSD, my expectations were of less potential for abreaction under hypnosis. To examine this hypothesis further, I adminis-tered the SHCS to 11 veterans. Of this group, only two achieved high scores on this test. These two men were exposed to the combat soundtrack in hypnotic trance *prior* to their exposure to it during light barbiturate narcosis. While slight startle reactions were observed with the onset of combat sounds during hypnotic trance, no abreaction occurred in either man. The second man so exposed was slightly tearful when hypnotized. Under barbiturate alteration of consciousness, this latter patient immediately responded with time regression to a Vietnam combat scene and abreacted emotionally with sadness, fear, and aggression as he re-enacted the killing of his close suppor-ter and friend, a noncommissioned officer.

In the Redlich *et al.* (1951) experimental study of the validity of informa-tion obtained under barbiturate narcosis, only healthy subjects were able to maintain their lying cover story. Of the six subjects with neurotic diagnoses two revealed the true story, and another two made partial admissions consist-ing of a pattern of both fantasy and truth: one admitted what seemed a fantasy as truth, and one exhibited a parapractic distortion. Those who confessed readily were considered to have strong unconscious guilt drives.

At this time, the relative merits of hypnosis versus narcosynthesis in eliciting repressed or suppressed memories cannot be stated with any cer-tainty. All of the clinical investigations undertaken to examine the validity of data obtained under states of altered consciousness brought about by barbi-turate medication make it clear that fantasy may be reported as well as fact and may intrude upon and distort the factual material. But in this altered state of consciousness, more information as to motivation may be elicited.

Soskis (1976), in a single-case study, compared the use of several uncovering techniques in obtaining a history from, and in clarifying the motivation for, self-mutilative acts in his subject. He demonstrated that recall of the traumatic incident occurred after amobarbital administration, but not through the use of interview, hypnosis, alcohol, or methylphenidate. Whether the potential for intrusion of fantasy occurs to a greater or lesser degree under hypnosis will remain unknown until more systematic comparisons are completed of the revelatory capacities of these differing techniques used to modify consciousness. From what is known now, it is clear that hypnosis and narcosynthesis differ in many respects, but that both are capable of bringing about derepression of highly cathectic memories and/or fantasies in appropriate subjects.

If hypnosis is less likely to lead to intense derepression of affect—as the Soskis report and one of my own clinical examples (Case 2) suggests—the conclusion one may reach in regard to elicitation of withheld information is that more conscious distortion may be possible in this state than under drug-induced alterations of consciousness. In my opinion, there does not exist sufficient scientific evidence to assure the validity in reality of information ascertained in altered states of consciousness induced by either hypnosis or drug administration. Nevertheless, the revelations obtained in such states shed important light upon the motivations that drive action in the fully conscious state, and thus become important as a therapeutic lever. In my patients, recurring "flashbacks" were terminated by the recovery of the dissociated and emotionally charged memories. However, the principal constant symptoms of the post-traumatic state continued.

In conclusion, the two cases presented herein illustrate the powerful process of repression in impairing memory for both intensively charged life-threatening incidents of real life and fantasies of life-threatening events connected with the emotion of terror. Uncovering of the repressed memories and fantasies by any means remains critical if personality reorganization and integration are to occur; it does not guarantee that a recovered emotionally charged memory accurately reflects a psychologically traumatic incident.

## REFERENCES

Blackwenn, W. J. (1931). The use of sodium amytal in catatonia. *Association for Research in Nervous and Mental Disease, 10*, 224.

Blanchard, E. B., Kolb, L. C., Pallmeyer, T. P., & Gerrardi, R. J. (1983). A psycho-physiologic study of post-traumatic stress disorder in Vietnam veterans. *Psychiatric Quarterly, 54*, 220–228.

Gerson, M. J., & Victoroff, V. M. (1948). Experimental investigation into the validity of confession obtained under sodium amytal narcosis. *Clinical Psychopathology, 9*(3), 359–375.

Grinker, R. R., & Spiegel, J. P. (1945). *Men under stress.* New York: McGraw-Hill.

Kolb, L. C. (1983). *The uses of videotape for therapeutic confrontation.* Paper presented at the World Congress of Psychiatry, Vienna.

Kolb, L. C. (1984a). Narcosynthesis. In T. B. Karasu (Ed.), *The psychiatric therapies: Part II. The psychosocial therapies* (pp. 737–746). Washington, DC: American Psychiatric Association.

Kolb, L. C. (1984b). The post-traumatic stress disorders of combat: A subgroup with a conditioned emotional response. *Military Medicine, 149,* 237–243.

Kolb, L. C., & Mutalipassi, L. R. (1983). The conditioned emotional response: A sub-class of the chronic and delayed post-traumatic stress disorder. *Psychiatric Annals, 11,* 531–545.

Redlich, F. C., Ravitz, L. J., & Dession, G. H. (1951) Narcoanalysis and truth. *American Journal of Psychiatry, 107,* 586–593.

Simmel, E. (1921). Chapter 3. In S. Freud, S. Ferenczi, E. Simmel, & E. Jones (Eds.), *Psychoanalysis and the war neurosis* (pp. 30–43). New York: International Psychoanalytic Press.

Soskis, D. A. (1976). Multiple drug interviews as a diagnostic technique: A clinical case study. *Neuropsychobiology, 2,* 127–133.

# SECTION FIVE

# OVERVIEW

# 11

## Hypnosis and Memory:
## Integrative Summary and Future Directions

HELEN M. PETTINATI
*Carrier Foundation and University of Medicine and Dentistry of
New Jersey–Robert Wood Johnson Medical School*

There has been a long-standing belief that hypnosis is a powerful tool for bringing back lost memories; this use of hypnosis has been termed "hypnotic hypermnesia." However, until the past decade, there had been relatively few serious attempts to validate such a claim. It was the introduction of hypnosis into the courtroom in the 1960s that provided the impetus for what is now a wealth of research investigations addressing the role of hypnosis in enhancing memory. Many of these studies have been summarized in this volume. At this juncture, it should be noted that the impressive body of work presented in this volume has not established a proven mechanism of action for hypnotic hypermnesia as distinct from nonhypnotic hypermnesia. However, it has been successfully demonstrated both by scientific research and through selected case material that distortions of memories can occur when remembering is attempted during hypnosis.

The issue of forensic hypnotic hypermnesia has generated tremendous controversy. It is no accident that many of the chapters deal directly with, or at least refer to, the forensic issues, carefully distinguishing them from therapeutic clinical uses of hypnosis for recovering forgotten memories; in the clinic, unlike the forensic setting, accuracy of memories is not critical for therapeutic effect. Importantly, there seems to be an overwhelming consensus among the contributors that forensic hypnosis carries potential dangers that can have major consequences in such a precarious setting.

The purpose of this concluding chapter is to integrate the findings and conclusions reached by the various authors, fitting them into a broader-based scientific and clinical perspective on the use of hypnosis for increasing memory.

## HOW OUR MEMORIES WORK

Bowers and Hilgard (Chapter 1) have provided the appropriate backdrop for a book on hypnotic effects on memory by highlighting our current understanding of how our memories normally work, irrespective of hypnosis. As the authors point out, the complexities of memory need to be defined without being confused with the complexities of hypnosis, and thus they provide this necessary service for the reader.

The unmistakable message is that normal memory production is inexact. That is, memory is not like a video recorder that can provide instant replays at the push of the appropriate buttons. Rather, following from the tradition of Sir Frederic Bartlett (1932), memory is reconstructive, not reproductive. In addition, Bowers and Hilgard underscore the point that confidence in our memories may not necessarily relate to the accuracy of those memories—another striking parallel to one of Bartlett's conclusions over half a century ago: "[W]hen visualisation is the primary method [of recall] employed, . . . it has the general effect of setting up an attitude of confidence which has nothing to do with objective accuracy" (1932, p. 61).

### Accuracy versus Confidence

As we read throughout this volume, accuracy and confidence in reporting lost memories are central issues to the study of hypnotic hypermnesia. Bowers and Hilgard describe a fourfold classification of normal remembering derived from the interface of accuracy and confidence. They use four hypothetical individuals as examples. To summarize these briefly, Alan has an excellent ("superior intact") memory; he is both accurate and confident in his recall. Dave has a poor ("failing") memory and he knows it; he is inaccurate and unsure. Betty has an accurate memory, but it is flawed by her belief that she is the novel source of her information when she actually acquired the information from someone else. Finally, Carol is labeled an "archetypal confabulator." She is inaccurate in her memories, but she is unaware that things did not quite happen the way she thinks they did. Rather, she is very confident that on "instant replay" *her* version would be played back.

We all know people like Alan, Dave, Betty, and Carol, and most of us have probably experienced on occasion each of the four scenarios described. As Bowers and Hilgard note, these individual differences in the experience of remembering that are all part of the generic construct of normal memory must be recognized before an evaluation can take place of what effect hypnosis can have on the accuracy and confidence of reporting when additional memories are recovered through hypnotic recall. We need also to ask how individual differences like those described affect the potential for memory recovery with hypnosis, although this question is not directly addressed in the chapter. For example, compared to a "superior intact" memory an "archetypal confabulator" may have additional material available for recovery with hypnosis. However, there may also be an increased potential for confabulation during hypnosis if one is an "archetypal confabulator" which may not be the case for one who has a "superior intact" memory.

### Nonhypnotic Hypermnesia

Memory can be enhanced and increased without hypnosis—an obvious comment in the context of the typical experience of suddenly remembering information that we thought we had totally forgotten. This ability is simply another characteristic example of how our memories work. It is interesting how this fact of nature can easily be overlooked when we are studying increases in memory through hypnosis. We are reminded by Erdelyi's findings (Chapter 3) that free association, fantasy, prolonged concentration, and even simple repeated recall efforts will often bring forgotten material to conscious recall. The lesson, then, is that we should not too quickly attribute hypermnesia during hypnosis to the hypnotic state per se, as the increase in recall may have come about merely through repeated retelling of the events. Erdelyi's work points to the need to distinguish whether there is anything unique about hypnosis in generating increases in recall.

Erdelyi mentions that the memory reports derived through the use of fantasy and free association have an intriguing similarity to memory reports derived through hypnosis, but they are not as comparable to reports derived from prolonged concentration. Enhanced recall with fantasy and free association, according to Erdelyi, does not appear to represent a genuine enhancement of memory like that found for pictorial material using prolonged concentration. Rather, subjects seem more willing to guess and to mention information that ordinarily would be critically judged too vague to report as having occurred. Therefore, Erdelyi concludes that a lowering of the response criterion, rather than a genuine enhancement of memory, accompanies hypermnesia in a free-association condition. He goes on to speculate that this is a likely explanation for hypnotic hypermnesia, given its shared qualities with fantasy and free association. Since hypnosis also includes prolonged concentration, however, we need to know the relative role each may play in the hypnosis condition. We also need to know more about the overlap among these various strategies (taking each separately) for *efficient* memory enhancement—that is, memory production with minimal distortion.

## HYPNOTIC HYPERMNESIA: THE FORENSIC SETTING

Hypnosis has been used in the forensic setting primarily to recover additional details from witnesses and victims in criminal and civil actions. It has also been used as an investigative or discovery tool to obtain leads when such information can be subsequently corroborated by independent evidence. Hypnosis in the forensic setting has, to date, been accompanied by intense debate about its usefulness and potential misuses.

## Usefulness of Hypnosis?

The usefulness of investigative hypnosis to law enforcement agencies has been enthusiastically described. For example, Reiser (1976) has reported "a 60% increment of success of hypnotic interrogation over traditional techniques in cases involving homicide, kidnap, and rape" (Relinger, 1984, p. 217). (See also Kroger & Douce, 1979; Schafer & Rubio, 1978.) However, this perspective has been tempered by the recent report of a panel established by the Council of Scientific Affairs of the American Medical Association (1985), whose task was to review the scientific evidence for hypnosis to improve memory. This panel, which included a number of the contributors to this volume, concluded "that recollections obtained during hypnosis can involve confabulations and pseudomemories and not only fail to be more accurate, but actually appear to be less reliable than nonhypnotic recall" (p. 1918). Partly responsible may be the fact that "hypnotized subjects tend to be more suggestible [and] . . . become more vulnerable to incorporating any cues given during hypnosis into their recollections" (p. 1922). The report mentions, too, that new memories recovered under hypnosis are curiously accompanied by an increased confidence on the part of the person remembering, with no differentiation between accurate and inaccurate memories. This will be confusing for jurors, who typically base decisions not only on the plausibility of the information but also on the confidence exuded by the witness. Of note is the fact that "the U.S. Supreme Court has cited self-confidence as one of five factors to be considered in assessing the competence and hence the admissibility of eyewitness identification evidence. . . . [In addition,] the citizenry from which jurors are selected commonly believes that eyewitness confidence is a valid sign of credibility" (Kassin, 1985, p. 878).

## Hypnotic Hypermnesia: Consensus of Findings

There now appear to be a number of specific findings that can easily be derived from this volume regarding hypnotic hypermnesia that represent a consensus across the relevant contributors (the following are also mentioned in the Council on Scientific Affairs report):

1. Hypermnesia during hypnosis occurs using a free-recall format (not recognition) for primarily meaningful material, particularly for pictures. Thus, studies that question the reliable occurrence of the phenomenon must evaluate the conditions under which memories are elicited.

2. Hypnosis facilitates normal reconstructive processes of memory.

When fantasies and confabulations occur, they can easily become confused with actual memories in the reconstruction process. Hypnosis appears to increase the likelihood of incorporating into memory production external influences from leading questions, particularly in highly hypnotizable individuals.

3. There appears to be no subjective discrimination between errors and accurate material recalled during hypnosis. Thus, confidence that the new memories are factual generally occurs, regardless of error.

As can be surmised from these points, the controversy no longer centers on whether or not hypnotic hypermnesia exists as a phenomenon, but has shifted to how much the potential distortions and increased false confidence that occur in hypnotic hypermnesia may actually pose a danger in permanently contaminating eyewitness testimony and/or contributing to destroying evidence. While the authors of each chapter provide an opinion, the extensive scholarly reviews of the hypnotic hypermnesia research provided by Orne, Whitehouse, Dinges, and Orne (Chapter 2), Erdelyi (Chapter 3), Sheehan (Chapter 4), and Perry, Laurence, D'Eon, and Tallant (Chapter 5) allow readers to draw their own conclusions.

*Hypnotic hypermnesia: More Selected Findings*

The review of the hypnotic hypermnesia literature by Orne and his colleagues (Chapter 2) is quite comprehensive and has been purposely selected to be the forerunner for the chapters that follow. It anticipates the various areas that are covered in depth by the other contributors: nonhypnotic hypermnesia (Chapter 3), confidence (Chapter 4), hypnotic age regression (Chapter 5), laboratory-induced and functional amnesias (Chapters 6, 7, and 8), and therapeutic usage (Chapters 9 and 10). In addition to the three main conclusions just summarized, there are a number of highlights derived from the chapters centering on forensic issues (Chapters 2–5) that warrant additional attention.

Increase in Memory versus Reporting

When hypnosis enhances recall, what actually may be occurring is a lowering of the criterion one uses for reporting information, rather than a true increment in memory production. That is, given the relaxed state during hypnosis in which critical judgment is temporarily suspended, an individual may be more willing to guess and report information that he or she ordinarily would be too uncertain about to mention. Even so, errors in reporting may occur with either genuine enhancement or lowering of the response criterion (or both). However, understanding the exact mechanism may be useful in minimizing memory distortion.

## Context versus Process

Exactly how much of a role does the hypnotic context, as opposed to the hypnosis process, contribute to memory distortion? Two potential influences are primary in this discussion. First, the willingness to guess or a lowering of the criterion for reporting memories may be due to a relaxed setting and expectations for hypnotic recall, *or* may be intrinsic to the hypnotic state that relaxes critical judgment. Second, the increased confidence in memories may be context-related, as indicated by the increased confidence in reports obtained from simulators (Sheehan, Chapter 4); or, as we know from Bartlett (1932), increased confidence can occur with intense visual imagery—one of the inherent characteristics of the hypnotic state (Crawford & Allen, 1983). While imagery can sometimes be very useful in remembering, it also facilitates reconstruction and can be associated with undue confidence in normal memory reports: "The visualisers, on the whole, were consistently confident in their attitude, and when a subject who was not naturally of the visualising type was able to use a visual image, he at once got an access of certainty" (Bartlett, 1932, p. 59).

If the biases that create distortion are conceptualized as context variables, there is possibly some alteration in context (beliefs, particularly) that might help minimize distortions. However, the alternative "process" explanations that are aspects inherent in the hypnotic state can only mean that altering those aspects (reducing imagery or reinstating critical judgment) would probably be tantamount to discouraging a hypnotic state.

## Age Regression for Memory Enhancement

Perry and his colleagues (Chapter 5) summarize the current knowledge about age regression, one of the hypnotic techniques used for remembering in the forensic setting. Age regression is a procedure in which an individual is asked to relive an experience that may not be consciously recalled. Perry *et al.* indicate that the report is not to be taken as a literal revivification of an earlier time frame. With age regression, there are all of the recall problems just described: confabulation, creation of pseudomemories, and inadvertent responses to environmental cues from the hypnotist and internal cues resulting from the subject's own beliefs.

As an aside, Perry and his colleagues, who are expert historians, do not leave us without discussing reports of age regression to another life—that is, reincarnation experiences under hypnosis. They attribute this phenomenon to "source amnesia"—accurate memory for information, but forgetting where the material was acquired (Evans, in Chapter 6, discusses source amnesia in depth). This explanation for reincarnation experiences seems very plausible in the context of Bowers and Hilgard's discussion of "cryptomnesia" (Reed,

1974), illustrated by an elaborate discussion of Helen Keller's "unconscious plagiarism" in writing her story "The Frost King" without realizing she had heard Margaret Canby's almost exactly similar story "The Frost Fairies" some years earlier.

## Alternative Memory Enhancement Strategies

Orne and his colleagues (Chapter 2) mention, but are skeptical of, some of the alternative interrogation techniques such as "guided memory" (Malpass & Devine, 1981) and the "cognitive interview" (Geiselman *et al.*, 1985). While it is foolhardy to assume that there is less distortion with nonhypnotic techniques simply because these are initiated outside the context of hypnosis, the Geiselman *et al.* (1985) study may be the best to date in support of a true hypermnesia effect when hypnosis was used.

## Misuse of Hypnosis in Forensic Case Reports

The anecdotal field reports provided by Perry and his colleagues (Chapter 5) merely reinforce the agreement among the contributors to this volume. The actual court calamities that have occurred due to the introduction of hypnosis into a civil or criminal case, while not constituting rigorous scientific data, complete a picture with the laboratory research findings of memory distortion.

Some of the abuses clearly result from the inexperience and/or unrealistic expectations of the hypnotechnician investigators in obtaining a report. Perry and his colleagues, for example, provide a description of a witness asked under hypnosis to pretend she could see the assailant's face and describe what he looked like when she would never actually have seen his face because he had always been behind her. Thus, any description given under these conditions had to stem solely from her imagination.

However, Perry and his colleagues (and other contributors—e.g., Orne *et al.*) go beyond a consideration of the misuse of hypnosis by naive interrogators. They cogently discuss the dangers that can occur due to what might be called the iatrogenic effects of hypnosis in obtaining additional recall (i.e., the increased fantasy, uncritical reporting, and false confidence that seem to accompany the hypnotic state/context). The contributors on the issue of forensic hypnosis have themselves pointed out the limitations of their work, suggesting that a number of directions remain open for potentially fruitful study, particularly the need for more controlled field studies. However, while the laboratory research has its limitations, the creativity and thoroughness of the methodology employed and the resultant findings by the reports contained in the chapters on forensic hypnosis cannot summarily be dismissed.

While Orne and his colleagues (Chapter 2) leave us with the fact that the "vagaries" of normal human memory are "considerably more reliable" than memories recalled under hypnosis, Sheehan (Chapter 4) is somewhat less pessimistic in that he, while documenting memory distortion during hypnosis, concludes that hypnosis per se has "no inherent distortion." Nevertheless, in both chapters there is an unmistakable concern about the implications of memory distortion for the forensic setting. Since normal memory seems tenuous enough, Orne and his colleagues (Chapter 2) are persuasive in their conclusion with respect to the forensic setting: "Hypnotically induced memories should *never* be permitted to form the basis for testimony by witnesses or victims in a court of law."

## *Future for Forensic Hypnosis?*

With all the knowledge we now possess about hypnotic hypermnesia, is it possible to control some of the biases outlined in the respective chapters and eventually successfully use hypnosis in forensic situations? The fact that additional errors and increased confidence occur during hypnosis and can contribute significantly to changing a report is of serious concern for a setting where inaccuracy can have the maximal potential for negative consequences. If the effects of hypnosis on recall are context-related, it may be within the realm of possibility to minimize biases by "demythifying" hypnotic hypermnesia through educating observers and hypnotic subjects to such factors; that is, a context could be created that discounts the confidence the subject himself or herself holds and that does not reinforce guessing. However, if the effects described are inherent to the hypnotic state, the additional reforming and reshaping effects of hypnosis on memory over and above what occurs in normal remembering can only be eliminated by not using hypnosis.

Meanwhile, none of the contributors appear to object to employing hypnosis to provide leads that can then be corroborated by independent sources. (Of course, considering the unpredictability in the accuracy of reports, criminal interrogators should determine the cost–benefit ratio involved in following up multiple false leads.) Orne (1979; see also Orne, Soskis, Dinges & Orne, 1984) has elsewhere provided guidelines designed to minimize unwanted biases for the forensic use of hypnosis.

Before this section is concluded, little has been mentioned in this volume about allowing suspects to undergo hypnosis (similar to submitting to a lie detector test). While there are court cases that have utilized hypnosis for this purpose, one can deliberately lie under hypnosis, and so hypnosis cannot be used as a truth-seeking device. Hypnosis can easily be simulated. Most people believe that an expert can detect whether or not a subject is truly hypnotized, but this is not the case (Orne, 1959). Feigning a deep hypnotic state can be impressive and is convincing (Council on Scientific Affairs, American Medical Association, 1985; Udolf, 1983).

## THE RELEVANCE OF AMNESIA TO HYPNOTIC HYPERMNESIA

No volume on hypnosis and memory can be complete without a discussion of using hypnosis to aid forgetting (posthypnotic amnesia), a field of study in its own right. However, while amnesia (failure to remember) appears to be the opposite of hypermnesia (increase in memory), in point of fact, it is not. Understanding the reversal of an amnesia seen in such laboratory studies as those studies of posthypnotic amnesia reviewed by Evans (Chapter 6) can be a useful approach to studying memory enhancement. In this regard, the second section of the book brings together three variant models for understanding amnesia.

### Inaccessible versus Available Material

Evans (Chapter 6) reviews, from a perspective of cognitive processing, the scientific work on posthypnotic amnesia—amnesia induced by a suggestion given during hypnosis to forget. Much of the chapter focuses on recall strategies (e.g., temporal sequencing) that appear to have consequences for enhancing memory under certain controlled circumstances. A theme derived from this chapter is that the inaccessibility of this material does not imply that the material remains dormant. Rather, it is likely to be active and can affect behavior without the subject's being aware of its effects.

This theme continues in Bennett's (Chapter 7) summary of a program of research aimed at discovering whether patients retain and can recall information heard during major surgery under adequate anesthesia. His astounding discovery is that while these memories are not available at a conscious level, patients appear at a nonverbal, behavioral, physiological level to comprehend personally relevant language and conversations held during anesthesia. Interestingly, as in the literature on hypnotic hypermnesia, only paradigms that use meaningful material have been successful in demonstrating subsequent nonverbal recall of material learned under anesthesia. But nothing as yet, including hypnosis, has been successful in consciously recovering these memories.

The implication from Bennett's chapter summary is that derogatory comments by clinical surgical staff members who assume that the patient cannot hear during surgery may have serious consequences that range from lengthening recovery time to causing severe postoperative medical complications. More systematic study of a large number of cases, and multicenter independent scientific investigations, are clearly warranted.

### Reversible versus Irreversible Memories

A striking difference between the two types of amnesia discussed by Evans and Bennett is that while posthypnotic amnesia is reversible and some material will be consciously recalled later, those memories encoded under anesthesia (with only very rare exceptions) seem not to be transmittable to conscious awareness. The issue of reversible versus irreversible memory loss is central to the last chapter in the section on amnesia, that by Hollender (Chapter 8) on hysteria and memory. He presents clinical case material that serves to illustrate different memory impairments accompanying different kinds of hysterical conditions. He describes the functional amnesias, or the Dissociative Disorders of the *Diagnostic and Statistical Manual of Mental Disorders*, third edition (DSM-III), as having the potential to be reversed. By contrast, in DSM-III Histrionic Personality Disorder, poor memory is a common descriptor but no reversibility of memory occurs; this is true because of the narrowed perspective and degree of distractibility that accompanies a character disorder (hence, limited material is encoded in memory to begin with).

In thinking back to Bowers and Hilgard's model of four different normal memory scenarios, one also necessarily needs to consider cognitive styles acquired through psychological trauma or character disorders. Just as Bowers and Hilgard make a plea for understanding normal memory, Hollender's discussion implies that identifying aspects of psychopathological memory conditions may be relevant before hypnotic effects on memory can be evaluated. Hence, a new variable for consideration has been introduced: the psychological state and character of the individual about to undergo hypnosis for refreshing memory. In the forensic setting, "witnesses and victims . . . are not selected for their mental health" (Council on Scientific Affairs, American Medical Association, 1985, p. 1921); thus, might more severe distortions of memory occur in an individual with Histrionic Personality Disorder whose perspective already deviates from reality?

## HYPNOTIC HYPERMNESIA: THE CLINICAL SETTING

The last section of the book illustrates the tremendous therapeutic benefit that can be gained from using hypnosis (Frankel, Chapter 9) and narcosynthesis (Kolb, Chapter 10) to allow the patient to reconnect with lost memories and emotions. Because it is both relaxing and likely to help dissociate emotion from cognition, hypnosis may minimize the psychic pain that normally accompanies the remembering of traumatic, forgotten events.

Both Frankel and Kolb indicate that the accuracy of these memories is not necessary for deriving therapeutic benefit. In fact, Kolb points out that it may be "the intense emotion rather than insight from the memory" that accounts for the therapeutic benefit. Frankel enumerates in some detail the possible therapeutic benefits of hypnotic hypermnesia in the clinical setting. A common theme in both Frankel's and Kolb's chapters is that all the factors that contribute unintentionally to memory distortion in hypnosis, that are problematic in the forensic setting, may be centrally important in the clinical setting and contribute in a major way to the healing process. If this proves true, it may account for why some clinicians use hypnosis in preference to other strategies, such as the prolonged concentration described by Erdelyi (Chapter 3), to deal with traumatic experiences.

Kolb's chapter is a fitting end to this volume, in that aspects of the two narcosynthesis case studies described are unmistakably similar to characteristics that have been observed during hypnotic recall. The reports given by Kolb's patients in the drug-induced state were vivid, lifelike recounting of a time past. However, the incidents reported may never have actually occurred. In Case 1, a 35-year-old combat Vietnam veteran under sodium amytal, was "living out" a feared, repressed fantasy of being captured and killed by the Viet Cong. The experience had not actually happened to him. Thus, drug-induced recall may create additional memory distortion; like hypnotic recall, it is untrustworthy and must therefore also be scrutinized. But the courts are already aware of this: The use of sodium amytal or similar drugs (Pentothal, Brevital), formerly called "truth serum," has been significantly restricted in the forensic setting, but the benefits of these drugs are still advocated for specific clinical situations. Will hypnosis share the same fate?

## FUTURE DIRECTIONS

The research directions are clear.

### More Field Research

Although the field-simulating studies have multiplied in recent years (these are comprehensively reviewed by Orne *et al.*, Chapter 2) more systematic forensic field research is needed before all of the dimensions of forensic hypnosis are known. A good example of such research was provided in a recent review by Kihlstrom (1985), in which he describes a dissertation by Sloan (1981):

> Actual witnesses and victims were interviewed in the normal waking state, and then randomly assigned to one of four treatment conditions for a second interview. Half of these were conducted in hypnosis, and half in the normal waking state; within each of these conditions, half employed a conventional interrogation format, while the remainder employed special instructions for visual imagery (the "television technique"; Reiser & Nielson, 1980). All interviews were conducted by police investigators specially trained in forensic hypnosis. The information obtained in both interviews was objectively recorded, and the police were given 60 days to verify each item. Contrary to the earlier

report, and the enthusiastic claims of individual case studies, there were no effects of hypnosis on memory—overall productivity, accurate recollection, or error—either as a main effect or in interaction with interview technique. (p. 396)

As evidenced by the conclusions of many of the contributors to this book, there is strong motivation to design studies that are applicable outside the experimental laboratory—studies that will permit an examination of real-life behavior in naturalistic settings.

## More Clinical Research

Clinical research on hypnotic hypermnesia in the therapeutic setting has not simply been overlooked by the contributors; it is completely lacking. While systematic investigation in the clinic will undoubtedly be met with some resistance (and is probably part of the reason why so little to date has been done), good clinical research on this topic is needed and can serve to benefit the treatment setting.

In addition, research in the clinical setting may provide some important advantages that have applications in the forensic setting. For example, in the clinic, deliberate efforts at memory recovery are ususally made for traumatic, highly emotionally charged forgotten memories. It is likely that the patient is very motivated to remember and has previously tried to recall the forgotten events a number of times. These conditions are not easily duplicated in the laboratory setting, as Orne and his colleagues (Chapter 2) have pointed out. Therefore, well-designed clinical research could have the dual purpose of improving current treatment and of teaching us more about recall under emotion-laden conditions.

While accuracy is not at issue in the clinic, as underscored by all the contributors, it did appear to be useful information in the clinical case work presented by Kolb (Chapter 10), in which, without compromising therapeutic benefit, he sought some verification from the patient in Case 1 as to whether or not certain experiences could have occurred. Kolb used this knowledge in summarizing the need of the patient to face a feared fantasy (being a prisoner of war—an event that did not actually occur). The analysis of the case would have differed if Kolb had assumed that the events recalled had actually transpired.

## More Systematic Case Compilation

While nothing quite compares with conclusions that can be drawn from systematic paradigms both from laboratory and clinical research, historical verification and follow-up of independent case reports like those presented by Perry *et al.* (Chapter 5) are important in completing a picture and can be highly persuasive to supporting laboratory findings if compiled systematically.

## Hypnotic versus Nonhypnotic Interrogation Techniques

We want to know more about other interviewing techniques, particularly ones such as guided memory (Malpass & Devine, 1981) and cognitive interviews (Geiselman *et al.*, 1985), and how they compare with hypnotic interviews. When no differences in output are found between such techniques and hypnosis for recall, speculation can be made that these techniques significantly overlap in some way (e.g., Nogrady, McConkey, & Perry, 1985). Perhaps hypnotizable subjects may simply be in hypnosis when such nonhypnotic techniques are applied (see Orne *et al.*, Chapter 2).

Finding out what aspects or combinations of factors, contribute to the successful use of hypnosis to enhance memory may eventually provide the key to determining which of the memory enhancement factors (free association, fantasy, imagery, beliefs, sustained concentration, etc.) are most responsible for the memory distortion that occurs. We need to study whether rearranging the relative amounts of these ingredients that make up the hypnotic recall strategy can lead to any alteration in the ability of hypnosis to distort memories. Thus, knowing the recipe may help us to learn ways to minimize or eliminate excessive memory distortion, and/or may allow us to predict more reliably under what circumstances accurate hypermnesia will occur. At the very least, active comparison of such strategies for enhancing recall will allow us to prioritize such strategies, ordering them according to the degree to which they yield efficient, accurate increases in memory as opposed to memory distortions. More broadly, the needs for future research include an improved technology for fully understanding and classifying various aids in improving memory, so that we may better comprehend how the dimensions of each overlap, and where hypnosis falls in relation to alternative techniques.

## Individual Differences

Individual differences in accuracy and confidence in normal remembering, as well as such characteristics as concomitant psychopathology, could use (and undoubtedly will receive) more explanation in future results. In addition, the ways in which individual differences in affect and anxiety at the time of recall interface with the ability to retrieve traumatic events under conditions such as hypnosis could benefit from more systematic research.

## CONCLUSIONS

The results of the plethora of research reviewed in this volume indicate that hypnosis can enhance the recall of meaningful material, but that the act of recalling during hypnosis may permanently alter memories for future recall. The inconsistency in the accuracy of the memories is unsettling when it has legal consequences.

While an abundance of studies now exists, the compelling interest and controversial nature of the topic are likely to provide the impetus for generating further data, with the methodologies of the laboratory being applied creatively in the clinical and field settings. We may hope that in the next decade we will also see a parallel interest in initiating hypnosis research that will complement the important clinical work that is taking place with respect to hypnotic hypermnesia. Regardless of focus, forensic or clinical, a close interaction between basic and applied research holds the key to resolving critical issues.

## ACKNOWLEDGMENTS

This work was supported in part by the Carrier Foundation. I would like to thank John F. Kihlstrom, Frederick J. Evans and Julie Wade for their helpful comments and Mary Anne Hinz for technical assistance.

## REFERENCES

Bartlett, F. C. (1932). *Remembering: A study in experimental and social psychology*. Cambridge, England: Cambridge University Press.

Council on Scientific Affairs, American Medical Association. (1985). Scientific status of refreshing recollection by the use of hypnosis. *Journal of the American Medical Association, 253*, 1918–1923.

Crawford, H. J., & Allen, S. N. (1983). Enhanced visual memory during hypnosis as mediated by hypnotic responsiveness and cognitive strategies. *Journal of Experimental Psychology: General, 112*, 662–685.

Geiselman, R. E., Fisher, R. P., MacKinnon, D. P., & Holland, H. L. (1985). Eyewitness memory enhancement in the police interview: Cognitive retrieval mnemonics versus hypnosis. *Journal of Applied Psychology, 70*, 401–412.

Kassin, S. M. (1985). Eyewitness identification: Retrospective self-awareness and the accuracy–confidence correlation. *Journal of Personality and Social Psychology, 49*, 878–893.

Kihlstrom, J. F. (1985). Hypnosis. *Annual Review of Psychology, 36*, 385–418.

Kroger, W. S., & Doucé, R. G. (1979). Hypnosis in criminal investigation. *International Journal of Clinical and Experimental Hypnosis, 27*, 358–374.

Malpass, R. S., & Devine, P. G. (1981). Guided memory in eyewitness identification. *Journal of Applied Psychology, 66*, 343–350.

Nogrady, H., McConkey, K. M., & Perry, C. (1985). Enhancing visual memory: Trying hypnosis, trying imagination, and trying again. *Journal of Abnormal Psychology, 94*, 195–204.

Orne, M. T. (1959). The nature of hypnosis: Artifact and essence. *Journal of Abnormal and Social Psychology, 58*, 277–299.

Orne, M. T. (1979). The use and misuse of hypnosis in court. *International Journal of Clinical and Experimental Hypnosis, 27,* 311–341.

Orne, M. T., Soskis, D. A., Dinges, D. F., & Orne, E. C. (1984). Hypnotically induced testimony. In G. L. Wells & E. F. Loftus (Eds.), *Eyewitness testimony: Psychological perspectives* (pp. 171–213). New York: Cambridge University Press.

Reed, G. (1974). *The psychology of anomalous experience.* Boston: Houghton Mifflin.

Reiser, M. (1976). Hypnosis as a tool in criminal investigation. *Police Chief, 43,* 39–40.

Reiser, M., & Nielson, M. (1980). Investigative hypnosis: A developing specialty. *American Journal of Clinical Hypnosis, 23,* 75–83.

Relinger, H. (1984). Hypnotic hypermnesia: A critical review. *American Journal of Clinical Hypnosis, 26,* 212–225.

Schafer, D. W., & Rubio, R. (1978). Hypnosis to aid the recall of witnesses. *International Journal of Clinical and Experimental Hypnosis, 26,* 81–91.

Sloane, M. C. (1981). A comparison of hypnosis versus waking state and visual versus non-visual recall instructions for witness/victim memory retrieval in actual major crimes. *Dissertation Abstracts International, 42,* 2551B. (University Microfilms No. 81-25873)

Udolf, R. (1983). *Forensic hypnosis.* Lexington, MA: Lexington Books.

# Index